Hypertension and Hypertensive Heart Disease

Guest Editor

GEORGE A. MENSAH, MD, FACC, FACP, FACN

CARDIOLOGY CLINICS

www.cardiology.theclinics.com

Consulting Editor
MICHAEL H. CRAWFORD, MD

November 2010 • Volume 28 • Number 4

SAUNDERS an imprint of ELSEVIER, Inc.

W.B. SAUNDERS COMPANY
A Division of Elsevier Inc.

1600 John F. Kennedy Blvd. • Suite 1800 • Philadelphia, PA 19103-2899

http://www.theclinics.com

CARDIOLOGY CLINICS Volume 28, Number 4
November 2010 ISSN 0733-8651, ISBN-13: 978-1-4377-2431-8

Editor: Barbara Cohen-Kligerman
Developmental Editor: Donald Mumford

Cardiology Clinics (ISSN 0733-8651) is published quarterly by Elsevier Inc., 360 Park Avenue South, New York, NY 10010-1710. Months of issue are February, May, August, and November. Business and Editorial Offices: 1600 John F. Kennedy Blvd., Ste. 1800, Philadelphia, PA 19103-2899. Customer Service Office: 3251 Riverport Lane, Maryland Heights, MO 63043. Periodicals postage paid at New York, NY and additional mailing offices. Subscription prices are $282.00 per year for US individuals, $458.00 per year for US institutions, $139.00 per year for US students and residents, $345.00 per year for Canadian individuals, $569.00 per year for Canadian institutions, $400.00 per year for international individuals, $569.00 per year for international institutions and $196.00 per year for Canadian and international students/residents. To receive student/resident rate, orders must be accompanied by name of affiliated institution, data of term, and the *signature* of program/residency coordinator on institution letterhead. Orders will be billed at individual rate until proof of status is received. Foreign air speed delivery is included in all *Clinics* subscription prices. All prices are subject to change without notice. **POSTMASTER:** Send address changes to *Cardiology Clinics*, Elsevier Health Sciences Division, Subscription Customer Service, 3251 Riverport Lane, Maryland Heights, MO 63043. **Customer Service: 1-800-654-2452 (U.S. and Canada); 314-447-8871 (outside U.S. and Canada). Fax: 314-447-8029. E-mail: journalscustomerservice-usa@elsevier.com (for print support); journalsonlinesupport-usa@elsevier.com (for online support).**

Reprints. For copies of 100 or more, of articles in this publication, please contact the Commercial Reprints Department, Elsevier Inc., 360 Park Avenue South, New York, NY 10010-1710. Tel.: 212-633-3812; Fax: 212-462-1935; E-mail: reprints@elsevier.com.

Cardiology Clinics is also published in Spanish by McGraw-Hill Interamericana Editores S. A., P.O. Box 5-237, 06500, Mexico D. F., Mexico; in Portuguese by Reichmann and Alfonso Editores Rio de Janeiro, Brazil; and in Greek by Dimitrios P. Lagos, 8 Pondon Street, GR115-28 Ilissia, Greece.

Cardiology Clinics is covered in *MEDLINE/PubMed (Index Medicus), Excerpta Medica, The Cumulative Index to Nursing and Allied Health Literature* (CINAHL).

Printed and bound by CPI Group (UK) Ltd, Croydon, CR0 4YY
Transferred to Digital Print 2011

Contributors

CONSULTING EDITOR

MICHAEL H. CRAWFORD, MD
Professor of Medicine, University of California, San Francisco; Lucie Stern Chair in Cardiology and Chief of Clinical Cardiology, University of California San Francisco Medical Center, San Francisco, California

GUEST EDITOR

GEORGE A. MENSAH, MD, FACC, FACP, FACN
Director, Heart Health and Global Health Policy, Global Research and Development, PepsiCo, Inc, Purchase, New York

AUTHORS

MARIA CZARINA ACELAJADO, MD
Post-Doctoral Fellow, Vascular Biology and Hypertension Program, Division of Cardiovascular Disease, Department of Medicine, University of Alabama at Birmingham, Birmingham, Alabama

GEORGE BAKRIS, MD
Professor of Medicine and Director, Hypertensive Diseases Unit, University of Chicago Pritzker School of Medicine, Chicago, Illinois

HAYDEN B. BOSWORTH, PhD
Associate Director, Center for Health Services Research in Primary Care, Durham Veterans Affairs Medical Center; Professor, Division of General Internal Medicine, Department of Medicine, Duke University, Durham, North Carolina

JAVED BUTLER, MD, MPH
Division of Cardiology, Emory University, Atlanta, Georgia

DAVID A. CALHOUN, MD
Medical Director, Vascular Biology and Hypertension Program; Professor, Division of Cardiovascular Disease, Department of Medicine, University of Alabama at Birmingham, Birmingham, Alabama

STEPHEN R. DANIELS, MD, PhD
Professor and Chairman, Department of Pediatrics, University of Colorado School of Medicine; Pediatrician in Chief and L. Joseph Butterfield Chair of Pediatrics, The Children's Hospital, Aurora, Colorado

BRENT M. EGAN, MD
Medical University of South Carolina, Charleston, South Carolina

KEITH C. FERDINAND, MD, FACC, FAHA
Cardiology Division, Department of Medicine, Morehouse School of Medicine, Emory University, Atlanta, Georgia

JOHN M. FLACK, MD, MPH, FAHA, FACP
Division of Translational Research and Clinical Epidemiology, Department of Medicine, Detroit Medical Center, Wayne State University, Detroit, Michigan

JOSEPH T. FLYNN, MD, MS
Professor of Pediatrics, Division of Nephrology, Seattle Children's Hospital, Seattle, Washington

VASILIKI V. GEORGIOPOULOU, MD
Division of Cardiology, Emory University, Atlanta, Georgia

DANIEL W. JONES, MD
University of Mississippi, Oxford, Mississippi

ANDREAS P. KALOGEROPOULOS, MD
Division of Cardiology, Emory University, Atlanta, Georgia

RAE-ELLEN W. KAVEY, MD, MPH
Professor, Department of Pediatrics, Division of Cardiology, Golisano Children's Hospital, University of Rochester Medical Center, Rochester, New York

DANIEL T. LACKLAND, DrPH
Medical University of South Carolina, Charleston, South Carolina

GEORGE A. MENSAH, MD, FACC, FACP, FACN
Director, Heart Health and Global Health Policy, Global Research and Development, PepsiCo, Inc, Purchase, New York

SAMAR A. NASSER, PA-C, MPH
Division of Translational Research and Clinical Epidemiology, Department of Medicine, Detroit Medical Center, Wayne State University, Detroit, Michigan

EUGENE Z. ODDONE, MD, MHSc
Director, Center for Health Services Research in Primary Care, Durham Veterans Affairs Medical Center; Professor, Division of General Internal Medicine, Department of Medicine, Duke University, Durham, North Carolina

GBENGA OGEDEGBE, MD
Associate Professor of Medicine and Director, Center for Healthful Behavior Change, Division of General Internal Medicine, Department of Medicine, New York University School of Medicine, New York, New York

†THOMAS PICKERING, MD, DPhil
Professor of Medicine, Center for Behavioral Cardiovascular Health, Columbia University, New York, New York

BENJAMIN J. POWERS, MD, MHSc
Faculty Member, Center for Health Services Research in Primary Care, Durham Veterans Affairs Medical Center; Assistant Professor, Division of General Internal Medicine, Department of Medicine, Duke University, Durham, North Carolina

PAOLO RAGGI, MD
Division of Cardiology, Emory University, Atlanta, Georgia

NOREEN F. ROSSI, MD
Division of Nephrology, Department of Medicine, Detroit Medical Center, Wayne State University, Detroit, Michigan

UCHECHUKWU K.A. SAMPSON, MB, BS, MBA, MPH, MSc(Oxon)
Assistant Professor of Medicine, Division of Cardiovascular Medicine, Vanderbilt University Medical Center; Department of Medicine, Meharry Medical College, Nashville, Tennessee

MUKESH SINGH, MD
Senior Fellow in Nephrology, University of Chicago Pritzker School of Medicine, Chicago, Illinois

MICHELLE L. SLIMKO, MPH, RD
Licensed Dietitian Nutritionist; Principal Nutrition Scientist, Global Research and Development, PepsiCo, Inc, Barrington; DrPH Student, School of Public Health, University of Illinois-Chicago, Chicago, Illinois

† Deceased.

Contents

Foreword xi

Michael H. Crawford

Preface: Hypertension and Hypertensive Heart Disease xiii

George A. Mensah

Pathogenesis and Clinical Physiology of Hypertension 545

Mukesh Singh, George A. Mensah, and George Bakris

Significant advances have been made in understanding the pathogenesis and clinical physiology of primary hypertension. This article presents an overview of the physiology of normal blood pressure control and the pathophysiologic mechanisms that predispose individuals and populations to primary hypertension. The role of genetics, environment, and the gene-environment interaction is discussed. The spectrum of changes in physiologic states that result in chronic increases of arterial blood pressure are reviewed. The nature and characteristics of feedback loops and the primary modulating systems, the central and peripheral nervous systems, and circulating and tissue hormones are reviewed. The role of the endothelium of the artery and its production of endothelin, nitric oxide, angiotensin II, as well as other vasoactive substances in response to various stimuli, is also discussed. A unifying pathway for the development of hypertension and the practical implications for the prevention and control of hypertension are discussed.

Prehypertension: An Opportunity for a New Public Health Paradigm 561

Brent M. Egan, Daniel T. Lackland, and Daniel W. Jones

From 2005 to 2006, approximately 3 of 8 adults in the United States had blood pressure (BP) in the prehypertensive range of 120 to 139/80 to 89 mm Hg and roughly 1 in 8 adults had BP in the range of 130 to 139/85 to 89 mm Hg, which is referred to as high normal BP or stage 2 prehypertension. Adults with stage 2 prehypertension are also roughly twice as likely as adults with normotension to suffer cardiovascular disease. The Seventh Report of the Joint National Committee on Hypertension recommended only lifestyle changes for most prehypertensive patients. BP in the range of 120 to 129/80 to 84 mm Hg is also associated with increased risk but roughly half of that of stage 2 prehypertension.

Principles and Techniques of Blood Pressure Measurement 571

Gbenga Ogedegbe and Thomas Pickering

Although the mercury sphygmomanometer is widely regarded as the gold standard for office blood pressure measurement, the ban on use of mercury devices continues to diminish their role in office and hospital settings. To date, mercury devices have largely been phased out in United States hospitals. This situation has led to the proliferation of nonmercury devices and has changed (probably forever) the preferable modality of blood pressure measurement in clinic and hospital settings. In this article, the basic techniques of blood pressure measurement and the technical issues associated with measurements in clinical practice are discussed. The devices currently available for hospital and clinic measurements and their important sources

of error are presented. Practical advice is given on how the different devices and measurement techniques should be used. Blood pressure measurements in different circumstances and in special populations such as infants, children, pregnant women, elderly persons, and obese subjects are discussed.

Initial Clinical Encounter with the Patient with Established Hypertension 587

Uchechukwu K.A. Sampson and George A. Mensah

The initial encounter with the patient with hypertension presents the opportunity to reprogram the trajectory of overall cardiovascular risk in the patient with suspected or established hypertension. The practicing clinician should strive to recognize other important considerations beyond drug prescription and treatment guidelines, such as the patient's level of health literacy, social and economic implications of lifelong drug therapy and health care costs, and readiness for and effectiveness of patient self-management. This should be followed by delivery of patient education that is appropriate for literacy level. Self-monitoring should be a tool to engage patients in active participation. Comprehensive risk stratification should be encouraged in all patients. Careful clinician adherence to established practice guidelines in overall risk assessment and treatment and control of blood pressure to target levels remain crucial.

Management of High Blood Pressure in Children and Adolescents 597

Rae-Ellen W. Kavey, Stephen R. Daniels, and Joseph T. Flynn

Hypertension in childhood is now recognized to be a common and serious problem with a prevalence of 2% to 5%. Large epidemiologic studies have established normative tables for blood pressure beginning in early childhood based on age, gender, and height. Making a diagnosis of hypertension in a child or adolescent identifies an individual at increased risk for early-onset cardiovascular disease who requires specific treatment. Routine blood pressure measurement is recommended at every health care encounter beginning at 3 years of age, but often this is not being accomplished. This measurement is especially important in relation to the obesity epidemic, because approximately one-third of obese children have high blood pressure. Hypertension can be effectively managed with effective lifestyle change and medication when necessary.

Treatment and Control of High Blood Pressure in Adults 609

George A. Mensah and George Bakris

Hypertension and prehypertension are major public health challenges. Prevention and control of prehypertension through lifestyle changes and the treatment of hypertension to goal blood pressure (BP) are important objectives. In most patients, 2 or more medications with complementary mechanisms of action should be used in combination. Referral for evaluation of resistant hypertension should be made when goal BP is not attained while patients are adherent on 3 or more appropriately dosed antihypertensive medications, including a diuretic. There are compelling indications for the use of specific drugs in patients with underlying ischemic heart disease, chronic heart failure, diabetes, chronic kidney disease, stroke, peripheral arterial disease, left ventricular hypertrophy, obesity, and metabolic syndrome. Adverse drug effects should be identified early and managed promptly to address patient safety and adherence. Other factors that affect adherence include the patient's health literacy level and ability to self-manage. The social, environmental, cultural, and financial sources of support in care must be addressed to achieve the full benefits of treatment and control of hypertension and prehypertension.

The benefits of appropriate blood pressure (BP) control include reductions in proteinuria and possibly a slowing of the progressive loss of kidney function. Overall, medication therapy to lower BP during pregnancy should be used mainly for maternal safety because of the lack of data to support an improvement in fetal outcome. The major goal of hypertension treatment in those with baroreceptor dysfunction is to avoid the precipitous, severe BP elevations that characteristically occur during emotional stimulation. The treatment of hypertension in African Americans optimally consists of comprehensive lifestyle modifications along with pharmacologic treatments, most often with combination, not single-drug, therapy.

Hypertension is a very common modifiable risk factor for cardiovascular morbidity and mortality. Patients with hypertension represent a diverse group. In addition to those with primary hypertension, there are patients whose hypertension is attributable to secondary causes, those with resistant hypertension, and patients who present with a hypertensive crisis. Secondary causes of hypertension account for less than 10% of cases of elevated blood pressure (BP), and screening for these causes is warranted if clinically indicated. Patients with resistant hypertension, whose BP remains uncontrolled in spite of use of 3 or more antihypertensive agents, are at increased cardiovascular risk compared with the general hypertensive population. After potentially correctible causes of uncontrolled BP (pseudoresistance, secondary causes, and intake of interfering substances) are eliminated, patients with true resistant hypertension are managed by encouraging therapeutic lifestyle changes and optimizing the antihypertensive regimen, whereby the clinician ensures that the medications are prescribed at optimal doses using drugs with complementary mechanisms of action, while adding an appropriate diuretic if there are no contraindications. Mineralocorticoid receptor antagonists are formidable add-on agents to the antihypertensive regimen, usually as a fourth drug, and are effective in reducing BP even in patients without biochemical evidence of aldosterone excess. In the setting of a hypertensive crisis, the BP has to be reduced within hours in the case of a hypertensive emergency (elevated BP with evidence of target organ damage) using parenteral agents, and within a few days if there is hypertensive urgency, using oral antihypertensive agents.

Cardiovascular diseases (CVDs) have become the leading cause of death and disability in most countries in the world. This article addresses how patient self-management is a crucial component of effective high-quality health care for hypertension and CVD. The patient must be a collaborator in this process, and methods of improving patients' ability and confidence for self-management are needed. Successful self-management programs have often supplemented the traditional patient-physician encounter by using nonphysician providers, remote patient encounters (telephone or Internet), group settings, and peer support for promoting self-management. Several factors need to be considered in self-management. Given the health care system's inability to achieve several quality indicators using traditional office-based physician visits, further consideration is needed to determine the degree to

Cardiology Clinics

FORTHCOMING ISSUES

February 2011

Catheterization Hemodynamics
Michael Lim, MD,
Guest Editor

May 2011

Cardiovascular Disease Prevention
Prakash Deedwania, MD,
Guest Editor

August 2011

Peripheral Vascular Disease
Sanjay Rajagopalan, MD,
Guest Editor

RECENT ISSUES

August 2010

Diabetes, the Kidney, and Cardiovascular Risk
George L. Bakris, MD,
Guest Editor

May 2010

Controversies in Diseases of the Aorta
John A. Elefteriades, MD,
Guest Editor

February 2010

Advanced Applied Interventional Cardiology
Samin K. Sharma, MD, FSCAI, FACC, and
Annapoorna S. Kini, MD, MRCP, FACC,
Guest Editors

ISSUES OF RELATED INTEREST

Cardiac Electrophysiology Clinics, September 2010 (Vol. 2, No. 3)
Advances in Antiarrhythmic Drug Therapy
Peter R. Kowey, MD, FACC, FHRS, FAHA, and
Gerald V. Naccarelli, MD, FACC, FHRS, FAHA, *Guest Editors*
Available at: http://www.cardiacep.theclinics.com/

Heart Failure Clinics, April 2010 (Vol. 6, No. 2)
Genetics of Cardiomyopathy and Heart Failure
Calum A. MacRae, MD, PhD, *Guest Editor*
Available at: http://www.heartfailure.theclinics.com/

Foreword

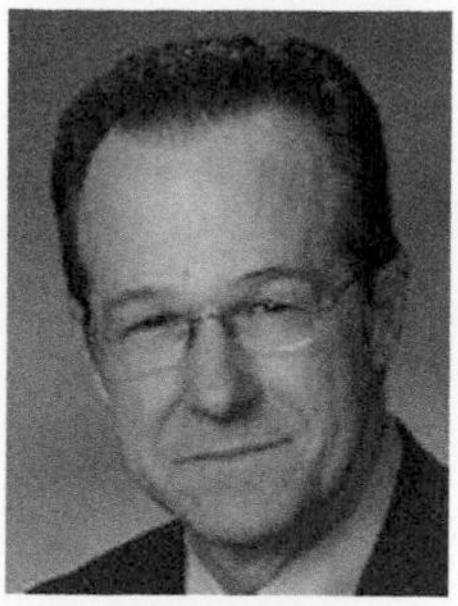

Michael H. Crawford, MD
Consulting Editor

I am very pleased that Dr George Mensah again agreed to guest edit an issue of *Cardiology Clinics* on Hypertension. Despite recent advances, it remains a major public and personal health issue. Also, it remains a challenge for physicians since the perfect therapy has not been discovered. In addition, there is a constant stream of new drugs and clinical information for the clinician to keep up with. Thus, the time is overdue for another issue on this topic.

Dr Mensah and the authors he assembled for this issue are world experts on hypertension. They cover everything from practical topics such as how to measure blood pressure to a cutting-edge discussion of the pathogenesis of hypertension. Many articles are devoted to difficult clinical issues we all face in managing hypertensive patients such as resistant hypertension and the role of dietary modification in hypertension control. I am convinced that all practicing cardiologists and primary care physicians will learn much from this issue of *Cardiology Clinics*.

Michael H. Crawford, MD
Division of Cardiology
Department of Medicine
University of California
San Francisco Medical Center
505 Parnassus Avenue
Box 0124
San Francisco, CA 94143-0124, USA

E-mail address:
crawfordm@medicine.ucsf.edu

Cardiol Clin 28 (2010) xi
doi:10.1016/j.ccl.2010.09.002
0733-8651/10/$ – see front matter

Preface
Hypertension and Hypertensive Heart Disease

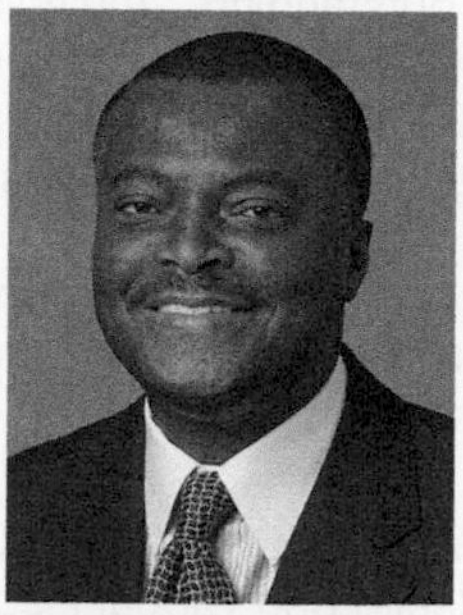

George A. Mensah, MD, FACC, FACP, FACN
Guest Editor

Hypertension is a powerful predictor of cardiovascular mortality and death from all causes. In fact, it is the leading risk factor for global mortality and accounted for 13% of worldwide deaths in 2004, far exceeding the contribution from tobacco use (9%), diabetes (6%), physical inactivity (6%), or overweight and obesity (5%).[1] Hypertension is also a major risk factor for nonfatal events, including stroke, end-stage kidney failure, myocardial infarction, and hypertensive heart disease. Through these nonfatal events, hypertension contributes significantly to outpatient doctor visits, repeat hospitalizations, reduced quality of life, and a substantial global economic burden.[2] The prevention and control of hypertension therefore takes on tremendous clinical, public health, and economic significance around the globe.

In 2002, the last time an issue of *Cardiology Clinics* addressed clinical hypertension, we lamented the disappointingly low hypertension control rates worldwide despite the wide availability of safe and effective medications. At that time, four of five hypertensive patients in the United States were not controlled; in the United Kingdom, only 6% of hypertensive patients had their blood pressure (BP) lowered below 140/90 mm Hg. Elsewhere in Europe, BP control rates ranged from 5% in Spain to 24% in France.[3] In most developing countries where resources for health care are more limited, BP control rates were even lower. That issue of *Cardiology Clinics* called for increased investments in hypertension awareness and education; a renewed commitment to refine strategies for hypertension prevention and treatment; and importantly, a renewed determination to set and achieve goal BP.

Since that time, much progress has been made. The most recent results from national surveys in the US demonstrate improvements in the rates of hypertension awareness (80.7%), treatment (72.5%), and control (50.1%).[4] Thus, for the first time in the US, more than half of all hypertensive patients in the 2007–2008 survey achieved goal BP.[4] Similarly, substantial progress has also been reported from two large surveys from Canada.[5,6] These are definitely encouraging reports; however, for most of the developed world, progress in hypertension control has only been modest. Especially in low- and middle-income countries where competing health care priorities are high and resources are relatively low, hypertension awareness, prevention, treatment, and control rates remain dismal.

In this issue of *Cardiology Clinics*, we focus on the prevention, treatment, and control of hypertension to goal BP and address the major sequelae of hypertensive heart disease. We take advantage of the major clinical practice guidelines published since the 2002 issue on clinical hypertension. In particular, the seventh report of the Joint National Committee on Prevention, Detection, Evaluation, and Treatment of High Blood Pressure (JNC 7)[7]

Cardiol Clin 28 (2010) xiii–xiv
doi:10.1016/j.ccl.2010.09.001

is referenced extensively, and, where appropriate, key lessons from other recently published guidelines are cited.

First, Singh et al address the pathophysiological basis for raised blood pressure and the complex spectrum of mechanisms responsible for maintaining a chronically elevated BP level. Egan et al then present the clinical epidemiology of prehypertension and examine the evidence suggesting that this condition is a major contributor to new cases of hypertension and overall cardiovascular risk, thus justifying a more aggressive approach for its prevention and control. Ogedegbe and Pickering review the basic techniques of BP measurement and discuss the important issues associated with measurements in special populations such as infants, children, pregnant women, elderly persons, and obese subjects in clinical practice.

Subsequent articles discuss the comprehensive assessment indicated at the initial clinical encounter with the patient who has established or suspected hypertension, and the strategies for treatment and control of hypertension to goal BP in children and adolescents as well as in adults. In particular, Kavey et al summarize the series of randomized trials in the most recent pediatric BP Task Force report from the National Heart, Lung, and Blood Institute that demonstrate the safety and efficacy of BP-lowering drugs in children and adolescents.

Several population groups that merit special attention in the treatment and control of hypertension are discussed by Flack et al. Acelajado and Calhoun present pearls in the evaluation and treatment of patients with secondary hypertension, resistant hypertension, or hypertensive crisis. Bosworth et al review concepts of patient self-management as a crucial component of effective, high-quality health care for chronic diseases and emphasize the need to incorporate strategies that allow patients to take more control in their care. The important role that diet, foods, and nutrients (especially sodium, potassium, and excess calories) play in the prevention and control of hypertension and prehypertension is then addressed. In the final article, Butler et al address the evaluation and treatment of hypertensive heart disease and suggest strategies for both the prevention as well as the regression of structural and functional cardiovascular abnormalities in the setting of long-standing hypertension.

Overall, the articles in this issue of *Cardiology Clinics* demonstrate the substantial progress as well as the persisting global challenges we face in the prevention and control of hypertension and hypertensive heart disease. I remain deeply indebted to the outstanding, multidisciplinary group of experts who helped make this endeavor successful. I am also very grateful to Dr Michael Crawford for his guidance and to Ms Barbara Cohen-Kligerman and the dedicated team at Elsevier for their unfailing commitment and support. I hope you find this issue useful in your practice.

George A. Mensah, MD, FACC, FACP, FACN
Heart Health and Global Health Policy
Global Research and Development
PepsiCo, Inc
700 Anderson Hill Road, Building 6-2
Purchase, NY 10755, USA

E-mail address:
george.mensah@pepsico.com

REFERENCES

1. World Health Organization. Global health risks: mortality and burden of disease attributable to selected major risks. Geneva: World Health Organization; 2009.
2. Gaziano TA, Bitton A, Anand S, et al. The global cost of nonoptimal blood pressure. J Hypertens 2009; 27(7):1472–7.
3. Mensah GA. The global burden of hypertension: good news and bad news. Cardiol Clin 2002;20(2): 181–5, v.
4. Egan BM, Zhao Y, Axon RN. US trends in prevalence, awareness, treatment, and control of hypertension, 1988-2008. JAMA 2010;303(20):2043–50.
5. Leenen FH, Dumais J, McInnis NH, et al. Results of the Ontario survey on the prevalence and control of hypertension. CMAJ 2008;178(11):1441–9.
6. Wilkins K, Campbell NR, Joffres MR, et al. Blood pressure in Canadian adults. Health Rep 2010;21(1): 37–46.
7. Chobanian AV, Bakris GL, Black HR, et al. The Seventh Report of the Joint National Committee on Prevention, Detection, Evaluation, and Treatment of High Blood Pressure: The JNC 7 Report. JAMA 2003;289(19):2560–72.

Pathogenesis and Clinical Physiology of Hypertension

Mukesh Singh, MD[a],
George A. Mensah, MD, FACC, FACP, FAHA[b],
George Bakris, MD, FASH, FASN, FAHA[a,*]

KEYWORDS

- Hypertension • Pathogenesis • Clinical physiology
- Pathophysiologic mechanisms

Although the definitive cause of primary hypertension remains unknown, significant advances have been made in understanding its pathogenesis and its clinical physiology. This article presents an overview of the physiology of normal blood pressure (BP) control and the pathophysiologic mechanisms that predispose individuals and populations to primary hypertension. The role of genetics, environment, and the gene-environment interaction is discussed. The spectrum of changes in physiologic states that result in chronic increases of arterial BP are briefly reviewed. In particular, the nature and characteristics of feedback loops and the primary modulating systems are presented. The key roles played by the central and peripheral nervous systems, renin-angiotensin-aldosterone system (RAAS), and other circulating and tissue hormones are reviewed. The role of the vessel wall and its interaction with the endothelium, endothelin, nitric oxide, angiotensin II (AII), as well as other vasoactive substances is also discussed. A unifying pathway for the development of hypertension and the practical implications for the prevention and control of hypertension are discussed.

THE PHYSIOLOGY OF NORMAL BP CONTROL

The product of cardiac output (CO) and total peripheral resistance (TPR) determines the mean arterial BP level. These 2 principal determinants are influenced by many physiologic factors, as shown in **Fig. 1**. CO depends primarily on heart rate and stroke volume. Heart rate is governed by β-1 and cholinergic receptors under the control of sympathetic and parasympathetic stimulation, respectively. The ventricular force of contraction (also under autonomic control) and the filling pressure, which is in turn determined by the intravascular fluid volume status and the venous capacitance, determines the stroke volume. The systemic vascular resistance is influenced by multiple vasoactive mechanisms under the control of local, regional, and systemic neural, humoral, and renal factors.[1–3] All of these physiologic determinants of flow and resistance are interdependently governed by rapid-, intermediate-, and late-acting mechanisms that maintain the arterial BP within the normal range despite significant variations in the individual parameters.[4–6]

The complex systems and mechanisms that constitute the feedback and reflex control of BP have been extensively studied and characterized. The most clinically relevant ones are depicted in **Fig. 2**. Rapid responses occurring within seconds after an acute increase in BP include the baroreceptor system, vagus nerve, and the central vasomotor center of the brainstem.[6] The arterial baroreceptor reflex pathway is a control system made up of a *neural arm*, including the arterial

A version of this article was originally appeared in *Cardiology Clinics*, Volume 20, issue 2.
[a] University of Chicago Pritzker School of Medicine, 5841 South Maryland Avenue, MC 1027, Chicago, IL 60637, USA
[b] Heart Health and Global Health Policy, Global Research and Development, 700 Anderson Hill Road, PepsiCo, Inc, Building 6-2, Purchase, NY 10755, USA
* Corresponding author.
E-mail address: gbakris@gmail.com

Cardiol Clin 28 (2010) 545–559
doi:10.1016/j.ccl.2010.07.001
0733-8651/10/$ – see front matter

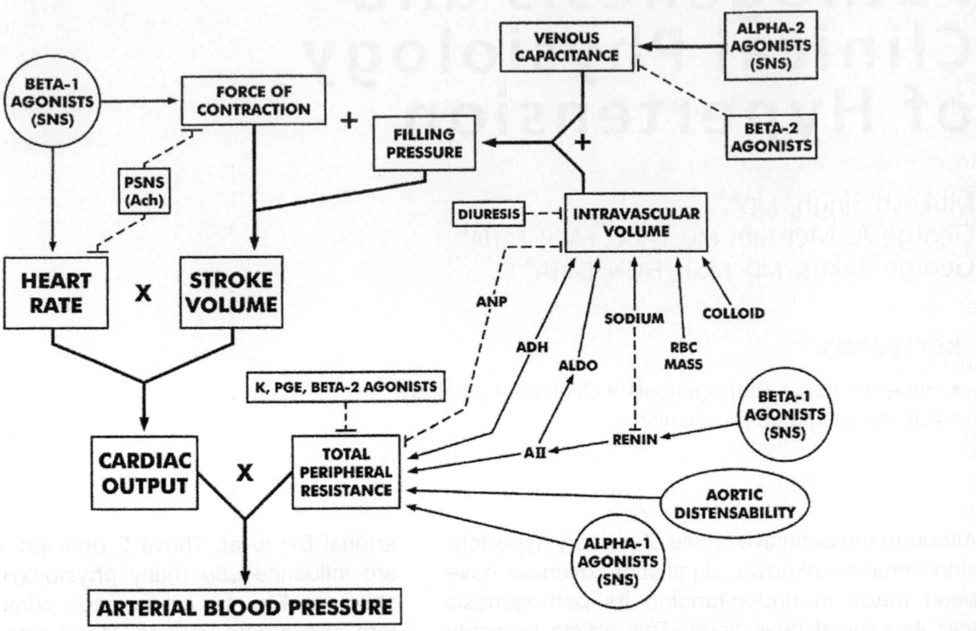

Fig. 1. Factors that determine arterial BP. Ach, acetylcholine; ADH, antidiuretic hormone; ALDO, aldosterone; AI, angiotensin I; AII, angiotensin II; ANP, atrial natriuretic peptide; i, inhibitory (negative influence); K, potassium; PGE, prostaglandin E; PNS, parasympathetic nervous system; RBC, red blood cells; SNS, sympathetic nervous system; →, stimulatory (positive) influence. (*From* Sobel BJ, Bakris GL. Hypertension: a clinician's guide to diagnosis and treatment. Philadelphia: Hanley & Belfus; 1999; with permission.)

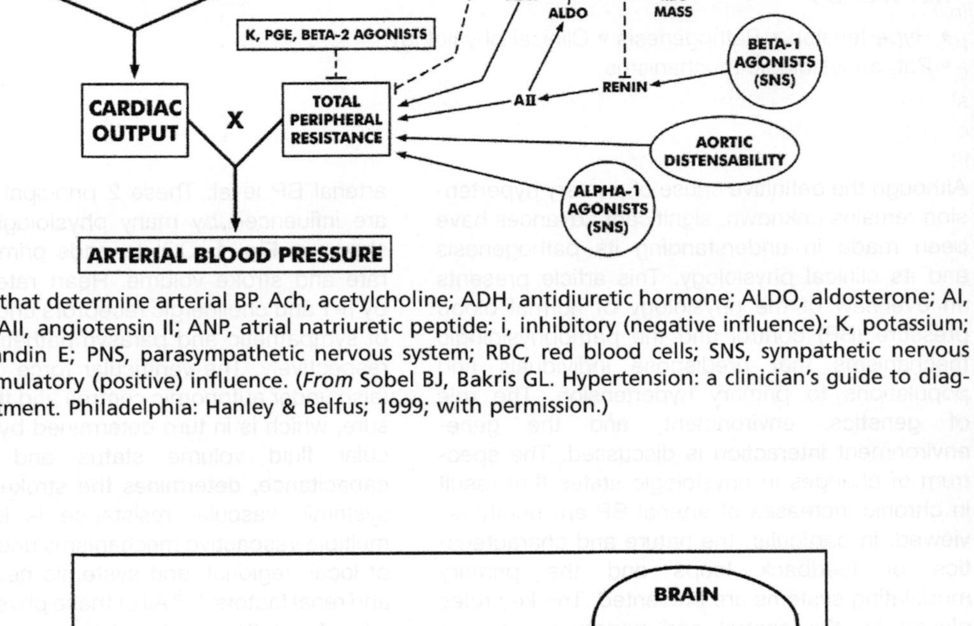

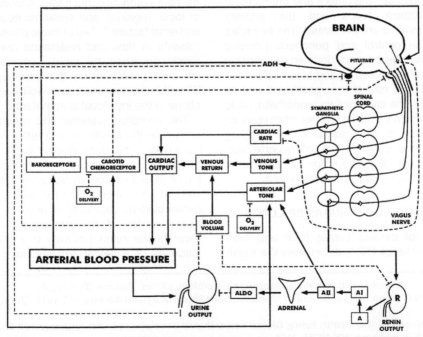

Fig. 2. Feedback mechanisms in the control of BP. A, angiotensinogen; ADH, antidiuretic hormone; AI, angiotensin I; AII, angiotensin 11; O_2, oxygen; ‖, inhibitory (negative) influence; →, stimulatory (positive) influence. (*From* Bakris GL, Mensah GA. Pathogenesis and clinical physiology of hypertension. Cardiol Clin 2002;20 (2):195–206; with permission.)

baroreceptors, their afferent nerve fibers, the medullary cardiovascular centers, and the efferent sympathetic and parasympathetic fibers and an *effector arm*, including the heart and peripheral blood vessels. Mean arterial pressure is the *input* to the neural arm and the *output* of the effector arm of this reflex pathway. Similarly, the activity of the sympathetic (and parasympathetic) cardiovascular nerves is the *output* of the neural arm of the arterial baroreceptor control system and, at the same time, the *input* to the effector arm.[7] An increase in arterial BP leads to a reflex decrease in the sympathetic traffic to the arterioles and veins, resulting in a decrease in peripheral resistance and cardiac filling pressure, respectively. In addition, slowing of the heart rate and reduced myocardial contractility occur because of simultaneous increases in parasympathetic outflow and decreased sympathetic tone to the heart.

Chemoreceptors acting at the vasomotor center also play a role in responding to acute changes in BP. This response is in addition to BP changes that result from chemoreceptor responses to blood oxygen tension and carbon dioxide tension. Thus, the rapid-acting reflex and feedback mechanisms in response to acute changes in BP are almost entirely mediated by changes in activity of the autonomic nervous system.[8] The adrenergic receptors, their associated agonists, and their physiologic actions, as well as the clinically useful antagonists, are shown in **Table 1**. However well the baroreceptor reflex counteracts temporary disturbances in arterial pressure, it cannot effectively regulate arterial pressure in the long-term, because the baroreceptor firing rate adapts to prolonged changes in arterial pressure.

Intermediate-acting responses to changes in arterial BP occur over minutes and hours, involve the RAAS, antidiuretic hormone (ADH), and the renal juxtaglomerular apparatus (**Fig. 3**). Both local and circulating RAASs play important roles in this feedback mechanism. Systemically, a reduction in BP stimulates renin release via afferent arteriole baroreceptor mechanisms and increased activity of the renal sympathetic nerves. A local macula densa mechanism of renin release also exists.[9–11] The available evidence suggests that there is significant interaction between the renal sympathetic nerve activity and the baroreceptor and macula densa mechanisms in the control of renin secretion.[10] Renin released by these mechanisms acts by converting angiotensinogen (synthesized in the liver and also produced locally) to angiotensin I, which is converted to AII by angiotensin-converting enzyme (ACE) produced in the lungs and locally. ACE is a nonspecific kininase that degrades vasodilatory kinins. The relevant actions of AII include (1) potent vasoconstriction; (2) stimulation of adrenal release of aldosterone, which leads to sodium retention and volume expansion; and (3) directly increasing proximal sodium chloride reabsorption. In addition, the RAAS also has a role in the long-term regulation of BP.[3,12,13]

ADH activity and capillary filtration are also intermediate-acting mechanisms for BP regulation (see **Fig. 3**). Acute reduction in BP leads to increased ADH secretion principally because of a decrease in the normal inhibitory tone from the baroreceptors to the hypothalamus. Conversely, an increase in BP causes increased baroreceptor activity to the hypothalamus, resulting in increased inhibition of the activity of hypothalamic ADH-releasing neurons. In the setting of acute, severe hypotension, ADH acts as part of the rapid response and serves as a pressor agent. However, during periods of prolonged decrease in BP, ADH also becomes a part of the late-acting response in continuing to conserve water (**Fig. 4**).

Late-acting mechanisms operate in days to weeks and are important because of their long-term efficiency in BP regulation.[14] Pressure natriuresis and diuresis are the key mechanisms[3,15,16] An increase in BP level beyond the normal set point leads directly to an increase in salt and water excretion. Guyton and colleagues[2] stated that none of the mechanisms discussed earlier can operate effectively to regulate BP without the participation of this kidney function, a phenomenon they termed the "overriding dominance of the kidneys" in the long-term regulation of arterial BP. Thus, in the long-term, arterial pressure is regulated by changes in blood volume because arterial pressure has a strong influence on urinary output rate via control of sodium and water excretion by the kidney.

Together, these complex interrelated mechanisms help regulate BP. Significant flexibility is built into the normal level at which BP is regulated. This feature permits significant transient increases in BP level through marked variations in CO and TPR to meet physiologic needs. Nevertheless, counter-regulatory and compensatory mechanisms contained in these feedback loops help to restore BP level to within normal limits after the end of the acute physiologic demands. The crucial difference between this normal pattern of BP regulation and chronic primary hypertension is an adverse neurohormonal activation, impaired renal handling of sodium, and an increased TPR, the characteristic hallmark of primary hypertension that helps to maintain hypertension and the progression to target-organ damage.

Table 1
Adrenergic receptors in the modulation of arterial BP

Receptors	Agonist Actions	Agonists	Antagonists
α-1	Vasoconstriction[a]	Norepinephrine ⋙ dopamine> dobutamine	Prazosin, labetalol
α-2, central effect	Vasodilation	Clonidine, norepinephrine	
α-2, peripheral effect	Venoconstriction	Clonidine, norepinephrine	
α-1, α-2	Net vasoconstriction; reflex decreased CO	Ergot, midodrine norepinephrine>epinephrine	Phentolamine, phenoxybenzamine
β-1	Increased CO, lipolysis, increased renin	Epinephrine, norepinephrine, low-dose dopamine, dobutamine[a]	Atenolol, metroprolol
β-2	Vasodilation[b]; bronchodilation	Albuterol, epinephrine ≫ norepinephrine[a]	
β-1, β-2	Net increased CO	Epinephrine, isoproterenol	Propranolol, pindolol
α-1, β-1	Vasoconstriction and increased CO	Epinephrine, high-dose dopamine	Labetalol
Parasympathetic	Decreased CO, decreased heart rate	Acetylcholine	Atropine
V_1	Increased peripheral resistance	Arginine vasopressin	Selective V_1 receptor antagonist (not commercially available) or calcium antagonist

[a] Predominantly arteriolar.
[b] Without chronotropic effects (unlike dopamine and isoproterenol).
Data from Sobel BJ, Bakris GL. Hypertension: a clinician's guide to diagnosis and treatment. Philadelphia: Hanley & Belfus; 1999.

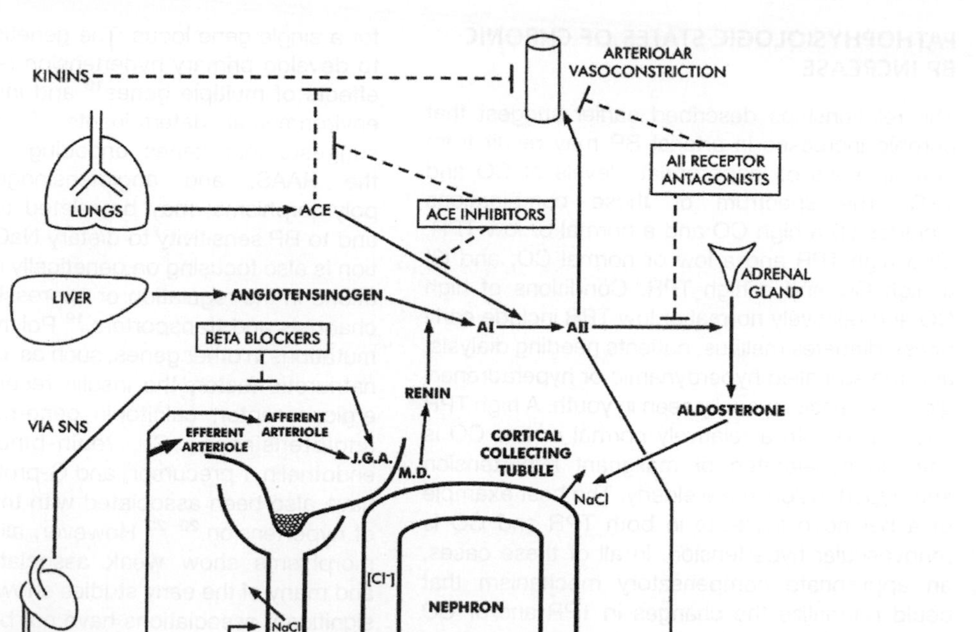

Fig. 3. The renin-angiotensin system in the control of BP. ACE, angiotensin-converting enzyme; AI, angiotensin I; AII, angiotensin II; JGA, juxtaglomerular apparatus; [C1⁻], luminal chloride concentration; MD, macula densa; SNS, sympathetic nervous system; →, positive influence; ‖, negative influence. (*From* Bakris GL, Mensah GA. Pathogenesis and clinical physiology of hypertension. Cardiol Clin 2002;20(2)195–206; with permission.)

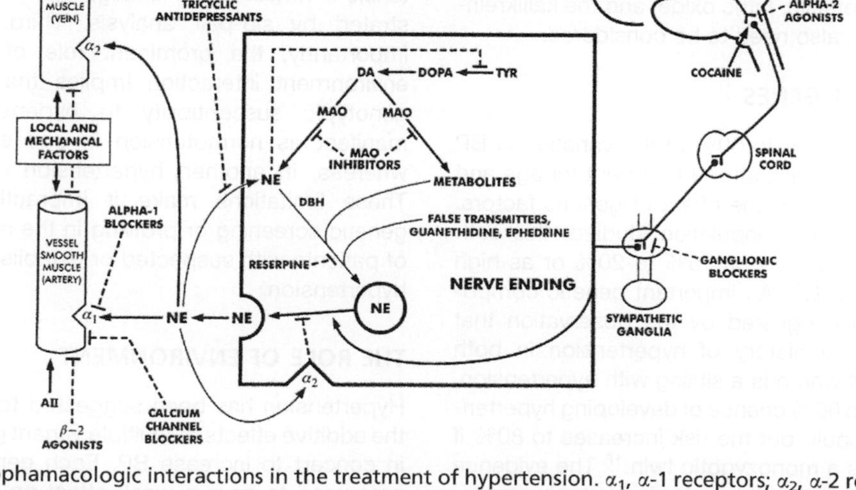

Fig. 4. Neurophamacologic interactions in the treatment of hypertension. α_1, α-1 receptors; α_2, α-2 receptors; AII, angiotensin II; DA, dopamine; DBH, dopamine hydroxylase; DOPA, dihydroxyphenylalanme; MAO, monoamine oxidase; NE, norepinephrine; TYR, tyrosine; ---|, inhibitory (negative) influence; →, stimulatory (positive) influence. (*From* Bakris GL, Mensah GA. Pathogenesis and clinical physiology of hypertension. Cardiol Clin 2002;20 (2):195–206; with permission.)

PATHOPHYSIOLOGIC STATES OF CHRONIC BP INCREASE

The relationships described earlier suggest that chronic increases in arterial BP may result from combinations of inappropriate levels of CO and TPR. The spectrum of these combinations includes (1) a high CO and a normal or low TPR, (2) a high TPR and a low or normal CO, and (3) a high CO and a high TPR. Conditions of high CO and relatively normal or low TPR include early phase diabetes mellitus, patients needing dialysis, and the so-called hyperdynamic or hyperadrenergic hypertension usually seen in youth. A high TPR associated with a relatively normal or low CO is seen in accelerated or malignant hypertension and hypertension in the elderly. The best example of a balanced increase in both TPR and CO is renovascular hypertension. In all of these cases, an appropriate compensatory mechanism that could normalize the changes in TPR and/or CO to return BP level to the normal range is missing.

PATHOGENESIS OF PRIMARY HYPERTENSION

Although the definitive cause of primary hypertension remains unknown, it is generally believed that genes and the environment, as well as their interactions, play important roles. Superimposed on this gene-environment predisposition to hypertension, a large number of hypotheses have been proposed to explain the development of hypertension. In almost any hypothesis, at least 3 major areas need to be addressed. These areas include the role of the sympathetic nervous system (SNS), the RAAS, and the kidney, particularly as it relates to the handling of sodium. Other factors, such as endothelin, nitric oxide, and the kallikrein-kinin system, also need to be considered.

THE ROLE OF GENES

An estimated 30% to 60% of the variation in BP between individuals, after adjustment for age and sex, is attributed to the effect of genetic factors. Depending on the population studied, this estimate may be as low as 15% to 20% or as high as 65% to 70%.[17] An important genetic component is also suggested by the observation that a child with a history of hypertension in both parents, and who has a sibling with hypertension, has a 40% to 60% chance of developing hypertension as an adult, but the risk increases to 80% if the sibling is a monozygotic twin.[18] The evidence so far suggests that it is unlikely for the hypertensive phenotype to be caused by a single gene. In addition, the inheritance patterns in primary hypertension do not follow classic Mendelian genetics for a single gene locus. The genetic susceptibility to develop primary hypertension results from the effects of multiple genes[19] and involves multiple environmental determinants. Current evidence suggests that genes encoding components of the RAAS, and angiotensinogen and ACE polymorphisms, may be related to hypertension and to BP sensitivity to dietary NaCl. Much attention is also focusing on genetically mediated alterations in the regulation or expression of renal ion channels and transporters.[19] Polymorphisms and mutations in other genes, such as α-adducin, atrial natriuretic factor, the insulin receptor, β_2-adrenergic receptor, calcitonin gene-related peptide, angiotensinase C, renin-binding protein, endothelin-1 precursor, and G-protein β_3-subunit, have also been associated with the development of hypertension.[20–23] However, all of these polymorphisms show weak associations with BP, and many of the early studies showing statistically significant associations have not been confirmed. Preliminary evidence suggests that there may also be genetic determinants of target-organ damage attributed to hypertension.

Despite these advances in our understanding of the genetic susceptibility to hypertension and the elucidation of the roles of these candidate genes, genetic profiling should not be considered in the routine evaluation and management of patients with primary hypertension. First, candidate gene polymorphisms associated with the hypertension phenotype in one population have not been consistently associated with hypertension in other populations of a different ethnic background. Second, there are cases in which candidate gene polymorphisms have been associated with hypertension; however, no linkage could be demonstrated by sib-pair analysis. Third, and most importantly, the prominent role of the gene-environment interaction implies that the same genotypic susceptibility to hypertension may manifest as normotension in one environment, whereas, in another, hypertension is observed. These limitations make it impractical to use genetic screening or profiling in the management of patients with suspected or established primary hypertension.

THE ROLE OF ENVIRONMENT

Hypertension has been suggested to result from the additive effects of multiple variant genes acting in concert to increase BP. Each gene variant is presumed to have a weak effect on BP but may produce significant hypertension when they act together in the presence of the necessary environmental conditions. These environmental influences on BP phenotype have been well described.[24–27] The environmental contribution to the variation in BP between individuals has been estimated to be at least 20%; however, as pointed out by Harrap,[24] environmental effects are most demonstrable between populations rather than between individuals presumably because of larger and more numerous differences. Key environmental factors include geography; dietary intake of sodium, calcium, potassium, and other micro- and macronutrients; physical activity; psychosocial stress; socioeconomic status; alcohol intake; cigarette smoking and other lifestyle choices.

Among these factors, dietary intake of sodium and salt (NaCl) have been the most studied. Epidemiologic and interventional studies have strongly linked salt intake with hypertension. Populations with a high-sodium content in their diet (>4 g/d), such as those in northern Japan and the southeastern United States, have a high prevalence of hypertension. Conversely, populations consuming a low-sodium diet, such as the Alaskan Eskimo or the Yanamao Indians from the Amazon, have an almost negligible prevalence of hypertension. However, in contrast to between-population and migration studies, most within-population studies have not found any close relationship between BP and sodium intake. A difference of only 2.2 mm Hg in systolic BP can be expected for a difference of 100 mmol sodium per day.[28] The susceptibility to increased BP in response to sodium loading is highly variable. The salt sensitivity of BP has a familial character and can be identified in the prehypertensive state.[29] Low birth weight has been associated with increased BP in children and with hypertension in adult.[30] This association may be caused by an inborn deficit in nephron number and an ensuing increased renal retention of sodium.[31]

Diets low in calcium or potassium have also been associated with a higher prevalence of hypertension.[32,33] Increasing potassium intake has been found to lower BP in both experimental and human studies. Migration as well as between- and within-population studies have shown an inverse relationship between potassium intake and the prevalence of hypertension.[34] In the United States, African Americans ingest less potassium than white people do and this may partly explain the continuing greater prevalence of hypertension in the former. This may also partly explain the tendency for a higher prevalence of severe hypertension observed in the African Americans. Low potassium intake may contribute to salt sensitivity.[35,36]

Obesity is perhaps the most salient risk factor for phenotypic expression of hypertension. There is a strong positive correlation between body fat and BP levels, and human obesity and hypertension frequently coexist.[37] Excess weight gain is a consistent predictor for subsequent development of hypertension.[38] The proportion of obese individuals as a function of the total population is continuing to grow in all westernized societies. This growth parallels the incidence of hypertension in these societies. Obesity may cause hypertension by various mechanisms.[39–42] An activation of sympathetic nerve activity leading to renal sodium retention seems to play a pivotal role. Hyperleptinemia and hyperinsulinemia represent 2 mechanisms by which obesity might increase sympathetic nerve activity. Other factors possibly contributing to renal sodium retention in obesity are increased AII and aldosterone production and raised intrarenal pressures caused by fat surrounding the kidneys.

Certain metabolic features are associated with the development of high BP, such as hyperglycemia (insulin resistance), increased hematocrit, and hyperuricemia. Increased serum uric acid has been shown to predict the development of hypertension as well as to be present in 25% of people with untreated hypertension. However, controversy exists as to whether uric acid is an independent risk factor or simply a marker for other conditions associated with higher cardiovascular risk. It has been implicated in the development of hypertension and is seen in obesity, insulin resistance, dyslipidemia, and high degrees of alcohol use.

There are other important demographic factors for the development of hypertension. Primary hypertension is uncommon in young adults but increases with age, with 65% prevalence in the population at age 65 years, and 75% at 75 years. This age-related increase in prevalence of hypertension has been observed in most Western countries but has not been uniformly observed in all populations. Second, the prevalence of hypertension is greater in men. Although the prevalence in women approaches that of men in the postmenopausal years, certain racial/ethnic groups are also at increased risk based on environmental influences and gene-environment interactions, particularly African Americans. Obesity, insulin resistance, gout, and sleep apnea are also associated with an increased risk, as are low socioeconomic status and increased stress at work. Certain physical features, such as increased heart rate, or an increased BP response to exercise, are also predictive.[43]

THE SNS

The SNS plays a pivotal role in the regulation of vascular tone. It modulates CO and peripheral vascular resistance, the 2 determinants of BP. Heart rate and stroke volume are increased, at least in the early, labile phase of BP increase, and at least part of the increased vascular resistance of the established phase of hypertension may be caused by the increased sympathetic tone.

Guyton and colleagues[2] have shown that much of the short-term arterial pressure control is mediated by the central and autonomic nervous system. High-pressure baroreceptors in the carotid sinus and aortic arch respond to acute increases in pressure by causing a reflex vagal bradycardia and inhibition of sympathetic output from the central nervous system (CNS), and the opposite occurs when BP suddenly decreases. Low-pressure cardiopulmonary receptors in the atria and ventricles respond to increases in atrial filling by increasing heart rate (via inhibition of the cardiac SNS), increasing atrial natriuretic peptide release, and inhibiting vasopressin release. These reflexes are largely controlled centrally, particularly in the nucleus tractus solitarius of the dorsal medulla. This vasomotor center also receives input from the limbus and hypothalamus in response to emotional or psychological stress.

Numerous studies have documented that the SNS is often hyperactive in essential hypertension, particularly in patients who are young or borderline hypertensive.[44] Many patients with newly diagnosed hypertension have increased plasma norepinephrine levels with increased heart rate and cardiac indices. These patients often show increases of BP with stress, exercise, or emotion. Some of these patients also have increased plasma renin levels, which may reflect β-adrenergic stimulation of renin secretion. Many of them also have increased vascular reactivity, systemic vascular resistance, and low blood volume.

The mechanisms involved in the stimulation of the SNS in hypertension have been an area of intense study. However, despite years of investigations, the mechanisms responsible for the adrenergic overactivity characterizing human hypertension remain undefined. A defect in baroreceptor sensitivity[45] has been postulated and may contribute to the increased BP variability noted in some patients with hypertension. The observation that some patients have an increase in SNS response to emotional or work-related stress also suggests this as a contributing factor. It has also been suggested that the metabolic alterations frequently detectable in hypertension, such as hyperinsulinemic state and the related insulin resistance, may be the triggering factors. This hypothesis is based on the evidence that insulin may have central sympathoexcitatory effects that may thus be enhanced in the adrenergic drive of patients who are hypertensive (this drive frequently displays insulin resistance).[45] Increased SNS activity is associated with primary hypertension in certain high-risk groups, such as African Americans, people who are obese, people who are insulin resistant, and users of certain drugs (eg, nicotine, alcohol, cyclosporine, cocaine) associated with hypertension. There may be a subset of patients in whom compression of the lateral medulla by cranial nerves and/or vessels may result in increased SNS activity and hypertension, and, in some of these patients, selective decompression may ameliorate the hypertension. Activation of the CNS/SNS may result from renal afferent sympathetics from hypertensive kidneys. In several experimental models of hypertension, renal sympathectomy can cause a reduction in BP.[46] Moreover, studies have shown that AII exerts central sympathoexcitatory effects and pharmacologic blockade of the RAAS via ACE inhibitors or AII receptor blockers exerts sympathomodulatory effects.[45,47,48]

The consequences of SNS stimulation are peripheral vasoconstriction, an increase in heart rate, release of norepinephrine from the adrenals, and a resultant increase in systemic BP. The increase in SNS also has been shown to exert prohypertrophic effects on the myocardial tissues and plays a crucial role in mediating vascular hypertrophy and increased vascular stiffness leading to reduced arterial distensibility and compliance.[45] This prohypertrophic effect, coupled with the evidence that the degree of sympathetic activation detected in hypertension is potentiated when left ventricular hypertrophy is observed at the echocardiographic examination,[45] strongly supports the hypothesis that the increase in cardiac wall thickness seen in hypertension depends not only on the hemodynamic overload but also on sympathetic factors.[49] Renal efferent sympathetics are also activated and cause intrarenal vasoconstriction with a decrease in renal blood flow and an increase in renal vascular resistance. The renal SNS also directly stimulates sodium reabsorption and renin release from the juxtaglomerular apparatus. Sympathetic neural factors may also promote the metabolic abnormalities frequently detected in the clinical history of patients with hypertension.[45] In particular, it has been shown that an increase in adrenergic activity may trigger an insulin resistance state via a series of hemodynamic and nonhemodynamic effects, causing massive vasoconstriction at the level of the skeletal muscle and organs involved in the development of insulin resistance.[45,49]

THE RAAS

The RAAS is one of the most important mechanisms in the regulation of blood volume and pressure. Renin is a proteolytic enzyme, initially synthesized as prorenin, cleaving off the decapeptide angiotensin I from angiotensinogen, a protein substrate produced by the liver and circulating in the blood. Angiotensin I does not have any vasoactive effects by itself, and is further degraded in the presence of ACEs to AII. Most of the angiotensin I is converted to AII during its passage through the pulmonary circulation, but ACE is ubiquitous at the surface of endothelial cells.[50] Two subtypes of AII receptors have been characterized in humans: AT_1 and AT_2. AII exerts most of its effects via AT_1 receptors.[51–55] The AT_1 receptor is G-protein coupled and contains 359 amino acids. AII causes stimulation of vascular smooth muscle contraction and hypertrophy, increases cardiac contractility, stimulation of the SNS in the central and peripheral nervous system (by activating receptors located on sympathetic nerve endings to facilitate norepinephrine release), increases thirst and vasopressin release, and stimulates aldosterone synthesis. Within the kidney, stimulation of the AT_1 receptor by aII also causes renal vasoconstriction (especially of the efferent arteriole and vasa rectae), a decrease in renal blood flow, and an increase in renal vascular resistance. AII also increases sodium reabsorption, not only through aldosterone but also by direct effects on the proximal tubules and also by increasing the sensitivity of the tubuloglomerular (TG) feedback response. An important effect mediated by the AT_1 receptor is the activation of membrane-reduced nicotinamide adenine dinucleotide phosphate (NADPH) oxidase, thereby increasing the generation of reactive oxygen species in the vasculature and facilitating the atherosclerotic process.[56] The vascular and cardiac effects of AT_2 receptor stimulation seem to counterbalance those exerted by the AT_1 receptor.[51,55,57,58] The vasodilation induced by the stimulation of the AT_2 receptor may involve bradykinin and nitric oxide.[59] In addition to the systemic RAAS, there is evidence that local RAASs are present in blood vessels, the heart, and the kidney, where they may mediate local effects (such as tissue remodeling) independently of circulating renin or angiotensinogen levels.

The role of the RAAS in essential hypertension is complex. Although plasma renin activity is increased in 20% of patients, renin activity is either normal (50%) or low (30%) in most. In the early phase of hypertension, the high renin levels may be secondary to an increased autonomic activity.[60] Renin secretion decreases with age, both in people who are normotensive and hypertensive, presumably reflecting sodium retention associated with a progressive decline in functional nephrons.[61] Racial differences exist in renin secretion. Thus, plasma renin activity is generally lower in blacks than in whites.[62] However, in many of the patients with normal renin activity, the plasma renin may be inappropriately high in relation to the total body sodium. This has been suggested by the observation that saline depletion or infusion results in blunted changes in renin levels in these patients, and by the observation that BP in these patients frequently responds to ACE inhibitors.[63] Sealey and colleagues[63] suggested that the reason for the widely varying renin levels may be nephron heterogeneity within individual kidneys, in which there are some ischemic nephrons making excess renin and other hyperfiltering nephrons in which renin secretion is suppressed. According to these investigators, the increased renin release from the ischemic nephrons enters the circulation, leading to AII generation that causes inappropriate vasoconstriction and sodium reabsorption in the other, hyperfiltering nephrons, and this results in sodium retention and the development of hypertension.

VASCULAR REMODELING, HYPERTROPHY, AND INCREASED PERIPHERAL RESISTANCE

Since the original observation by Folkow[64,65] that resistance vessels from hypertensive animals had greater vascular resistance than in control animals, the importance of peripheral vascular resistance as a hallmark of hypertension has always been recognized. Although partly considered an adaptive response to normalize increased wall stress, this structural remodeling in resistance vessels plays an important role in the maintenance of hypertension via its vascular amplifying effect. Recent advances in the biology of the vessel wall and its interaction with the endothelium and vasoactive substances have significantly advanced our understanding of the growth and remodeling of these resistance vessels. Many of the vasoactive substances considered important for their pressor effects also have significant trophic influences on the vascular smooth muscle. For example, AII, the potent vasoconstrictor and pressor agent, is also a powerful mediator of vascular remodeling through direct stimulation of protein synthesis in vascular smooth muscle cells,[66] induction of growth factor genes,[67] alteration of the extracellular matrix,[68] and promotion of vascular cellularity.[69] These vascular growth promotion and remodeling properties have also been described for other vasoconstrictors, including endothelin and norepinephrine. However, endogenous vasodilators tend to be inhibitors of growth promotion and remodeling. Thus, nitric oxide, natriuretic peptides, bradykinin, and prostacyclin all inhibit growth of vascular smooth muscle cells.[70] Persistent perturbations in the normal balance of endogenous vasoconstrictors and vasodilators leading to a relative excess of growth promoters compared with growth inhibitors, as may be seen in settings of endothelial dysfunction, set the stage for adverse vascular remodeling and hypertrophy that contribute to sustained hypertension.

HYPERINSULINEMIA AND INSULIN RESISTANCE

Patients who are hypertensive often exhibit some degree of hyperinsulinemia. Hyperinsulinemia-associated hypertension has a strong genetic component. Mechanisms by which hyperinsulinemia can cause hypertension include (1) increased renal sodium reabsorption, (2) stimulation of SNS, and (3) insulin acting as a growth factor.

Several factors might be implicated in the pathogenesis of insulin resistance. Free fatty acid concentrations are increased in patients with metabolic syndrome,[71] which has an inhibitory influence on insulin signaling, resulting in a reduction in insulin-stimulated glucose muscle transport. In addition, the adipose tissue produces several proteins, called adipocytokines, which alter insulin sensitivity.[72,73] Studies have also shown a link between insulin resistance and endothelial dysfunction.[74]

THE KIDNEY AND PRIMARY HYPERTENSION

Guyton and colleagues[2] noted that, although the SNS and RAAS are important for short-term changes in BP, ultimately it is the kidney that is responsible for long-term blood-volume and pressure control. Dahl and Heine[75] were the first to show that hypertension can be transferred from the hypertensive Dahl salt-sensitive rat to the non-hypertensive Dahl salt-resistant rat by transplantation of the kidney, and this has been subsequently verified in 4 different genetic strains of rats with hypertension. Patients with essential hypertension-associated renal failure have also been cured of their underlying hypertension by renal transplantation from a normotensive donor.

Most authorities believe that the mechanism by which the kidney causes hypertension derives from impairment in the excretion of salt. Epidemiologic studies have linked the relative sodium content in the diet with the prevalence of hypertension in various populations, and intervention studies with salt restriction or loading has also revealed that the BP response in many patients with hypertension is salt-sensitive. In addition, several studies have shown that salt loading of patients with essential hypertension results in some net total body sodium accumulation. Further evidence has been provided by the observation that 3 genetic diseases associated with hypertension in childhood (Liddle syndrome, the syndrome of apparent roineralocorticoid excess, and glucocorticoid remediable aldosteronism) are also associated with increased reabsorption of salt by the kidney.[76] This has led to many investigators to search for genetically mediated alterations in the regulation or transport of salt in the nephrons of patients with hypertension. Another possibility, proposed by Mackenzie and colleagues,[77] is that a genetic reduction in nephron number may be the key initiating event, in that, over time, the hyperfiltration and increased glomerular pressure damage the kidney and affect its ability to excrete salt.

However, the concept of a genetically mediated defect in the ability of the kidney to excrete salt does not explain all observations. Young patients with hypertension seem to excrete salt normally or supernormally, and people with borderline or early hypertension may have low blood volume. As many as 40% of people with hypertension do not show a change in BP with salt loading (salt resistance), and this is primarily observed in younger patients. With aging, salt sensitivity increases both in frequency and in degree, such that, by 70 years of age, almost all patients with hypertension are salt sensitive. Meta-analyses have suggested that salt restriction may not be important either in people who are normotensive or in young patients with hypertension.[78,79] All of these findings are most consistent with the possibility that the defect in sodium excretion in patients with hypertension is acquired.[80]

A UNIFYING PATHWAY FOR THE DEVELOPMENT OF HYPERTENSION

The unifying pathway proposes that the kidneys are normal in the prehypertensive state, but that renal injury is initiated in most circumstances by repeated and intermittent renal vasoconstriction induced by a variety of factors.[81,82] These factors include a hyperactive SNS induced by stress or a genetic mechanism,[83,84] alterations in the RAAS (from genetic polymorphisms, oral contraceptives, or secondary to activation of the renal SNS, renal ischemia, hypokalemia, and so forth) resulting in increased circulating all[85] or hyperuricemia induced by diet, genetics, or activation of the SNS.[86,87]

In the early phase of hypertension, the increases in BP may be intermittent and the levels may only be in the prehypertension range. However, unlike patients who are normotensive, the BP variability is likely to be greater and with higher and more frequent levels above normal. Norepinephrine and AII have sodium-retaining properties, but the increases in BP caused by these agents result in a pressure natriuresis and lead to sodium loss and a normal or low blood volume state. During this phase, the hypertension tends to be salt resistant, because the ischemia is frequently intermittent (because of intermittent activation of the SNS or fluctuating uric acid levels from diet) and the kidney relatively uninjured, so that the pressure natriuresis mechanism remains largely intact.[88] Sodium loading in these patients would be likely to increase renal blood flow[89] and to have a brisk or exaggerated natriuresis.[90]

The intermittent activation of the SNS and/or RAAS eventually results in acquired injury to the kidney, with impairment in its ability to excrete salt. Normally, the kidney responds to increases in BP by a process of renal autoregulation. In this situation, the afferent arteriole and interlobular artery vasoconstrict secondary to a myogenic reflex (mediated by calcium channels) and by TG feedback *in* an attempt to prevent transmission of pressure distally to the sensitive structures in the glomerulus and per tubular capillaries. Presumably, this autoregulatory response explains why arteriolosclerosis of the afferent arteriole is the classic renal biopsy finding in patients with essential hypertension. Goldblatt and others interpreted arteriolosclerosis of the afferent arteriole as the primary disease of the renal arterioles that caused essential hypertension. This observation resulted from arteriosclerosis of this arteriole being both sensitive (observed in >95% of cases) and specific (observed in <30% in other organs) for essential hypertension.[91] However, according to the hypothesis mentioned earlier, this vasoconstriction could be considered a protective, secondary response. Gradually, the vasoconstrictive response leads to the development of a preglomerular arteriolopathy that is not mediated by the hypertension, but by the effects of uric acid, AII, or a loss of local NO.[82]

In time, injury to the kidney could occur via one of 2 mechanisms. The first mechanism is transmission of systemic pressure into the glomerulus caused by an imperfect renal autoregulatory response,[92,93] likely secondary to the deposition of extracellular matrix within the arteriole that results in making it stiff. There is evidence for reduced renal autoregulation in conditions associated with a reduction in nephron number, in obesity, and in African Americans. Micropuncture studies have confirmed that norepinephrine infusion can increase glomerular and peritubular capillary pressures in the rat.[94] The consequence is that some increase in pressure can be transmitted and could lead lo glomerular damage (sclerosis) and tubulointerstitial injury. Bohle and Ratschck[95] described a population of patients with hypertension in which the renal biopsy showed a decompensated nephrosclerosis with glomerulosclerosis and tubulointerstitial damage. This pattern is similar to what is observed in hypertensive African Americans, in obesity, and with aging, (all conditions associated with salt-sensitive hypertension).

The second mechanism of renal injury is by ischemia caused by preglomerular arteriopathy. As the afferent arteriole thickens in response to the increases in BP, the arteriolar lumen becomes progressively smaller. Eventually, the pressure within the narrowed arteriole cannot support the tension in the afferent arteriole, and the arteriole collapses, leading to distal glomerular and peritubular ischemia. The ischemia attracts leukocytes (both T cells and macrophages) with the local expression of oxidants by inflammatory and possibly resident cells, which have been shown to scavenge the local intrarenal nitric oxide, causing further renal vasoconstriction.[96,97] The microvascular disease may also lead to different degrees of relative renal ischemia, leading to a heterogeneous renin response.[63] This process leads to a reduction in sodium filtration (by reducing cortical filtration coefficient and glomerular filtration rate) and increased tubular reabsorption of sodium, leading to increased BP. As renal perfusion pressure increases, the ischemia is partially relieved, allowing sodium handling to return toward normal, but at the expense of a shift in pressure natriuresis and an increase in systemic BP. Other alterations in vasoconstrictors and activation of the renal sympathetics could be postulated, because renal injury is known to activate renal afferent sympathetics.[98] The consequence is sodium retention caused by both glomerular and tubular mechanisms, resulting in a volume-dependent increase in BP.[2] In addition, the vasoactive properties of both norepinephrine and AII cause prominent vasoconstriction of the arterioles and vasa rectae, resulting in a decrease in blood flow to the peritubular capillaries. Evidence of tubular ischemia can be found in most biopsies of patients with essential hypertension.[99]

This pathway suggests that hypertension may shift from a salt-resistant, renin-dependent type of hypertension to a salt-sensitive, kidney-dependent, and volume-dependent hypertension in time. This is consistent with the progressive increase in salt sensitivity that occurs with aging[80] and obesity.[100]

IMPLICATIONS FOR CLINICAL MANAGEMENT OF HYPERTENSION

Regardless of the specific cause of primary hypertension, target-organ damage occurs in patients with hypertension because of the chronically increased BP. Therefore, the clinician's first priority must be the control of BP, improvement in the quality of life, and prevention of premature death and disability in patients with established hypertension. In patients with prehypertension, or normotensive individuals with parental history of hypertension, aggressive attention must be paid to environmental factors and lifestyle choices to help prevent the development of hypertension.[101,102]

In this regard, emphasis must be placed on evidence-based and outcomes-based guidelines for the prevention and optimal control of hypertension rather than treatment dictated by a presumed pathophysiologic profile. However, in the absence of compelling evidence from randomized, controlled clinical trials, the pathophysiologic mechanisms described earlier provide a rational basis for drug selection. For example, the complexity of the interrelated mechanisms of BP control suggests that combination drug therapy is more likely to be successful than monotherapy in moderate to severe hypertension, and that 2 drugs that target both intravascular volume and peripheral resistance are likely to be more successful in controlling BP than drugs that target peripheral resistance alone. Similarly, the prominent role of the kidney and sodium excretion in the regulation of hypertension also suggests that, in any patient taking 3 or more drugs for hypertension, one of the drugs must be a diuretic.[101,102]

SUMMARY

Although the definitive cause of primary hypertension remains unknown, several important advances have been made in the pathogenesis and clinical history of this common disease. Genes, environment, and the gene-environment interaction play important roles in the development of hypertension. Genetic susceptibility, operating through complex polygenic influences, accounts for 30% to 50% of the variation in BP between individuals. Environmental influences and lifestyle choices account for another 20% of variation in BP. Alterations in multiple BP-regulatory systems, including the central and peripheral nervous system, circulating and tissue RAAS, renal parenchyma and nervous mechanisms, and multiple feedback loops involving a wide spectrum of receptors and neurotransmitters also play key roles in the development and maintenance of hypertension. The endothelium and its interaction with vasoactive substances, including endothelin, nitric oxide, and AII, further affect BP levels.

Regardless of the underlying mechanisms of primary hypertension, the clinical course of the disease in the absence of effective treatment and control is that hypertension begets more hypertension, leading to target-organ damage, organ failure, and premature death. Although the mechanisms discussed in this article provide important clues in understanding the cause of hypertension, the rationale for combination drugs, and even the targeted design of specific antihypertensive drugs, is that proper management of patients with hypertension must be based on the clinical outcomes evidence rather than the pathophysiology alone. Where there is no compelling evidence for the use of a specific drug class, BP control guided by the underlying pathophysiologic profile becomes appropriate.

REFERENCES

1. Guyton AC. Dominant role of the kidneys and accessory role of whole-body autoregulation in the pathogenesis of hypertension. Am J Hypertens 1989;2:575–85.
2. Guyton AC, Coleman TG, Cowley AV Jr, et al. Arterial pressure regulation: overriding dominance of the kidneys in long-term regulation and in hypertension. Am J Med 1972;52:584–94.
3. Hall JE, Coleman TG, Guy ton AC. The renin-angiotensin system. Normal physiology and changes in older hypertensives. J Am Geriatr Soc 1989;37:801–13.
4. Guyton AC. Abnormal renal function and autoregulation in essential hypertension. Hypertension 1991;18:11149–53.
5. Izzo JL Jr, Taylor AA. The sympathetic nervous system and baroreflexes in hypertension and hypotension. Curr Hypertens Rep 1999;1:254–63.
6. Sobel BJ, Bakris GL. Hypertension: a clinician's guide to diagnosis and treatment. Philadelphia: Hanley & Belfus; 1999.
7. Mohrman DE, Heller LJ. Regulation of arterial pressure. In: Mohrman DE, Heller LJ, editors. Cardiovascular physiology. 6th edition. New York: McGraw Hill; 2006. p. 161–83. Chapter 9.
8. Krakoff LR, Dziedzic S, Mann SJ, et al. Plasma epinephrine concentration in healthy men:

correlation with systolic pressure and rate-pressure product. J Am Coll Cardiol 1985;5:352–6.
9. Itoh S, Carrelero OA. Role of the macula densa in renin release. Hypertension 1985;7:149–54.
10. Kopp UC, DiBona GF. Neural regulation of renin secretion. Semin Nephrol 1993;13:543–51.
11. Lorenz JN, Weihprecht H, Schnermann J, et al. Renin release from isolated juxtaglomerular apparatus depends on macula densa chloride transport. Am J Physiol 1991;260:F486–93.
12. Guyton AC. Long-term arterial pressure control: an analysis from animal experiments and computer and graphic models. Am J Physiol 1990;259:R865–77.
13. Lundie MJ, Friberg P, Kline RL, et al. Long-term inhibition of the renin-angiotensin system in genetic hypertension: analysis of the impact on blood pressure and cardiovascular structural changes. J Hypertens 1997;15:339–48.
14. Guyton AC. The surprising kidney-fluid mechanism for pressure control–its infinite gain!. Hypertension 1990;16:725–30.
15. Guyton AC, Manning RD Jr, Hall JE, et al. The pathogenic role of the kidney. J Cardiovasc Pharmacol 1984;6(Suppl I):S151–61.
16. Hall JE, Guyton AC, Coleman TG, et al. Regulation of arterial pressure: role of pressure natriuresis and diuresis. Fed Proc 1986;45:2897–903.
17. Triel B, Weder AB. Genes for essential hypertension: hype, help, or hope? J Clin Hypertens (Greenwich) 2000;2:187–93.
18. Slocks P. A biometric investigation of twins and their brothers and sisters. Ann Eugen 1930;4:49–62.
19. Lifton RP, Gharavi AG, Geller DS. Molecular mechanisms of human hypertension. Cell 2001;104:545–56.
20. Luft FC. Geneticism of essential hypertension. Hypertension 2004;43:1155–9.
21. Barlassina C, Lanzani C, Manunta P, et al. Genetics of essential hypertension: from families to genes. J Am Soc Nephrol 2002;13(Suppl 3):S155–64.
22. Luft FC. Molecular genetics of human hypertension. J Hypertens 1998;16:1871–8.
23. Williams RR, Hunt SC, Hopkins PN, et al. Tabulations and expectations regarding the genetics of human hypertension. Kidney Int 1994;45(Suppl 44):S57–64.
24. Harrap SB. Hypertension: genes versus environment. Lancet 1994;344:169–71.
25. Pausova Z, Tremblay J, Harriet P. Gene-environment interactions in hypertension. Curr Hypertens Rep 1999;1:42–50.
26. Sims J, Hewitt JK, Kelly KA, et al. Familial and individual influences on blood pressure. Acta Genet Med Gemellol (Roma) 1986;35:7–21.
27. Sing CF, Boerwinkle E, Turner ST. Genetics of primary hypertension. Clin Exp Hypertens A 1986;8:623–51.
28. Stamler J, Rose G, Elliott P, et al. Findings of the International Cooperative INTERSALT Study. Hypertension 1991;17(Suppl):9–15.
29. Luft FC, Miller JZ, Weinberger MH, et al. Genetic influences on the response to dietary salt reduction, acute salt loading, or salt depletion in humans. J Cardiovasc Pharmacol 1988;12(Suppl 3):49–55.
30. Sallout B, Walker M. The fetal origin of adult diseases. J Obstet Gynaecol 2003;23:555–60.
31. Keller G, Zimmer G, Mall G, et al. Nephron number in patients with primary hypertension. N Engl J Med 2003;348:101–8.
32. Whelton PK, He J, Cutler JA, et al. Effects of oral potassium on blood pressure. Meta-analysis of randomized controlled clinical trials. JAMA 1997;277:1624–32.
33. Campese VM. Calcium, parathyroid hormone, and blood pressure. Am J Hypertens 1989;2:34S–44S.
34. Langford HG. Dietary potassium and hypertension: epidemiologic data. Ann Intern Med 1985;98:770.
35. Aviv A, Hollenberg NK, Weder A. Urinary potassium excretion and sodium sensitivity in blacks. Hypertension 2004;43:707–13.
36. Delgado MC. Potassium in hypertension. Curr Hypertens Rep 2004;6:31–5.
37. Hall JE. The kidney, hypertension, and obesity. Hypertension 2003;41:625–33.
38. Vasan RS, Larson MG, Leip EP, et al. Assessment of frequency of progression to hypertension in non-hypertensive participants in the Framingham Heart Study: a cohort study. Lancet 2001;358:1682–6.
39. Egan BM. Insulin resistance and the sympathetic nervous system. Curr Hypertens Rep 2003;5:247–54.
40. Rahmouni K, Correia ML, Haynes WG, et al. Obesity-associated hypertension: new insights into mechanisms. Hypertension 2005;45:9–14.
41. Goodfriend TL, Calhoun DA. Resistant hypertension, obesity, sleep apnea, and aldosterone: theory and therapy. Hypertension 2004;43:518–24.
42. Hall JE, Hildebrandt DA, Kuo J. Obesity hypertension: role of leptin and sympathetic nervous system. Am J Hypertens 2001;14:103S–15S.
43. Lauer MS, Okin PM, Larson MG, et al. Impaired heart rate response to graded exercise. Prognostic implications of chronotropic incompetence in the Framingham Heart Study. Circulation 1996;93:1520–6.
44. Juliti S, Schork MA. Predictors of hypertension. Ann N Y Acad Sci 1978;304:38–58.
45. Grassi G, Mancia G. Hyperadrenergic and labile hypertension. In: Lip GH, Hall J, editors. Comprehensive hypertension. Philadelphia: Mosby Elsevier; 2007. p. 719–26.
46. Muirhead EE. Renal vasodepressor mechanisms: the medullipin system. J Hypertens 1993;5:S53–8.
47. Grassi G. Renin-angiotensin-sympathetic cross-talks in hypertension: reappraising the relevance

of peripheral interactions. J Hypertens 2001;19: 1713–6.
48. Grassi G, Cattaneo BM, Seravalle G, et al. Effects of chronic ACE inhibition on sympathetic nerve traffic and baroreflex control of circulation in heart failure. Circulation 1997;96:1173–9.
49. Grassi G, Quarti-Trevano F, Dell'Oro R, et al. Essential hypertension and the sympathetic nervous system. Neurol Sci 2008;29:S33–6.
50. Erdos EG. Angiotensin I converting enzyme and the changes in our concepts through the years. Lewis K. Dahl memorial lecture. Hypertension 1990;16:363–70.
51. Chung O, Stoll M, Unger T. Physiologic and pharmacologic implications of AT1 versus AT2 receptors. Blood Press Suppl 1996;2:47–52.
52. Zimmerman BG, Sybertz EJ, Wong PC. Interaction between sympathetic and renin-angiotensin system. J Hypertens 1984;2:581–7.
53. Touyz RM. The role of angiotensin II in regulating vascular structural and functional changes in hypertension. Curr Hypertens Rep 2003;5: 155–64.
54. Burns KD, Li N. The role of angiotensin II-stimulated renal tubular transport in hypertension. Curr Hypertens Rep 2003;5:165–71.
55. Kaschina E, Unger T. Angiotensin AT1/AT2 receptors: regulation, signalling and function. Blood Press 2003;12:70–88.
56. Dzau VJ. Theodore Cooper Lecture: tissue angiotensin and pathobiology of vascular disease: a unifying hypothesis. Hypertension 2001;37:1047–52.
57. Hannan RE, Widdop RE. Vascular angiotensin II actions mediated by angiotensin II type 2 receptors. Curr Hypertens Rep 2004;6:117–23.
58. Widdop RE, Jones ES, Hannan RE, et al. Angiotensin AT2 receptors: cardiovascular hope or hype? Br J Pharmacol 2003;140:809–24.
59. Carey RM, Wang ZQ, Siragy HM. Update: role of the angiotensin type-2 (AT(2)) receptor in blood pressure regulation. Curr Hypertens Rep 2000;2: 198–201.
60. Julius S. Interaction between renin and the autonomic nervous system in hypertension. Am Heart J 1988;116:611–6.
61. Weidmann P, De Myttenaere-Bursztein S, Maxwell MH, et al. Effect on aging on plasma renin and aldosterone in normal man. Kidney Int 1975;8: 325–33.
62. Price DA, Fisher ND. The renin-angiotensin system in blacks: active, passive, or what? Curr Hypertens Rep 2003;5:225–30.
63. Sealey JE, Blumenfeld JD, Bell GM, et al. On the renal basis for essential hypertension: nephron heterogeneity with discordant renin secretion and sodium excretion causing a hypertensive vasoconstriction-volume relationship. J Hypertens 1988;6:763–77.
64. Tom B, Dendorfer A, Danser AH. Bradykinin, angiotensin-(1–7), and ACE inhibitors: how do they interact? Int J Biochem Cell Biol 2003;35: 792–801.
65. Folkow B. Physiological aspects of primary hypertension. Physiol Rev 1982;62:347–504.
66. Berk BC, Vekshtein V, Gordon HM, et al. Angiotensin H-stimulated protein synthesis in cultured vascular smooth muscle cells. Hypertension 1989;13:305–14.
67. Naftilan A, Pratt R, Dzau V. Induction of c-fos, C-myc and PDGF A-chain gene expressions by angiotensin II in cultured vascular smooth muscle cells. J Clin Invest 1989;83:1419–24.
68. Gibbons GH. Mechanisms of vascular remodeling in hypertension: role of autocrine-paracrine vasoactive factors. Curr Opin Nephrol Hypertens 1995;4:189–96.
69. Pollman MJ, Yamada T, Horiuchi M, et al. Vasoactive substances regulate vascular smooth muscle cell apoptosis. Countervailing influences of nitric oxide and angiotensin II. Circ Res 1996;79:748–56.
70. Dzau VJ. The role of mechanical and humoral factors in growth regulation of vascular smooth muscle and cardiac myocytes. Curr Opin Nephrol Hypertens 1993;2:27–32.
71. Boden G, Shulman GI. Free fatty acids in obesity and type 2 diabetes: defining their role in the development of insulin resistance and beta-cell dysfunction. Eur J Clin Invest 2002;32(Suppl 3):14–23.
72. Pittas AG, Joseph NA, Greenberg AS. Adipocytokines and insulin resistance. J Clin Endocrinol Metab 2004;89:447–52.
73. Matsuzawa Y, Funahashi T, Kihara S, et al. Adiponectin and metabolic syndrome. Arterioscler Thromb 2004;24:29–33.
74. Wheatcroft SB, Williams IL, Shah AM, et al. Pathophysiological implications of insulin resistance on vascular endothelial function. Diabet Med 2003; 20:255–68.
75. Dahl LK, Heine M. Primary role of renal homo-grafts in setting chronic blood pressure levels in rats. Circ Res 1975;36:692–6.
76. Lifton RP. Molecular genetics of human blood pressure variation. Science 1996;272:676–80.
77. Mackenzie HS, Lawler EV, Brenner BM. Congenital oligo nephropathy: the fetal flaw in essential hypertension? Kidney Int 1996;55(Suppl):S30–4.
78. Alam S, Johnson AG. A meta-analysis of randomised controlled (trials (RCT)) among healthy normotensive and essential hypertensive elderly patients to determine the effect of high salt (NaCl) diet of blood pressure. J Hum Hypertens 1999;13:367–74.
79. Midgley JP, Matthew AG, Greenwood CM, et al. Effect of reduced dietary sodium on blood pressure: a meta-analysis of randomized controlled trials. JAMA 1996;275:1590–7.

80. Weinberger MH, Fineberg NS. Sodium and volume sensitivity of blood pressure age and pressure change over time. Hypertension 1991;18:67–71.
81. Johnson RJ, Schreiner GF. Hypothesis: the role of acquired tubulointerstitial disease in the pathogenesis of salt-dependent hypertension. Kidney Int 1997;52:1169–79.
82. Johnson RJ, Rodriguez-Iturbe B, Kang DH, et al. A unifying pathway for essential hypertension. Am J Hypertens 2005;18:431–40.
83. Julius S. The evidence for a pathophysiologic significance of sympathetic overactivity in hypertension. Clin Exp Hypertens 1996;18:305–21.
84. Mancia G. Bjorn Folkow Award Lecture: the sympathetic nervous system in hypertension. J Hypertens 1997;15:1553–65.
85. Jeunemaitre X, Gimenez-Roqueplo AP, Celerier J, et al. Angiotensinogen variants and human hypertension. Curr Hypertens Rep 1999;1:31–41.
86. Johnson RJ, Titte SR, Cade JR, et al. Uric acid, evolution and primitive cultures. Semin Nephrol 2005;25(1):3–8.
87. Johnson RJ, Rideout BA. Uric acid and diet: insights into the epidemic of cardiovascular disease [editorial]. N Engl J Med 2004;350:1071–4.
88. Rodríguez-Iturbe B, Pons H, Quiroz Y, et al. Mycophenolate mofetil prevents salt-sensitive hypertension resulting from angiotensin II exposure. Kidney Int 2001;59:2222–32.
89. Williams GH, Hollenberg NK. Sodium-sensitive essential hypertension. Emerging insights into pathogenesis and therapeutic implications. Contemp Nephrol 1985;3:303–11.
90. Lowenstein J, Beranbaum ER, Chasis H, et al. Intrarenal pressure and exaggerated natriuresis in essential hypertension. Clin Sci 1970;38:359–74.
91. Moritz AR, Oldt MR. Arteriolar sclerosis 111 hypertensive and non-hypertensive individuals. Am J Pathol 1937;13:679–728.
92. Sánchez-Lozada LG, Tapia E, Avila-Casado C, et al. Mild hyperuricemia induces glomerular hypertension in normal rats. Am J Physiol Renal Physiol 2002;283:F1105–10.
93. Sánchez-Lozada LG, Tapia E, Santamaria J, et al. Mild hyperuricemia induces vasoconstriction and maintains glomerular hypertension in normal and remnant kidney rats. Kidney Int 2005;67(1):237–47.
94. Myers BD, Deen WM, Brenner BM. Effects of norepinephrine and angiotensin II on the determinants of glomerular ultrafiltration and proximal tubule fluid reabsorption in the rat. Circ Res 1975;25:663–73.
95. Bohle A, Ratschck M. The compensated and the decompensated form of benign nephrosclerosis. Pathol Res Pract 1982;174:357–67.
96. Vaziri ND. Roles of oxidative stress and antioxidant therapy in chronic kidney disease and hypertension. Curr Opin Nephrol Hypertens 2004;13:93–9.
97. Wilcox CS. Redox regulation of the afferent arteriole and tubuloglomerular feedback. Acta Physiol Scand 2003;179:217–23.
98. DiBona GF. Sympathetic nervous system and the kidney in hypertension. Curr Opin Nephrol Hypertens 2002;11:197–200.
99. Sommers SC, Relman AS, Smith wick RH. Histologic studies of kidney biopsy specimens from patients with hypertension. Am J Pathol 1958;34:715.
100. Egan BM, Stepniakowski KT. Adverse effects of short-term, very low-salt diets in subjects with risk-factor clustering. Am J Clin Nutr 1997;65(Suppl 2):671S–7S.
101. The sixth report of the Joint National Committee on prevention, detection, evaluation, and treatment of high blood pressure. Arch Intern Med 1997;57:2413–6.
102. Chobanian AV, Bakris GL, Black HR, et al. The seventh report of the Joint National Committee on prevention, detection, evaluation, and treatment of high blood pressure: the JNC 7 report. JAMA 2003;289(19):2560–72.

Prehypertension: An Opportunity for a New Public Health Paradigm

Brent M. Egan, MD[a,*], Daniel T. Lackland, DrPH[a], Daniel W. Jones, MD[b]

KEYWORDS

• Prehypertension • Hypertension • Cardiovascular disease
• Lifestyle change • Pharmacologic therapy

From 2005 to 2006, approximately 3 of 8 adults in the United States had blood pressure (BP) in the prehypertensive range of 120 to 139/80 to 89 mm Hg and roughly 1 in 8 adults had BP in the range of 130 to 139/85 to 89 mm Hg referred to as high normal BP or stage 2 prehypertension. The term stage 2 prehypertension may serve to more fully convey the actual risk of progression to hypertension and cardiovascular disease (CVD). Stage 2 prehypertension progresses to hypertension at a rate of about 8% to 14% annually, which is 2- to 3-fold higher than normotension (BP <120/80 mm Hg). Adults with stage 2 prehypertension are also roughly twice as likely as adults with normotension to suffer CVD. The Seventh Report of the Joint National Committee on Hypertension (JNC 7) recommended only lifestyle changes for most prehypertensive patients. Although hygienic measures are efficacious in controlled clinical trials, evidence for community-wide effectiveness is limited. BP in the range of 120 to 129/80 to 84 mm Hg is also associated with increased risk but roughly half of that of stage 2 prehypertension.

Most individuals with stage 2 prehypertension have 1 or more concomitant conditions associated with increased cardiovascular risk. These include, but are not limited to dyslipidemias, an early family history of CVD, cigarette use and abdominal obesity, hyperinsulinemia and insulin resistance, impaired fasting glucose, a prothrombotic state, endothelial dysfunction, and impaired vascular distensibility. The combination of multiple risk factors magnifies absolute risk. In fact, clinical epidemiology suggests that the benefits of treating stage 2 prehypertension and stage 1 hypertension are similar when both groups have additional risk factors.

This review examines evidence indicating that (1) prehypertension is a major contributor to incident hypertension and CVD, (2) although current public health and hygienic strategies are efficacious, they are largely ineffective in reducing prehypertension-related risk, and (3) a new public health paradigm for the prevention and management of prehypertension is needed and should include expanding the evidence base through comparative effectiveness research.

JNC 7 departed from previous reports by defining BP in the range of 120 to 139/80 to 89 mm Hg as prehypertension.[1] Although controversial, the designation for prehypertension was intended to strengthen the recommendation for therapeutic lifestyle changes among a group of individuals at significantly greater risk for progression to hypertension and clinical CVD when compared with normotensive individuals with BP less than 120/80 mm Hg.[1–7]

JNC 7 was not the original source for the term prehypertension or the BP range that defines it. In 1939, Robinson and Brucer[2] defined BP in the range of 120 to 139/80 to 89 mm Hg as prehypertensive. They observed that most hypertension

[a] Medical University of South Carolina, 135 Rutledge Avenue, RT1230, Charleston, SC 29425, USA
[b] University of Mississippi, Office of Chancellor, 123 Lyceum, Box 148, Oxford, MS, USA
* Corresponding author.
E-mail address: eganbm@musc.edu

Cardiol Clin 28 (2010) 561–569
doi:10.1016/j.ccl.2010.07.008
0733-8651/10/$ – see front matter

originated from prehypertension in individuals who also had roughly double the mortality of people with a normal BP less than 120/80 mm Hg.

When compared with normotensive individuals, prehypertensive individuals are more likely to be overweight and obese, to have other cardiovascular risk factors, to progress to established hypertension, and to experience premature clinical CVD.[1–7] Given these considerations, the American Society of Hypertension Writing Group[8] defined a subset of individuals with BP in the range of 120 to 139/80 to 89 mm Hg as hypertensive based on concomitant risk factors and vascular disease. The scientific evidence and expert opinion that BP in the range of 120 to 139/80 to 89 mm Hg and especially 130 to 139/85 to 89 mm Hg (stage 2 prehypertension) are not optimal for health are longstanding, impressive, and growing.

CLINICAL EPIDEMIOLOGY OF PREHYPERTENSION

A preliminary report from the National Health and Nutrition Examination Survey (NHANES) in 2005 to 2006 estimated that approximately 37% of US adults had prehypertension.[9] The number of adults with prehypertension was estimated to be approximately 83 million based on extrapolations from NHANES 2005-2006 and information from prior surveys.[9–12] Among this group, roughly 3 of 8, or approximately 31 million, US adults have stage 2 prehypertension. Prehypertension is associated not only with concomitant cardiovascular risk factors but also with several adverse health outcomes including new-onset diabetes and hypertension, cognitive impairment, and increased CVD events.

Prehypertension and Concomitant Cardiovascular-Metabolic Abnormalities

Individuals with stage 2 prehypertension are more likely than individuals with normotension to be overweight, hyperinsulinemic, insulin resistant[3,7] and to exhibit a complex dyslipidemia characterized by hypertriglyceridemia, low level of high-density lipoprotein cholesterol, and greater numbers of small low-density lipoprotein cholesterol particles. Stage 2 prehypertensive individuals frequently display other risk factors or markers, which include high levels of fibrinogen, plasminogen activator inhibitor 1, adipokines including leptin and tumor necrosis factor α, and inflammatory cytokines including C-reactive protein as well as endothelial dysfunction, greater vascular stiffness, left ventricular hypertrophy, diastolic dysfunction, decreased coronary flow reserve, and cognitive dysfunction.[13–20]

New-Onset Diabetes

A representative sample of 11,001 German men and women between the ages of 25 and 74 years and free of diabetes at baseline were followed up for a mean of 12.5 years.[21] Hypertension was associated with approximately 2-fold higher incident diabetes in men and women after adjusting for multiple covariates including age, family history of diabetes, physical activity, education, and body mass index. Stage 2 prehypertension was linked to a multivariate-adjusted approximately 1.8-fold (hazard ratio [HR], 1.76; 95% confidence interval [CI], 1.24–2.51) higher incidence of diabetes in men, whereas the adjusted risk was not significant in stage 2 prehypertensive women (HR, 1.07; 95% CI, 0.67–1.73). Although it is important to extend these observations to other racial or ethnic groups, the findings suggest that stage 2 prehypertension is associated with diabetes risk in men.

New-Onset Hypertension

Patients with prehypertension are at greater risk for developing hypertension than patients with normotension.[2,5,22–24] In the Framingham Heart Study, approximately 37% of patients younger than 65 years with stage 2 prehypertension (high normal BP) and 50% of patients older than 65 years progressed to hypertension in 4 years compared with 5% and 16% of patients with a normal BP less than 120/80 mm Hg, respectively.[25] In the Trial of Preventing Hypertension (TROPHY), around 52% of placebo-treated patients with stage 2 prehypertension progressed to clinical hypertension within 4 years with the conventional definition of 2 successive visits and a BP of 140/90 mm Hg or more.[26] The German Hypertension League Study on hypertension prevention reported a 43% incidence over 3 years of de novo hypertension among patients with stage 2 prehypertension randomized to placebo, which is similar to the rates observed in TROPHY and Framingham Study.[27]

Prehypertension and CVD Risk

Given the spectrum of risk factors associated with stage 2 prehypertension, this group has a higher incidence of CVD.[4,6,7,28–35] At least 7 cohort studies documented a significant contribution of stage 2 prehypertension to CVD risk (**Table 1**).[4,28–30,32–35] The adjusted hazard ratios in these studies ranged from approximately 1.4 to 2.3, with several studies documenting risk independent of progression to hypertension and other major risk factors. Given an estimated number of 31 million people with stage 2 prehypertension in

Table 1
Cardiovascular risk associated with stage 2 prehypertension and estimates of the number needed to treat to prevent a major CVD event in 10 years

Study	Total, N[b]	PHT2, N	Follow-Up Period, y	HR[a], 95% CI	Absolute Difference, %/y[c] PHT2 vs NT	NNT (10 y) 50%[e]	NNT (10 y) 100%[e]
Morbidity and Mortality							
ARIC[30]	8960	1279	11.6	2.33, 1.85–2.92	~0.42%	48	24
Framingham[28]	6859	1794	12	Men 1.6, 1.1–2.2	~0.54% (0.43%)[d]	37	19
				Women 2.5, 1.6–4.1	~0.51% (0.25%)[d]	39	20
NHANES I[29]	8986	2708[g]	18	1.42, 1.09–1.84	~0.53%	38	19
NHEFS 1[33]	12,269	1947	7–21		46(26)[f]23(13)[f]		
Strong Heart[32]	2629	1390[g]	12.6	1.80, 1.28–2.54	~0.61%	33	17
Women's Health[34]	60,785	23,596[g]	7.7	1.77, 1.52–2.06	~0.39%	51	26
Mortality only							
MRFIT[4]	347,978	77,248	15	CHD 1.66 (fatal only) CVA 2.14 (fatal only)	~0.09%[h]	222	111
Taiwan[35]	35,259	4655	15	1.96, 1.5–2.6	~0.1%	200	100

Abbreviations: ARIC, Atherosclerosis Risk in Communities; CHD, coronary heart disease; CVA, cerebrovascular accident; MRFIT, Multiple Risk Factor Intervention Trial; NHEFS, National Health Examination Follow-up Study; PHT2, stage 2 prehypertension; NT, normotension; NNT, number needed to treat.

[a] HR from cardiovascular risk factor–adjusted Cox proportional hazards regression model.

[b] Total study N. Stage 2 prehypertension comprised a subset of total N.

[c] Estimated absolute difference in CVD event rates, unadjusted unless otherwise specified.

[d] Age-adjusted absolute difference in CVD events. Non–age-adjusted rates were used to calculate NNT, because those rates reflect the actual risk for affected individuals.

[e] NNT assuming 50% or 100% efficacy of antihypertensive therapy in reducing excess CVD risk.

[f] Numbers in parenthesis represent adjustment for regression dilution bias from error in systolic BP measurement of 0.53.[33]

[g] All prehypertensive patients with BP in the range of 120 to 139/80 to 89 mm Hg are included, as the number with stage 2 hypertension was not provided. For NHANES I and Women's Health Initiative, mean HRs and 95% CIs were provided for stage 2 prehypertension. For Strong Heart study, mean HRs and 95% CIs were provided only for all prehypertensive patients; the HR for stage 2 prehypertensive patients was 2.1, but CIs were not provided.

[h] Fatal CHD only.

the United States and an absolute excess CVD risk ranging from 0.39% to 0.61% annually, this population contributes to between 121,000 and 189,000 excess cardiovascular events annually.

CLINICAL EPIDEMIOLOGY AND TREATMENT CONSIDERATIONS IN STAGE 2 PREHYPERTENSION

The potential benefits of intervening are worth considering in stage 2 prehypertension, given the individual and population attributable risk. Ogden and colleagues[33] estimated the benefits of treating stage 2 prehypertension, using National Health Examination Follow-Up Survey I data. These investigators projected that lowering BP by 12 mm Hg for 10 years in 13 individuals with stage 2 prehypertension and who had at least one other major cardiovascular risk factor would prevent a major CVD event. These findings apply to most prehypertensive patients who have 1 or more concomitant major cardiovascular risk factors.[31,33,36]

The projected number needed to treat for 10 years to prevent 1 CVD event were 11 for stage 1 hypertension and 13 for stage 2 prehypertension, when both groups had 1 or more additional cardiovascular risk factors.[33] Of note, more than 70% of patients with stage 2 prehypertension in this report had 1 or more additional cardiovascular risk factors, and an additional 15% of patients had diabetes, clinical CVD, or significant target organ damage. These estimates were based on the further assumption that the intervention was 100% effective in eliminating the risk associated with a 12 mm Hg higher BP and included a correction of 0.53 for regression dilution bias because of imprecision in BP measurement. Without correction for regression dilution bias, the estimated numbers needed to treat were 23 for stage 2 prehypertension and 19 for stage 1 hypertension. If it is further assumed that treatment reduced excess risk by 50% rather than by 100%, then the number needed to treat increases to 38 for stage 1 hypertension and 46 for stage 2 prehypertension. The projected numbers needed to treat from the various studies listed in **Table 1** that included both cardiovascular morbidity and mortality are similar in magnitude without adjustment for regression dilution bias. As expected, the 2 studies that reported CVD mortality only yielded higher estimates of the numbers needed to treat.

The Effect of Lifestyle Interventions on Progression to Hypertension and CVD Events

Because lifestyle changes are the only current recommendation by JNC 7 for most individuals with prehypertension,[1] the evidence for efficacy in reducing the progression to hypertension and preventing incident CVD is examined.

Progression to hypertension

The Trials of Hypertension Prevention, Phase II (TOHP II), included 2382 volunteers with a diastolic BP of 83 to 89 mm Hg and a systolic reading less than 140 mm Hg. Participants were randomized to usual care including weight loss, sodium restriction, or a combination of both.[37] A preintervention stage designed to foster a participant's commitment to the assigned lifestyle change was followed by an intensive intervention period including 14 weekly visits for the weight loss and combined intervention group and 10 weekly visits for the sodium restriction group. The subsequent transitional stage included 6 biweekly sessions for the weight loss and combined intervention group and 4 monthly sessions for the low sodium group. For the remainder of the trial, participants were seen 3 to 6 times annually to reinforce the assigned lifestyle intervention. Over 4 years, intensive lifestyle interventions reduced absolute risk of hypertension by 6% to 7% and relative risk by 13% to 15%.[38]

CVD events

The Oslo Diet and Antismoking Trial enrolled 1234 men aged 40 to 50 years and in the upper quartile of risk based on total cholesterol level, cigarette smoking, and BP.[38] Men with a systolic BP of 150 mm Hg or more were excluded. The intervention group reduced the proportion of fat calories from 44% to 28% ($P<.01$), increased polyunsaturated/saturated fat intake ratio to 1.01 from 0.39 ($P<.01$), raised fiber consumption from 4.4 to 6.0 g/d ($P<.05$), lowered total cholesterol level from 341 to 263 mg/dL ($P<.01$), decreased cigarette use from approximately 10 to 6 per day, and lost about 3.7 kg versus a gain of approximately 0.6 kg in the control group.[39,40] The intervention group had 47% less incidence of fatal and nonfatal coronary heart disease (CHD) including sudden death ($P = .03$) and approximately 42% fewer CVD events ($P = .04$).[39] This finding represents an impressive reduction in CVD, which rivals results with pharmacotherapy.

Lifestyle change is appropriate for all people with prehypertension. Aerobic exercise, sodium restriction, the dietary approaches to stop hypertension (DASH) eating plan, and weight loss, either individually or combined, are especially attractive based on controlled clinical trials documenting BP-lowering efficacy. These lifestyle changes may also reduce multiple risk factors, minimize progression to hypertension and diabetes, and decrease CVD events.[38–47] Yet, the US population is becoming progressively heavier and their diets less DASH-like over time,[48,49] which suggests that healthy lifestyles are becoming less common. Thus, if we are serious about public health and disease prevention, we need to implement more effective strategies for facilitating adoption and maintenance of healthy lifestyle patterns in the general population[41,42] and/or need to strongly consider pharmacotherapeutic options for a larger proportion of the population,[24,27] that is, a new public health paradigm.

Options for increasing effectiveness of lifestyle changes

In the 1960s, antismoking public health service announcements were so effective that the tobacco industry agreed to cease advertising on television. Together with changes in collective attitudes of the general public, limiting smoking in public places and higher tobacco taxes gained widespread support, and the per capita cigarette consumption, which peaked at around 1960, declined steadily from around 1965 to 2000.[41,42,50] Public health messaging on the dangers of saturated fat and cholesterol led to a greater than 50% reduction in saturated fat intake and a lowering of mean population cholesterol level by more than 10 mg/dL. Incidence of age-adjusted CHD in the United States decreased more than 30% between 1965 and 1978, and more than 50% of the decline was attributed to healthy lifestyle changes.[41,42] It is likely that a coordinated national campaign against the unhealthy foods provided by the fast food industry would yield similar results today. However, those efforts have been largely abandoned by public health agencies in the United States.

Individual liberty versus collective responsibility

Natural foods are generally healthy foods, and processing food rarely improves nutritional quality or health benefits and typically degrades them significantly.[51] Legislative initiatives to limit and/or tax unhealthy food processing practices, for example, the amount of added salt, sugar, and saturated fat, could have substantial health benefits.

Because public health has failed in primary disease prevention, we have loaded progressively more responsibility for managing the resulting avalanche of chronic diseases on our primary health care system and then criticized it for not being more prevention oriented. We talk about preventive medicine yet virtually ignore the most important component: healthy lifestyles. The cost of health care is soaring in part because Americans are being consumed by chronic diseases that are largely preventable through healthy lifestyles.[51–53] We are becoming progressively heavier and our nutritional patterns less DASH-like with time.[48,49] We are digging our graves with a knife and fork[54] and imposing an enormous financial burden on our country in the process. Obesity and poor physical fitness disqualify one-third of individuals aged 17 to 24 years from military service, which threatens military readiness and national security.[55] National and international security were a key theme of John F. Kennedy's inaugural address on January 21, 1961, nearly 50 years ago. His inspired words are relevant to our health problems today.

> *In the long history of the world, only a few generations have been granted the role of defending freedom in its hour of maximum danger. I do not shank from this responsibility—I welcome it. I do not believe that any of us would exchange places with any other people or any other generation. The energy, the faith, the devotion which we bring to this endeavor will light our country and all who serve it—and the glow from that fire can truly light the world.*
>
> *And so, my fellow Americans: ask not what your country can do for you - ask what you can do for your country. My fellow citizens of the world: ask not what America will do for you, but what together we can do for the freedom of man.*
>
> *Finally, whether you are citizens of America or citizens of the world, ask of us the same high standards of strength and sacrifice which we ask of you. With a good conscience our only sure reward, with history the final judge of our deeds, let us go forth to lead the land we love, asking His blessing and His help, but knowing that here on earth God's work must truly be our own.*
>
> *One of the best things that we can do for our country today is to be healthy and productive. While more and better health care for all citizens is a worthy and laudable national goal, we are deluding ourselves about the potential for real progress and true savings if healthier lifestyles are not the centerpiece. Our current lifestyle patterns are creating a national health, economic, and security catastrophe for present and future generations.*

The Case for Antihypertensive Therapy in Stage 2 Prehypertension

While a new and effective public health paradigm grounded in history and current realities is desperately needed, the burden of prehypertension-related cardiovascular risk and disease is growing. Thus, a complementary pharmacologic strategy deserves strong consideration. In fact, a scientific statement from the 3 councils of the American Heart Association (AHA) suggested a BP goal of less than 130/80 mm Hg for all patients with a 10-year CHD risk of 10% or more,[56] which includes many patients with stage 2 prehypertension. The recommendation is based largely on the clinical epidemiology of risk rather than evidence-based benefit from randomized controlled clinical trials. Nonetheless, it may be useful to review the evidence for pharmacologic treatment in stage 2 prehypertension to determine what is known about safety, antihypertensive efficacy, and cardiovascular outcomes.

Safety and efficacy of antihypertensive therapy in stage 2 prehypertension

In both TROPHY, which used an angiotensin receptor blocker (ARB), and prevention of hypertension with the angiotensin converting enzyme inhibitor ramipril in patients with high normal blood pressure (PHARAO) study, which used the angiotensin-converting enzyme (ACE) inhibitor, ramipril, in patients with high normal BP to reduce progression to hypertension, adverse effects were generally comparable to placebo.[24,27] In TROPHY, during the first 2 years of the study, BP was lowered by approximately 9/5 mm Hg in the group on candesartan (16 mg) compared with the placebo-treated group. BP was lowered by 3 to 5/2 to 3 mm Hg during the first year of ramipril, 5 mg, administration compared with placebo therapy in the PHARAO study, with narrowing of the BP differential with the placebo group thereafter. Both the studies documented that BP can be lowered safely in patients with stage 2 prehypertension.

Clinical outcomes with antihypertensive therapy in stage 2 prehypertension

In TROPHY, patients with stage 2 prehypertension randomized to candesartan, 16 mg, daily had an absolute reduction of 26.8% and a relative reduction of 66.3% in new-onset hypertension during the first 2 years compared with placebo-treated patients.[24] Two years after discontinuing the therapy, the group treated with candesartan had an absolute reduction of 9.8% and a relative reduction of 15.6% in new-onset hypertension. The benefits of candesartan at 2 and 4 years were comparable when the data were reanalyzed using the JNC 7 definition of hypertension.[26] Two years after discontinuing therapy, the absolute reduction in new-onset hypertension was greater and the relative reduction in hypertension was similar in TROPHY as in TOHP II with continued efforts at intensive lifestyle change.[38] In the PHARAO study, de novo hypertension over 3 years in patients with stage 2 prehypertension occurred in 42.9% of the placebo-treated group and 30.7% of the low-dose ramipril group; relative risk reduction of 34.4%, $P = .0001$.

A patient with a home systolic BP of 135 mm Hg or more has roughly an 80% chance of becoming hypertensive within 4 years.[24] These data suggest that masked hypertension, daytime out-of-office BP $\geq$135/$\geq$85 mm Hg, in subjects with stage 2 prehypertension unmasks quickly in the office. Subjects with masked hypertension are at significantly higher CVD risk than patients with normal office and home BP.[57,58] Because subjects with masked hypertension are at very high risk for progression to hypertension over a limited follow-up period and at nearly 2-fold higher risk for CVD events, the clinical epidemiology supports a treatment decision.

Antihypertensive therapy to reduce CVD events in stage 2 prehypertension

Stage 2 prehypertension contributes significantly and independently to CVD, even after adjusting for progression to hypertension and concomitant risk factors (see **Table 1**). The absolute excess risk related to stage 2 prehypertension with 1 or more additional cardiovascular risk factors is substantial, particularly when follow-up periods of more than 5 years are considered (see **Table 1**). Epidemiologic data suggest that the numbers needed to treat to prevent a CVD event are similar in patients with stage 2 prehypertension and stage 1 hypertension, when both have at least 1 additional major cardiovascular risk factor.[33]

Unlike stage 1 hypertension, there are no adequately powered trials examining the benefits of antihypertensive therapy on CVD outcomes in stage 2 prehypertension. Randomized clinical mortality trials for this group are expensive and difficult. This gap in evidence-based medicine could be most efficiently addressed by comparative effectiveness research on patients with stage 2 prehypertension conducted in representative practice settings. Such studies are needed to establish effectiveness and not simply efficacy, which is established by studies conducted in more research-intensive settings. Although efficacy studies are important, they are frequently difficult to translate into usual practice. Effectiveness, which is key to improving population health, is better addressed by practical clinical trials, that is, comparative effectiveness research.[59,60]

Initiating antihypertensive therapy in patients with stage 2 prehypertension at high risk for ischemic heart disease is an attractive option as suggested by the 3 councils of the AHA[56] and consistent with estimates of benefit from the clinical epidemiology.[33] There are not yet any official guidelines for pharmacotherapy of stage 2 prehypertension in the absence of diabetes, chronic kidney disease, or other compelling indication.[1] Nevertheless, future guidelines may endorse treatment in the absence of randomized controlled clinical trials in a fashion similar to the original National Cholesterol Education Program (NCEP) guidelines. The first NCEP expert panel recommended statin therapy for lowering cholesterol levels, based largely on evidence that these agents safely lowered cholesterol levels, although randomized controlled clinical outcome data were very limited at the time.[61]

If a concerned clinician decides to implement pharmacotherapy based on the absolute risk of an individual patient, for example, 10-year CHD risk of 10% or more,[56] there are several classes of medications, which are effective antihypertensive agents that have documented outcome benefits in patients with higher BP values.[1,56] An ACE inhibitor or ARB data may be considered, because both agents have been shown to safely lower BP and reduce the development of frank hypertension among individuals with stage 2 prehypertension.[24,27]

SUMMARY

Prehypertension or BP in the range of 120 to 139/80 to 89 mm Hg is a common public health problem affecting approximately 83 million adults in the United States alone.[9–12] Approximately 31 million adults have BP in the range of 130 to 139/85 to 89, which is referred to as stage 2 prehypertension. Stage 2 prehypertension is associated with an approximately 8% to 14% annual incidence of de novo hypertension, as documented from studies with 3 to 4 years follow-up,[25–27] and 50% to 130% greater risk for CVD events (see **Table 1**). Lifestyle changes, directed at reducing BP and overall cardiovascular risk, are appropriate for all prehypertensive patients (see **Table 1**). For patients with stage 2 prehypertension whose BP does not respond to a 3- to 6-month trial of lifestyle change, the concerned clinician may elect to initiate antihypertensive therapy, especially in those at high absolute risk for CVD complications. Regular follow-up of all patients with stage 2 prehypertension is appropriate for evaluation of BP responses to lifestyle change with or without antihypertensive therapy, progression to hypertension, changes in the cardiovascular risk factor profile, and target organ damage. Concomitant risk factors, especially lipid disorders, must be effectively managed to optimize outcomes in patients with elevated BP.[62,63]

Given the magnitude of population attributable risk of hypertension and CVD posed by stage 2 prehypertension, a new public health paradigm is urgently needed. The new prototype should emphasize public health strategies with proved effectiveness tailored to current realities and comparative effectiveness research using a factorial design to quickly provide the evidence base needed for optimal decision making. Progress in addressing the public health threat presented by stage 2 prehypertension could serve as a national template for more effective health promotion and disease prevention.

REFERENCES

1. Chobanian AV, Bakris GL, Black HR, et al. Seventh report of the joint national committee on prevention, evaluation, and treatment of high blood pressure. Hypertension 2003;42:1206–52.
2. Robinson SC, Brucer M. Range of normal blood pressure: a statistical and clinical study of 11,383 persons. Arch Intern Med 1939;64:409–44.
3. Greenlund KJ, Croft JB, Mensah GA. Prevalence of heart disease and stroke risk factors in persons with prehypertension in the United States, 1999–2000. Arch Intern Med 2004;164:2113–8.
4. Neaton JD, Kuller L, Stamler J, et al. Impact of systolic and diastolic blood pressure on cardiovascular mortality. In: Laragh JH, Brenner BM, editors. Hypertension, pathophysiology, diagnosis, and management. 2nd edition. New York: Raven Press, Ltd; 1995.
5. Levy RL, Hillman CC, Stoud WD, et al. Transient tachycardia: prognostic significance alone and in association with transient hypertension. JAMA 1945;129:585–8.
6. Julius S, Schork MA. Borderline hypertension—a critical review. J Chronic Dis 1971;23:723–54.
7. Julius S, Jamerson K, Mejia A, et al. The association of borderline hypertension with target organ changes and higher coronary risk. JAMA 1990; 264:354–8.
8. Giles TD, Berk BC, Black HR, et al. Expanding the definition and classification of hypertension. J Clin Hypertens 2005;7:505–12.
9. Ostchega Y, Yoon SS, Hughes J, et al. Hypertension awareness, treatment, and control—continued disparities in adults: United States, 2005–2006. NCHS Data Brief, No. 3, 2008.
10. Wang Y, Wang QJ. The prevalence of prehypertension and hypertension among US adults according to the new Joint National Committee Guidelines. Arch Intern Med 2004;164:2126–34.

11. Qureshi AI, Suri MF, Kirmani JF, et al. Prevalence and trends of prehypertension and hypertension in United States: National Health and Nutrition Examination Surveys 1976 to 2000. Med Sci Monit 2005; 11:CR403–9.
12. USA Quick Facts from the US Census Bureau. Available at: http://quickfacts.census.gov/qfd/states/00000.html. Accessed January 7, 2010.
13. Julius S, Jamerson K, Mejia A, et al. The association of borderline hypertension with target organ changes and higher coronary risk: Tecumseh Blood Pressure Study. JAMA 1990;265:354–8.
14. Eliasson M, Jansson JH, Nilsson P, et al. Increased levels of tissue plasminogen activator antigen in essential hypertension: a population-based study. J Hypertens 1997;15:349–56.
15. Toikka JO, Laine H, Ahotupa M, et al. Increased arterial intima-media thickness and in vivo LDL oxidation in young men with borderline hypertension. Hypertension 2000;36:929–33.
16. Palombo C, Kozakova M, Magagna A, et al. Early impairment of coronary flow reserve and increase in minimum coronary resistance in borderline hypertensive patients. J Hypertens 2000;18:453–9.
17. Millgard J, Hagg A, Sarabi M, et al. Endothelium-dependent vasodilation in normotensive subjects with a familial history of essential hypertension and in young subjects with borderline hypertension. Blood Press 2002;11:279–84.
18. Chrysohoou C, Pitsavos C, Panagiotakos DB, et al. Association between prehypertension status and inflammatory markers related to atherosclerotic disease. The Attica Study. Am J Hypertens 2004; 17:568–73.
19. Knecht S, Wersching H, Lohmann H, et al. High-normal blood pressure is associated with poor cognitive performance. Hypertension 2008;51:663–8.
20. Sehestedt T, Jeppesen J, Hansen TW, et al. Which markers of subclinical organ damage to measure in individuals with high normal blood pressure? J Hypertens 2009;27:1165–71.
21. Meisinger C, Döring A, Heier M. Blood pressure and risk of type 2 diabetes mellitus in men and women from the general population: the monitoring trends and determinants of cardiovascular diseases/cooperative health research in the region of Augsburg cohort study. J Hypertens 2008;26:1809–15.
22. Leitschuh M, Cuppies LA, Kannel W, et al. High-normal blood pressure progression to hypertension in the Framingham Study. Hypertension 1991;17: 22–7.
23. Winegarden CR. From "prehypertension" to hypertension? Additional evidence. Ann Epidemiol 2004; 15:720–5.
24. Julius S, Nesbitt SD, Egan BM, et al. Feasiblity of treating prehypertension with an angiotensin receptor blocker. N Engl J Med 2006;354:1685–97.
25. Vasan RS, Larson MG, Leip EP, et al. Assessment of frequency of progression to hypertension in non-hypertensive participants in the Framingham Heart Study: a cohort study. Lancet 2001;358:1682–6.
26. Julius S, Kaciroti N, Nesbitt S, et al. TROPHY revisited: outcomes based on the JNC 7 definition of hypertension. J Agric Saf Health 2008;2:39–43.
27. Lüders S, Schraderr J, Jürgen B, et al. The PHARAO study: prevention of hypertension with angiotensin-converting enzyme inhibitor ramipril in patients with high-normal blood pressure – prospective, randomized, controlled prevention trial of the German Hypertension League. J Hypertens 2008;26:1487–96.
28. Vasan RS, Larson MG, Leip EP, et al. Impact of high-normal blood pressure on the risk of cardiovascular disease. N Engl J Med 2001;345:1291–7.
29. Liszka HA, Mainous AG, King DE, et al. Prehypertension and cardiovascular morbidity. Ann Fam Med 2005;3:294–9.
30. Kshirsagar AV, Carpenter M, Bang J, et al. Blood pressure usually considered normal is associated with an elevated risk of cardiovascular disease. Am J Med 2006;119:133–41.
31. Egan BM. Should metabolic syndrome patients with prehypertension receive antihypertensive therapy? In: Bakris GL, editor. Therapeutic strategies in hypertension. Oxford (UK): Clinical Publishing; 2006. p. 9–25, Chapter 2.
32. Zhang Y, Lee ET, Devereux RB, et al. Prehypertension, diabetes, and cardiovascular disease risk in a population-based sample: the Strong Heart Study. Hypertension 2006;47:410–4.
33. Ogden LG, He J, Lydick E, et al. Long-term absolute benefit of lowering blood pressure in hypertensive patients according to the JNC VI risk stratification. Hypertension 2000;35:539–43.
34. Hsia J, Margolis KL, Eaton CB, et al. Prehypertension and cardiovascular disease risk in the Women's Health Initiative. Circulation 2007;115:855–60.
35. Tsai SP, Wen CP, Chan HT, et al. The effects of pre-disease risk factors within metabolic syndrome on all-cause and cardiovascular disease mortality. Diabetes Res Clin Pract 2008;82:148–56.
36. Nesbitt SN, Julius S, Leonard D, et al. Is low-risk hypertension fact or fiction? Cardiovascular risk profile in the TROPHY Study. Am J Hypertens 2005;18(7):979–84.
37. Lasser VI, Raczynski JM, Stevens VJ, et al. Trial of prevention, phase II: structure and content of the weight loss and dietary sodium reduction interventions. Ann Epidemiol 1995;5:156–64.
38. The Trials of Hypertension Prevention Collaborative Research Group. Effects of weight loss and sodium reduction intervention on blood pressure and hypertension incidence in overweight people with high-normal blood pressure. Arch Intern Med 1997;157: 657–67.

39. Hjermann I, Holme I, Vlve BK, et al. Effect of diet and smoking intervention on the incidence of coronary heart disease: report from the Oslo study group of a randomised trial in healthy men. Lancet 1981;2 (8259):1303–10.
40. Hjermann I. Smoking and diet intervention in healthy coronary high risk men. Methods and 5-year follow-up of risk factors in a randomized trial. The Oslo study. J Oslo City Hosp 1980;30:3–17.
41. Moser M. A decade of progress in the management of hypertension. Hypertension 1983;5:808–13.
42. Goldman L, Cook F. The decline in ischemic heart disease mortality rates: an analysis of the comparative effective of medical interventions and changes in lifestyle. Ann Intern Med 1984;101:825–36.
43. Appel LJ, Moore TJ, Obarzanek E, et al. A clinical trial of the effects of dietary patterns on blood pressure. N Engl J Med 1997;336:1117–24.
44. Esposito K, Marella R, Ciotaola M, et al. Effect of a Mediterranean-style diet on endothelial dysfunction and markers of vascular inflammation in the metabolic syndrome. JAMA 2004;292:1440–6.
45. Katzmarzyk PT, Church TS, Blair SN. Cardiorespiratory fitness attenuates the effects of the metabolic syndrome on all-cause and cardiovascular disease mortality in men. Arch Intern Med 2004;164: 1092–7.
46. The Diabetes Prevention Program Research Group. Reduction in the incidence of type 2 diabetes with lifestyle intervention or metformin. N Engl J Med 2002;346:393–403.
47. Fung TT, Chiuve SE, McCullough ML, et al. Adherence to a DASH-style diet and risk of coronary heart disease and stroke in women. Arch Intern Med 2008;168:713–20.
48. Ford ES, Zhao G, Li C, et al. Trends in obesity and abdominal obesity among hypertensive and nonhypertensive adults in the United States. Am J Hypertens 2008;21:1124–8.
49. Mellen PB, Gao SK, Vitolins MZ, et al. Deteriorating dietary habits among adults with hypertension. DASH dietary accordance, NHANES 1988–1994 and 1999–2004. Arch Intern Med 2008;168:308–14.
50. Merill RM, Timmreck TC. Introduction to epidemology. 4th edition. Sadbury (MA): Jones and Barlett Publishers; 2006. p. 128, Fig. 5.11.
51. Cordain L, Eaton SB, Sebastian A, et al. Origins and evolution of the Western diet: health implications for the 21st century. Am J Clin Nutr 2005;81:341–5.
52. Booth FW, Laye MJ, Lees SJ, et al. Reduced physical activity and risk of chronic disease: the biology behind the consequences. Eur J Appl Physiol 2008;102:381–90.
53. Kennedy ET. Evidence for nutritional benefits in prolonging wellness. Am J Clin Nutr 2006;83:410S–4S.
54. Huckabee M. Quit digging your grave with a knife and fork: a 12-stop program to end bad habits and begin a healthy lifestyle. Center Street. New York: Time Warner Book Group; 2005.
55. Davenport C, Brown E. The Washington Post, Girding for an uphill battle for recruits: obesity, poor education make many younger people unfit for military. Nov. 5, 2009.
56. Rosendorff C, Black HR, Cannon CP, et al. Treatment of hypertension in the prevention and management of ischemic heart disease. A scientific statement from the American Heart Association Council for High Blood Pressure Research and the Councils on Clinical Cardiology and Epidemiology and Prevention. Hypertension 2007;50:e28–55.
57. Bobrie G, Chatellier G, Genes N, et al. Cardiovascular prognosis of 'masked hypertension' detected by blood pressure self-measurement in elderly hypertensive patients. JAMA 2004;291:1342–9.
58. Mancia G, Facchetti R, Bombelli M, et al. Long-term risk of mortality associated with selective and combined elevation in office, home, and ambulatory blood pressure. Hypertension 2006;47:846–53.
59. Tunis SR, Stryer DB, Clancy CM. Practical clinical trials: increasing the value of clinical research for decision making in clinical and health policy. JAMA 2003;290:1624–32.
60. Luce BR, Kramer JM, Goodman SN, et al. Rethinking randomized clinical trials for comparative effectiveness research: the need for transformational change. Ann Intern Med 2009;151:206–9.
61. Report of the National Cholesterol Education Program expert panel on detection, evaluation and treatment of high blood cholesterol in adults. The expert panel. Arch Intern Med 1988;148: 36–69.
62. Wong ND, Pio JR, Franklin SS, et al. Preventing coronary events by optimal control of blood pressure and lipids in patients with the metabolic syndrome. Am J Cardiol 2003;91:1421–6.
63. Sever PS, Dahlof B, Poulter NR, et al. Prevention of coronary and stroke events in hypertensive patients who have average or lower-than-average cholesterol concentrations, in the Anglo-Scandinavian Cardiac Outcomes Trial—Lipid Lowering Arm (ASCOT-LLA): a multicentre randomised controlled trial. Lancet 2003;361:1149–58.

Principles and Techniques of Blood Pressure Measurement

Gbenga Ogedegbe, MD[a,*], Thomas Pickering, MD, DPhil[b,†]

KEYWORDS

- Blood pressure measurement • Self-monitoring
- Ambulatory blood pressure monitoring

BASIC TECHNIQUES OF BLOOD PRESSURE MEASUREMENT

Location of Measurement

The standard location for blood pressure measurement is the brachial artery. Monitors that measure pressure at the wrist and fingers have become popular, but it is important to realize that systolic and diastolic pressures vary substantially in different parts of the arterial tree, with systolic pressure increasing in more distal arteries, and diastolic pressure decreasing.

The Auscultatory Method

Although the auscultatory method using mercury sphygmomanometer is regarded as the gold standard for office blood pressure measurement, widespread implementation of the ban in use of mercury sphygmomanometers continues to diminish the role of this technique.[1] The situation is made worse by the fact that existing aneroid manometers, which use this technique, are less accurate and often need frequent calibration.[1] New devices known as "hybrid" sphygmomanometers have been developed as replacement for mercury devices. Basically these devices combine the features of both electronic and auscultatory devices such that the mercury column is replaced by an electronic pressure gauge, similar to oscillometric devices, but the blood pressure is taken in the same manner as a mercury or aneroid device, by an observer using a stethoscope and listening for the Korotkoff sounds.[1]

The Oscillometric Technique

This technique was first demonstrated by Marey in 1876,[2] and it was subsequently shown that when the oscillations of pressure in a sphygmomanometer cuff are recorded during gradual deflation, the point of maximal oscillation corresponds to the mean intra-arterial pressure.[3–5] The oscillations begin at approximately systolic pressure and continue below diastolic (**Fig. 1**), so that systolic and diastolic pressure can only be estimated indirectly according to some empirically derived algorithm. This method is advantageous in that no transducer need be placed over the brachial artery, and it is less susceptible to external noise (but not to low-frequency mechanical vibration), and that the cuff can be removed and replaced by the patient during ambulatory monitoring, for example, to take a shower. The main disadvantage is that such recorders do not work well during physical activity when there may be considerable movement artifact. The oscillometric technique has been used successfully in ambulatory blood pressure monitors and home

A version of this article originally appeared in *Cardiology Clinics* volume 20, issue 2.
This work was supported by Grant No. R01HL078566 from the National Institutes of Health.
[a] Center for Healthful Behavior Change, Division of General Internal Medicine, Department of Medicine, New York University School of Medicine, 423 East 23rd Street, 15N-168, New York, NY 10010, USA
[b] Center for Behavioral Cardiovascular Health, Division of General Medicine, Department of Medicine, Columbia University, 622 West 168th Street, New York, NY 10034, USA
[†] Deceased.
[*] Corresponding author.
E-mail address: olugbenga.ogedegbe@nyumc.org

Cardiol Clin 28 (2010) 571–586
doi:10.1016/j.ccl.2010.07.006

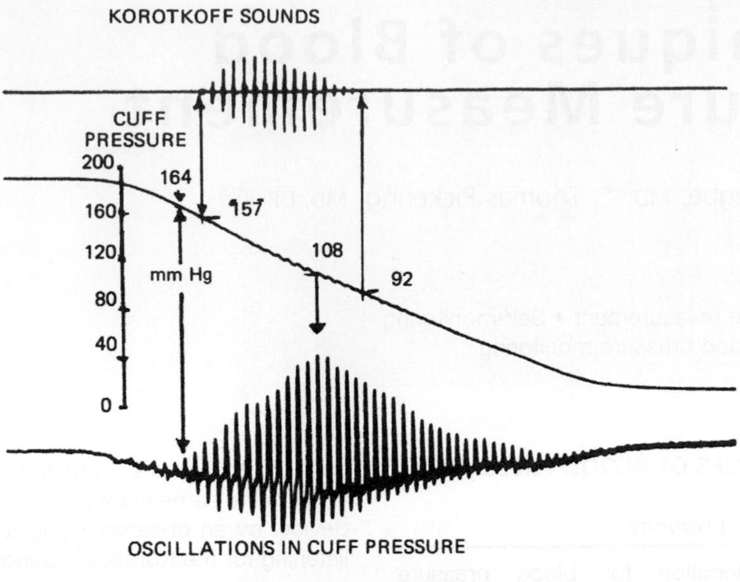

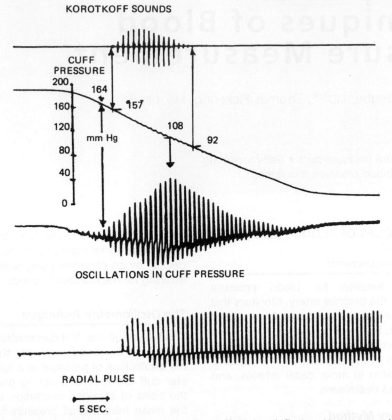

Fig. 1. Changes occurring distal to a sphygmomanometer cuff during deflation. Upper trace: Korotkoff sounds. Second trace: cuff pressure. Third trace: oscillations in cuff pressure. The maximal oscillation occurs at a pressure of 108 mm Hg, the mean arterial pressure. Bottom trace: radial pulse. *From* Pickering TG. Blood pressure variability and ambulatory monitoring. Curr Opin Nephrol Hypertens 1993;2:380; with permission.

monitors. It should be pointed out that different brands of oscillometric recorders use different algorithms, and there is no generic oscillometric technique. Comparisons of several different commercial models with intra-arterial and Korotkoff sound measurements, however, have shown generally good agreement.[6,7]

Ultrasound Techniques

Devices incorporating this technique use an ultrasound transmitter and receiver placed over the brachial artery under a sphygmomanometer cuff. As the cuff is deflated, the movement of the arterial wall at systolic pressure causes a Doppler phase shift in the reflected ultrasound, and diastolic pressure is recorded as the point at which diminution of arterial motion occurs. Another variation of this method detects the onset of blood flow at systolic pressure, which has been found to be of particular value for measuring pressure in infants and children.[8] In patients with very faint Korotkoff sounds (for example those with muscular atrophy), placing a Doppler probe over the brachial artery may help to detect the systolic pressure, and the same technique can be used for measuring the ankle-brachial index, in which the systolic pressures in the brachial artery and the posterior tibial artery are compared to obtain an index of peripheral arterial disease.

The Finger Cuff Method of Penaz

This interesting method was first developed by Penaz[9] and works on the principle of the "unloaded arterial wall." Arterial pulsation in a finger is detected by a photo-plethysmograph under a pressure cuff. The output of the plethysmograph is used to drive a servo-loop, which rapidly changes the cuff pressure to keep the output constant, so that the artery is held in a partially opened state. The oscillations of pressure in the cuff are measured and have been found to resemble the intra-arterial pressure wave in most subjects (**Fig. 2**). This method gives an accurate estimate of the changes of systolic and diastolic

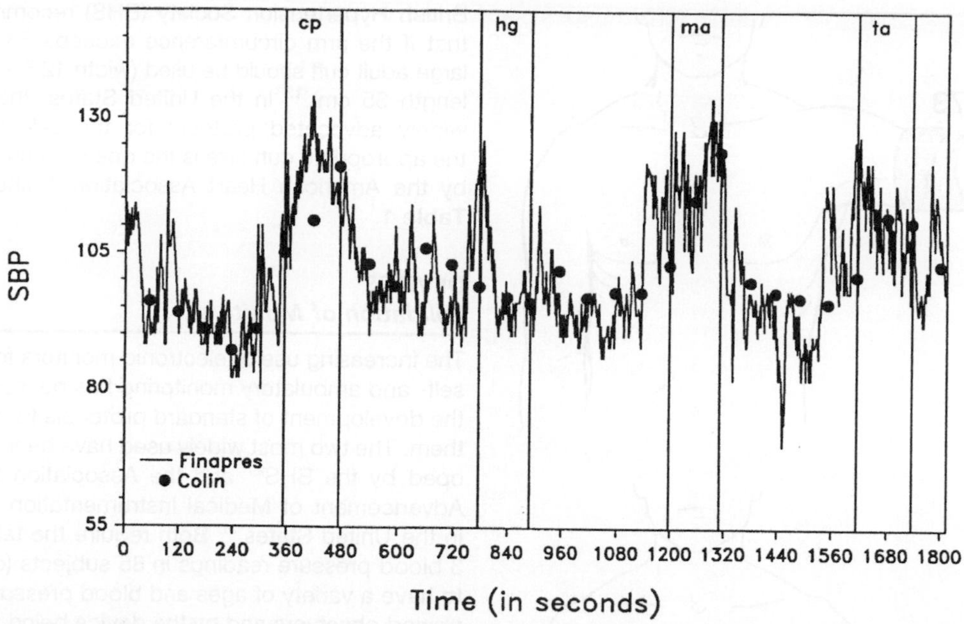

Fig. 2. Recording of systolic pressure (SBP) during laboratory stress testing, made simultaneously with a continuous beat-to-beat monitor (Finapres) and an intermittent oscillometric device (Colin). cp, cold pressor test; hg, handgrip; ma, mental arithmetic; ta, talking.

pressure in comparison with brachial artery pressures[9]; the cuff can be kept inflated for up to 2 hours. The technique is now commercially available as the Finometer and Portapres recorders, and has been validated in several studies against intra-arterial pressures.[10,11] The Portapres enables readings to be taken over 24 hours while the subjects are ambulatory, although it is somewhat cumbersome.[12]

Technical Issues with Measurement from the Arm

There are important potential sources of error with measurements from the upper arm, which are discussed in the following sections.

Effects of posture

There is no consensus as to whether blood pressure should be routinely measured while seated or supine, although most guidelines recommend sitting.[1,13] In a survey of 245 subjects of different ages, Netea and colleagues[14] found that systolic pressures were the same in both positions, but there was a systematic age-related discrepancy for diastolic pressure such that at the age of 30 years the sitting diastolic was about 10 mm Hg higher than the supine reading, whereas at the age of 70 the difference was only 2 mm Hg.

Body position

Blood pressure measurements are also influenced by the position of the arm.[15–18] As shown in **Fig. 3**, there is a progressive increase in the pressure of about 5 to 6 mm Hg as the arm is moved down from the horizontal to vertical position. These changes are exactly what would be expected from the changes of hydrostatic pressure. It is also important that the patient's back be supported during the measurement; if the patient is sitting bolt upright the diastolic pressure may be up to 6.5 mm Hg higher than if sitting back.[19]

Cuff-inflation hypertension

Although in most patients the act of inflating a sphygmomanometer cuff does not itself change the blood pressure, as shown by intra-arterial[20] and Finapres[21] recordings, in occasional patients there may be a transient but substantial increase of up to 40 mm Hg coinciding with cuff inflation.[22] This condition appears to be distinct from white-coat hypertension, in which the increase in pressure both precedes the act of inflation and outlasts it. It should also be differentiated from the transient increase of blood pressure that occurs during self-measurement, due to the muscular act of inflating the cuff.

Cuff size

The size of the cuff relative to the diameter of the arm is critical. The most common mistake is to use a cuff that is too small, which will result in an overestimation of the pressure.[23–25] In general, this error can be reduced by using a large adult-sized cuff for all except the thinnest arms. The

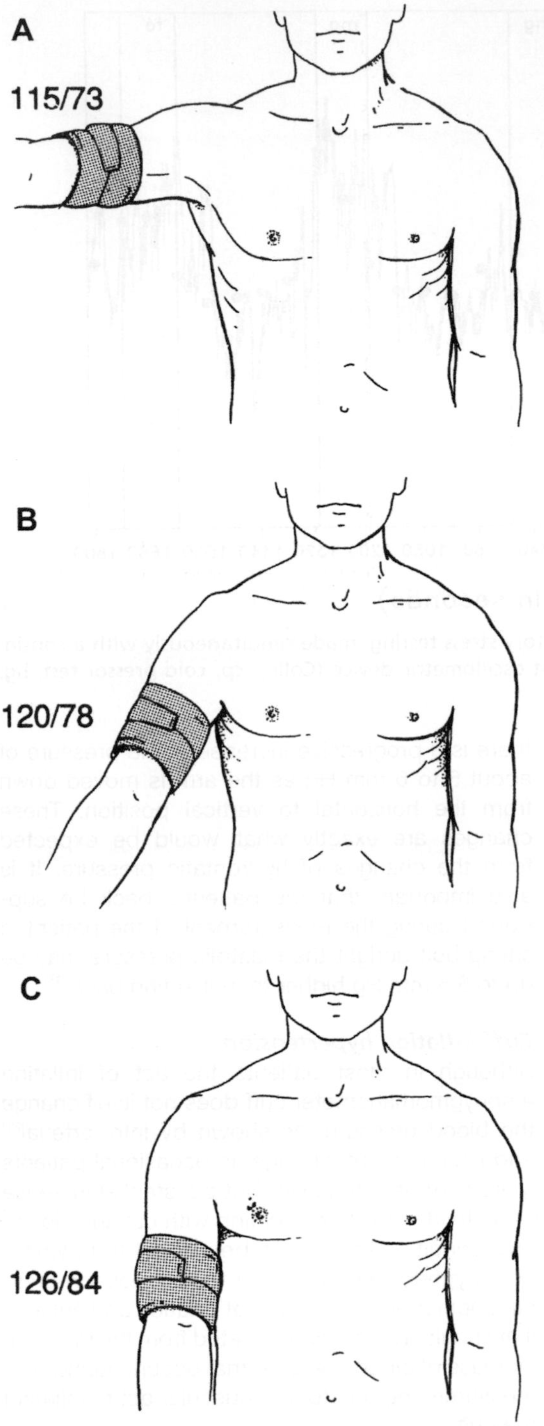

Fig. 3. (*A–C*) The effects of varying arm position on blood pressure recorded from the brachial artery. *From* Pickering TG. Blood pressure variability and ambulatory monitoring. Curr Opin Nephrol Hypertens 1993;2:380–5; with permission.

British Hypertension Society (BHS) recommends that if the arm circumference exceeds 33 cm, a large adult cuff should be used (width 12.5–13 cm, length 35 cm).[13] In the United States, the most widely advocated protocol for the selection of the appropriate cuff size is the one recommended by the American Heart Association,[26] shown in **Table 1**.

DEVICES

Validation of Monitors

The increasing use of electronic monitors for both self- and ambulatory monitoring has necessitated the development of standard protocols for testing them. The two most widely used have been developed by the BHS[27] and the Association for the Advancement of Medical Instrumentation (AAMI) in the United States.[28] Both require the taking of 3 blood pressure readings in 85 subjects (chosen to have a variety of ages and blood pressures) by trained observers and by the device being tested. The BHS protocol requires that a device must give at least 50% of readings within 5 mm Hg and 75% within 10 mm Hg with the 2 methods (grade B), and the AAMI requires that the average difference between the 2 methods not exceed 5 mm Hg with a standard deviation of less than 8 mm Hg. One of the limitations of the validation procedures is that they analyze the data on a population basis and pay no attention to individual factors. Thus, it is possible that a monitor will pass the validation criteria and still be consistently in error in a substantial number of individuals.[29]

Devices for Clinic and Hospital Measurement

Mercury sphygmomanometers

The design of mercury sphygmomanometers has changed little over the past 50 years, except that

Table 1
Cuff sizes recommended by the American Heart Association

Cuff	Arm Circumference (cm)	Bladder Width (cm)	Bladder Length (cm)
Newborn	<6	3	6
Infant	6–15	5	15
Child	16–21	8	21
Small adult	22–26	10	24
Adult	27–34	13	30
Large adult	35–44	16	38
Adult thigh	45–52	20	42

modern versions are less likely to spill mercury if dropped. As indicated earlier, although the use of mercury sphygmomanometer is widely regarded as the gold standard for office blood pressure measurement, widespread implementation of the ban in use of mercury devices continues to diminish their role in office and hospital settings. To date, mercury devices have largely being phased out in United States hospitals.[30] The reason is not because any more accurate device has been developed but because of concerns about the safety of mercury. At present the two alternatives for replacement of mercury are aneroid sphygmomanometer and electronic (oscillometric) devices.

Aneroid devices

The ban on mercury sphygmomanometers has created new interest in alternative methods, of which aneroid devices are the leading contenders. The error rates reported regarding accuracy of aneroid devices in older hospital surveys range from 1% in one survey[31] to 44% in another.[32] Validation studies conducted a decade ago indicated that these devices could be accurate.[33,34] A recent study, which compared the use of mercury versus aneroid device in the setting of a large clinical trial across more than 20 clinical sites, also found it to be accurate.[35] This evidence is the best to date attesting to the accuracy of aneroid devices.

Sources of Error with the Auscultatory Method

Some of the major causes of a discrepancy between the conventional clinical measurement of blood pressure and the true blood pressure are listed in **Table 2**. The measurement of blood pressure typically involves an interaction between the patient and the physician (or whoever is taking the reading), and factors related to both may lead to a tendency to either overestimate or underestimate the true blood pressure or to act as a source of bidirectional error. As shown in **Table 2**, there may be activities that precede or accompany the measurement that make it unrepresentative of the patient's "true" pressure. These activities include exercise and smoking before the measurement as well as talking during it.

The white-coat effect and white-coat hypertension

One of the main reasons for the growing emphasis on blood pressure readings taken outside the physician's office or clinic is the white-coat effect, which is conceived as the increase of blood pressure that occurs at the time of a clinic visit and dissipates soon thereafter. Recent studies indicate that the mechanisms underlying the white-coat effect may include anxiety, a hyperactive alerting response, or a conditioned response[36,37] In one of these studies, the authors assessed office blood pressure, ambulatory blood pressure, and anxiety scores on 3 separate occasions 1 month apart in 238 patients. The authors found the largest white-coat effect occurred in the physician's presence, and the noted that white-coat effect was a conditioned response to the medical environment and the physician's presence rather than a function of the patient's trait anxiety level (**Fig. 4**). The white-coat effect is seen to a greater or lesser extent in most if not all hypertensive patients, but is much smaller or absent in normotensive individuals. The effect usually has been defined as the difference between the clinic and daytime ambulatory pressure.[38] A closely linked but discrete entity is white-coat hypertension, which refers to a subset of patients who are hypertensive according to their clinic blood pressures but normotensive at other times. Thus, white-coat hypertension is a measure of blood pressure levels, whereas the white-coat effect is a measure of blood pressure change.

What distinguishes patients with white-coat hypertension from those with true or sustained hypertension is not that they have an exaggerated white-coat effect but that their blood pressure is within the normal range when they are outside

Table 2
Patient- and physician-related factors that lead to a discrepancy between clinic and true blood pressure (BP)

	Clinic BP Overestimates True BP	Bidirectional Error	Clinic BP Underestimates True BP
Physician	Inadequate cuff size	Digit preference	
Patient	White-coat effect/anxiety Talking Recent ingestion of pressor substances	Spontaneous BP variability	Smoker Recent exercise

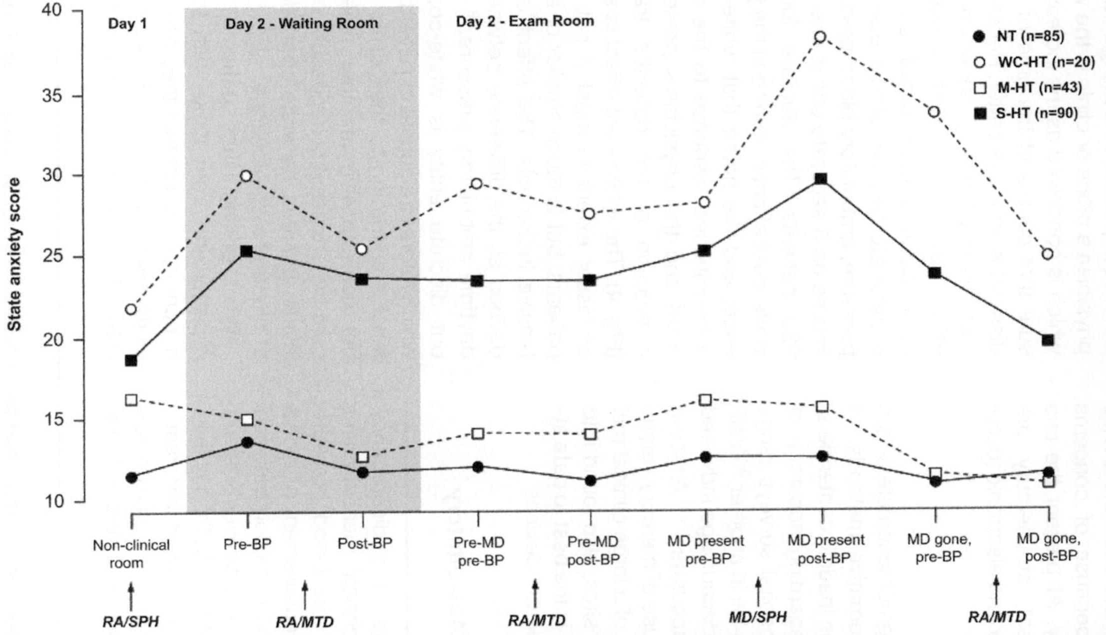

Fig. 4. On day 1, the research assistant (RA) measured blood pressure outside the medical environment using a mercury sphygmomanometer (SPH). On day 2, the RA measured blood pressure in the absence of a physician (MD) by manually triggering a device for ambulatory blood pressure measurement (MTD) first in the waiting room and next in the examination before and after the MD measured blood pressure using SPH. Anxiety scores were obtained in normotensive subjects (NT) and in patients with white-coat hypertension (WC-HT), masked hypertension (M-HT), and sustained hypertension (S-HT). (*Reproduced from* Ogedegbe G, Pickering TG, Clemow L, et al. The misdiagnosis of hypertension: the role of patient anxiety. Arch Intern Med 2008;168(22):2459–65; with permission.)

the clinic setting. White-coat hypertension is important clinically because it appears to be a relatively low-risk condition compared with sustained hypertension (defined by an elevated blood pressure in both the clinic and ambulatory settings).[39] White-coat hypertension can only be diagnosed reliably by ambulatory monitoring and home self-monitoring, as described later. Observer error and observer bias are important sources of error when sphygmomanometers are used. Differences of auditory acuity between observers may lead to consistent errors, and digit preference is very common, with most observers recording a disproportionate number of readings ending in 5 or 0.[40] An example is shown in **Fig. 5** of readings taken by hypertension specialists, who are clearly not immune to this error. The average values of blood pressure recorded by trained individual observers have been found to vary by as much as 5 to l0 mm Hg.[41] The level of pressure that is recorded may also be profoundly influenced by behavioral factors related to the effects of the observer on the subject, the best known of which is the presence of a physician. It has been known for more than 40 years that blood pressures recorded by a physician can be as much as 30 mm Hg higher than pressures taken by the patient at home, using the same technique and in the same posture.[42] Physicians also record higher pressures than nurses or technicians.[43,44] Other factors that influence the pressure recorded may include both the race and sex of the observer.[45,46]

Rate of cuff inflation and deflation

The rate of inflation has no significant effect on the blood pressure,[23] but with very slow rates of deflation (2 mm Hg/s or less) the intensity of the Korotkoff sounds is diminished, resulting in slightly higher

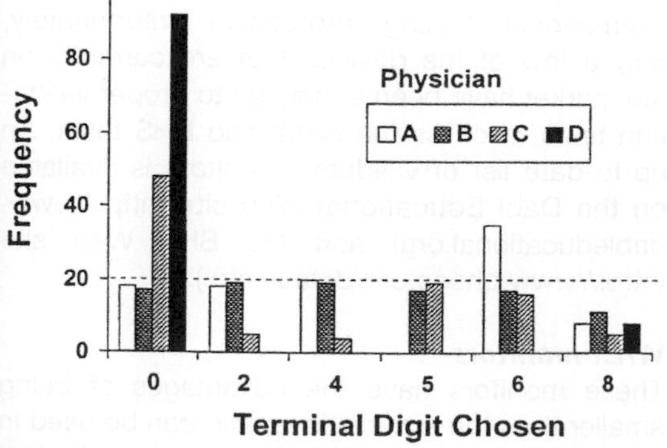

Fig. 5. The percentage of terminal digits chosen by 4 physicians in a hypertension clinic during routine blood pressure measurement. Note the marked preference for zeroes in physicians C and D.

diastolic pressures. This effect has been attributed to venous congestion reducing the rate of blood flow during very slow deflation.[47] The generally recommended deflation rate is 2 to 3 mm Hg/s. The rate of inflation and deflation is of crucial importance during self-monitoring of blood pressure, because the isometric exercise involved in inflating the cuff produces a transient elevation of pressure of about 10 mm Hg.[48] Although this lasts for only about 20 seconds, if the cuff is deflated too soon the pressure may not have returned to baseline, and a spuriously high systolic pressure will be recorded.

Auscultatory gap

This phenomenon can be defined as the loss and reappearance of Korotkoff sounds that occur between systolic and diastolic pressures during cuff deflation in the absence of cardiac arrhythmias. Thus, if its presence is not recognized, it may lead to the registration of spuriously high diastolic or low systolic pressures. the gap may occur either because of phasic changes of arterial pressure or in patients who have faint Korotkoff sounds (**Fig. 6**). The auscultatory gap may pose a problem for automatic recorders, which operate by the Korotkoff sound technique, and result in gross errors in the measurement of diastolic pressure.[47] Oscillometric devices are less susceptible to this problem.[47] The presence of the auscultatory gap is of clinical significance, because it is associated with an increased prevalence of target organ damage.[49]

Technical sources of error

There are also technical sources of error with the auscultatory method, although these are usually fewer when a mercury column is used than when many of the semiautomatic methods are in use (see later). These error sources include the position of the column, which should be at approximately the level of the heart. The mercury should read zero when no pressure is applied, and it should fall freely when the pressure is reduced (this may not occur if the mercury is not clean or if the pin-hole connecting the mercury column to the atmosphere is blocked). With aneroid meters, it is essential that they be checked against a mercury column both at zero pressure and when pressure is applied to the cuff. Surveys of such devices used in clinical practice frequently have shown them to be inaccurate.[50]

Electronic Monitors for Self-Monitoring of Blood Pressure

When home monitoring was introduced, most studies used aneroid sphygmomanometers.[51]

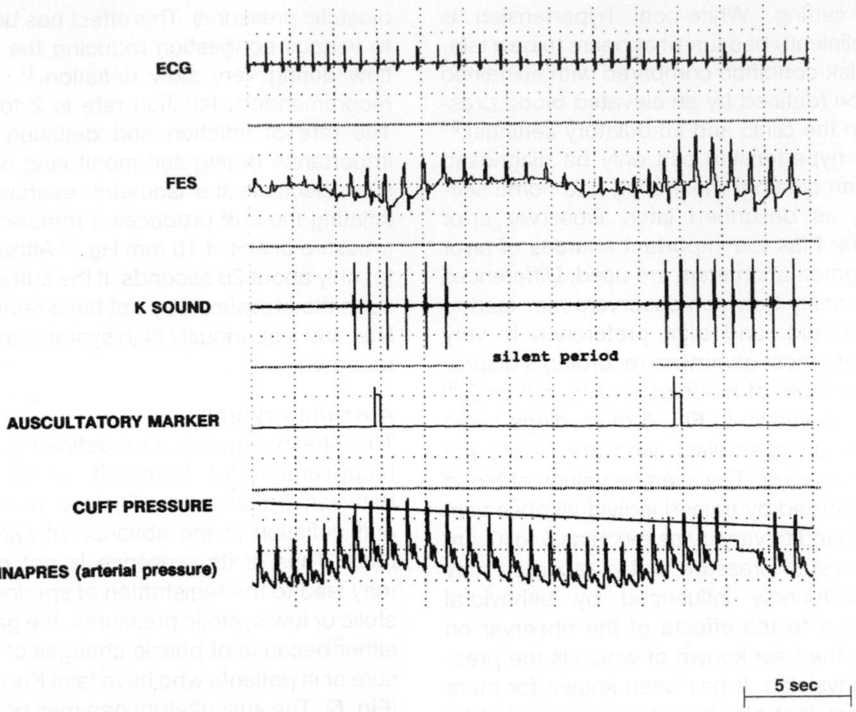

Fig. 6. The phenomenon of the auscultatory gap during cuff deflation. Upper trace: Electrocardiogram (ECG). Second trace: low frequency recording of sounds under the sphygmomanometer cuff. Third trace: Korotkoff sounds. Fourth trace: auscultatory marker pressed when systolic and diastolic sounds were heard. Fifth trace: cuff pressure. Sixth trace: Finapres recording of arterial pressure; note oscillations of pressure corresponding to silent period of K sounds. (*From* Pickering TG. Blood pressure variability and ambulatory monitoring. Curr Opin Nephrol Hypertens 1993;2:380–5; with permission.)

More recently, however, automatic electronic devices have become more popular. A Gallup poll conducted in 2005 indicated an increase in the number of patients monitoring their blood pressure at home from 38% in 2000 to 55% in 2005. Similarly, the proportion of patients owning a monitor increased from 49% in 2000 to 64% in 2005.[52] The standard type of monitor for home use is now an oscillometric device that records pressure from the brachial artery. These devices have the advantage of being easy to use, because cuff placement is not as critical as with devices that use a Korotkoff sound microphone, and the oscillometric method has in practice been found to be as reliable as the Korotkoff sound method. The early versions were mostly inaccurate[53] but the currently available ones are often satisfactory.[54,55]

The advantages of electronic monitors have begun to be appreciated by epidemiologists,[56] who have always been greatly concerned about the accuracy of clinical blood pressure measurement and have paid much attention to the problems of observer error, digit preference, and the other aforementioned causes of inaccuracy. Cooper and colleagues[56] have made the case that the ease of use of the electronic devices and the relative insensitivity to whom is actually taking the reading can outweigh any inherent inaccuracy when compared with the traditional sphygmomanometer method. Patients should be advised to use only monitors that have been validated for accuracy and reliability according to standard international testing protocols. Unfortunately, only a few of the devices that are currently on the market have been subjected to proper validation tests, such as the AAMI and BHS tests. An up-to-date list of validated monitors is available on the Dabl Educational Web site (http://www.dableducational.org) and the BHS Web site (http://www.bhsoc.org/default.stm).

Wrist monitors

These monitors have the advantages of being smaller than the arm devices, and can be used in obese people, as the wrist diameter is little affected by obesity. A potential problem with wrist monitors is the systematic error introduced by the hydrostatic effect of differences in the position of the wrist relative to the heart,[15] as shown in **Fig. 7**. This situation can be avoided if the wrist is always at heart level when the readings are taken, but there is no way of knowing retrospectively whether this was complied with when a series of readings are reviewed. Wrist monitors have potential but need to be evaluated further.[57,58]

Finger monitors

Although these monitors are convenient, they have so far been found to be inaccurate and therefore should not be used.[52]

Ambulatory Monitors

First developed almost 40 years ago, ambulatory blood pressure monitoring is only now beginning to find acceptance as a clinically useful technique. Recent technologic advances have led to the introduction of monitors that are small and relatively quiet, and that can take up to 100 readings of blood pressure over 24 hours while patients go about their normal activities. These devices are reasonably accurate while the patient is at rest but less so during physical activity. When last systematically surveyed (in 2001), only 24 had been validated according to the AAMI or BHS criteria, of which only 16 satisfied the criteria for accuracy.[55] Now many more monitors have been validated, and an updated list can be found on the Dabl Educational Web site (http://www.dableducational.org). Ambulatory monitors can in theory provide information about the 3 main measures of blood pressure: the average level, the diurnal variation, and short-term variability. Recordings in hypertensive patients show that in

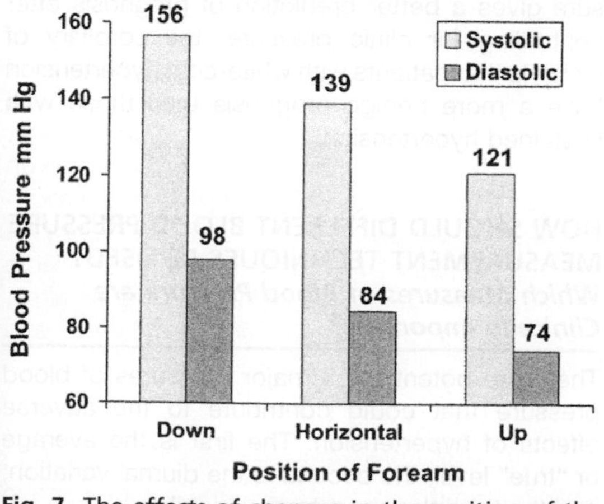

Fig. 7. The effects of changes in the position of the forearm on the blood pressure recorded by a wrist monitor. Ten readings were taken in each of 3 positions: vertically down, horizontal, and vertically up. The average values are shown at the top of each bar.

most patients the average ambulatory pressure is lower than the clinic pressure, and in some cases it may be within the normal range, leading to a diagnosis of white-coat hypertension, described later. Given that there is a discrepancy between the clinic and ambulatory pressure, it is reasonable to suppose that the prediction of risk will be different. There are now more than 30 cross-sectional studies relating the extent of cardiovascular damage to both clinic and ambulatory pressures.[59,60] Almost all have shown that the correlation coefficients are higher for ambulatory pressure, although in many instances the differences were small. The superiority of ambulatory pressure in this respect may be attributed at least in part to the greater number of readings and to their more representative nature.

Measurement in Different Situations

Clinic measurement

The recent interest in alternative methods of measuring blood pressure has served to emphasize some of the potentially correctable deficiencies of the routine clinic measurement of blood pressure. By increasing the number of readings taken per visit and the number of visits as well as by attempting to eliminate sources of error such as digit preference, the reliability of clinic pressure for estimating the true blood pressure and its consequences can be greatly increased. Despite this, it must be remembered that there are a substantial number of subjects with white-coat hypertension in whom clinic readings will continue to give unrepresentative values, no matter how many measurements are taken. Surveys of the techniques used by physicians and nurses in actual practice make depressing reading. One performed in a teaching hospital found that not one out of 172 workers followed the American Heart Association guidelines for measuring blood pressure in the clinic setting. Although 68% considered the mercury sphygmomanometer to be the most accurate, only 38% chose to use it when given a choice, and 60% were judged to be taking blood pressure inaccurately.[61]

Self-measurement

The potential advantages of having patients take their own blood pressure are twofold: the distortion produced by the white-coat effect is eliminated, and multiple readings can be taken over prolonged periods. Self-measurement of blood pressure at home has been shown to be useful in predicting target organ damage, cardiovascular events, and mortality.[52] Five prospective studies have compared the prediction of morbid events with the use of both conventional office and home blood pressure. Three were based on population samples and 2 recruited hypertensive patients. Four studies found that home blood pressure was the stronger predictor of risk. The fifth found that both blood pressure measures predicted risk.[62–66] The most recent population-based study of comparative prognosis of self-monitoring versus office blood pressure in predicting cardiovascular events and total mortality, among 2081 adults, was the Finn-Home Study.[67] Although home blood pressure and office blood pressure were strongly associated with cardiovascular events in separate Cox proportional hazard models, when both modalities were included in the model, home blood pressure (Hazard Ratio [HR], 1.22/1.15; 95% confidence interval [CI], 1.09–1.37/1.05–1.26) remained a strong predictor of cardiovascular events per 10/5 mm Hg increase in blood pressure, whereas office blood pressure was not predictive (HR, 1.01/1.06; 95% CI, 0.92–1.12/0.97–1.16). Similarly, home systolic blood pressure was the only predictor of total mortality (HR, 1.11; 95% CI, 1.01–1.23). This study is the second population-based study to conclusively confirm the superior prognostic value of home blood pressure versus office blood pressure on total mortality. The concern about the potential for observer error compared with physician readings can often be mitigated by use of automated devices with memory chips. These devices allow the physician to recall the blood pressure readings taken by their patients. Although exclusive reliance on self-monitored readings is not recommended, they can provide a useful adjunct to clinic readings, both for the initial evaluation of newly diagnosed patients and for monitoring their response to treatment.

Ambulatory blood pressure monitoring

There are 6 prospective studies to date showing that ambulatory blood pressure is a better predictor of risk than clinic pressure, and more are on the way. The first, published by Perloff and colleagues,[68,69] used noninvasive monitoring performed during the day only and reported that those whose ambulatory pressure was low in relation to their clinic pressure were at lower risk of morbidity. The second, by Verdecchia and colleagues,[70] followed a group of 1187 normotensive and hypertensive individuals for 3 years; hypertensive subjects were classified as having white-coat or sustained hypertension. The morbid event rate was 0.49 per 100 patient-years in white-coat hypertensive patients (similar to the rate of 0.47 in the normotensive subjects), whereas it was 1.79 in hypertensive dippers, who constituted the majority, and 4.99 in nondippers. The third study comprises the pilot results of a population study in Ohasama, Japan,[71] which reported that ambulatory pressure was a better predictor of morbidity than screening pressure; no attempt was made to classify individuals as having white-coat hypertension. The fourth[72] is a study of patients with refractory hypertension, defined as a diastolic pressure above 100 mm Hg while on 3 or more antihypertensive medications. Patients were classified in 3 groups according to their daytime ambulatory pressure; those in the lowest tertile (below 88 mm Hg) had a significantly lower rate of morbidity over the next 4 years, despite similar clinic pressures. A fifth study, from Northwick Park Hospital in London,[73] followed 479 patients for nearly 10 years, all of whom were initially evaluated with intra-arterial ambulatory blood pressure monitoring using the intra-arterial technique. Patients were classified as having white-coat or sustained hypertension, and a diagnosis of white-coat hypertension was found to be associated with one-third the risk of cardiovascular morbidity as sustained hypertension. The sixth study in this series is Syst-Eur, a large placebo-controlled study of the effects on cardiovascular morbidity of treating systolic hypertension of the elderly with a calcium channel blocker. A substudy of 808 patients used ambulatory blood pressure monitoring, and found that ambulatory blood pressure was a much more potent predictor of risk than office blood pressure.[74] The findings from these older studies were confirmed by more recent data in other prospective studies. Thus, although these prognostic studies differed widely in their design, ranging from a population study to one of refractory hypertensive subjects, the results all point in the same direction, namely that ambulatory pressure gives a better prediction of prognosis after controlling for clinic pressure, the corollary of which is that patients with white-coat hypertension have a more benign prognosis than those with sustained hypertension.

HOW SHOULD DIFFERENT BLOOD PRESSURE MEASUREMENT TECHNIQUES BE USED?

Which Measures of Blood Pressure are Clinically Important?

There are potentially 3 major measures of blood pressure that could contribute to the adverse effects of hypertension. The first is the average or "true" level, the second is the diurnal variation, and the third the short-term variability.

Average clinic blood pressure

At present, epidemiologic and clinical data are available only for the average level of blood pressure. In clinical practice, a patient's blood pressure is typically characterized by a single value of the systolic and diastolic pressures, to denote the average level. Such readings are normally taken in a clinic setting, but there is extensive evidence that in hypertensive patients, clinic pressures are consistently higher than the average 24-hour pressures recorded with ambulatory monitors.[75] This overestimation by clinic readings of the true pressure at high levels of pressure and underestimation at low levels has been referred to as the regression dilution bias, and means that the slope of the line relating blood pressure and cardiovascular morbidity should be steeper for the true blood pressure than for the clinic pressure.[76]

Diurnal variation in blood pressure

There is a pronounced diurnal rhythm of blood pressure, with a decrease of 10 to 20 mm Hg during sleep and a prompt increase on waking and rising in the morning. The highest blood pressures are usually seen between 6 AM and noon, which is also the time at which the prevalence of many cardiovascular morbid events tends to be highest.[77] The pattern of blood pressure during the day is to a large extent dependent on the pattern of activity, with pressures tending to be higher during the hours of work and lower while at home.[78] In hypertensive patients, the diurnal blood pressure profile is reset at a higher level of pressure, with preservation of the normal pattern in the majority. The short-term blood pressure variability is increased when expressed in absolute terms (mm Hg), but the percentage changes are no different. Thus, hypertension can be regarded as a disturbance of the set point or tonic level of blood pressure with normal short-term regulation. Antihypertensive treatment reverses these changes, again by resetting the set point toward normal, with little effect on short-term variability. The normal diurnal rhythm of blood pressure is disturbed in some hypertensive individuals, with loss of the normal nocturnal decrease of pressure. This occurrence has been observed in a variety of conditions, including malignant hypertension, chronic renal failure, several types of secondary hypertension, preeclampsia, and conditions associated with autonomic neuropathy.[76] There is ample evidence linking elevated nighttime blood pressure to increased cardiovascular morbidity and mortality compared with daytime blood pressure. In the Ohasama population-based study, a 5% reduction in nighttime blood pressure resulted in up to 20% higher risk of cardiovascular mortality.[79] Similarly, a 9 mm Hg increase in nighttime diastolic blood pressure was associated a 25% increased risk of congestive heart failure among elderly Swedish men.[80] In the Sys-Eur trial,[74] a large placebo-controlled study of the effects on cardiovascular morbidity of treating systolic hypertension of the elderly with a calcium channel blocker, a substudy of 808 patients used ambulatory blood pressure monitoring. Staessen and colleagues[74] found that nighttime blood pressure was a better predictor of cardiovascular morbidity and mortality than daytime blood pressure. Although these findings are not sufficiently well established to be applied to routine clinical practice, the clinical significance of nocturnal hypertension and nondipping status cannot be ignored for long, given the potential beneficial effect of the treatment of nocturnal hypertension on cardiovascular disease risk reduction in hypertensive patients.[81]

Blood pressure variability

Information on the clinical significance of blood pressure variability has accumulated over the past decade, with recent data suggesting that increased ambulatory blood pressure variability is associated with the development of early carotid arteriosclerosis[82] and a high rate of cardiovascular morbidity.[83] More recently, in a prospective ambulatory blood pressure study of an initially untreated sample of 2649 hypertensive patients, Verdecchia and colleagues[84] compared the independent prognostic value of daytime and nighttime blood pressure variability for cardiovascular events. These investigators found elevated nighttime systolic blood pressure to be an independent predictor of cardiac events. Similarly, among elderly patients in the Syst-Eur trial, increased nighttime systolic blood pressure variability on admission to the trial was an independent risk factor for stroke during the trial among those in the placebo arm of the trial.[85]

The Combined use of Clinic, Home, and Ambulatory Monitoring

The measurement of clinic blood pressure, either by use of automated devices or conventional sphygmomanometry, will continue to be the principal method of clinical evaluation. A cardinal rule is that the closer the blood pressure is to the threshold level at which treatment will be started, the more readings should be taken over more visits before a decision on treatment is made. In patients who have persistently elevated clinic pressure and evidence of blood pressure–related target organ damage, it is usually unnecessary to supplement the clinic readings with other types of measurement before reaching a therapeutic decision. When an elevated blood pressure is the only detectable abnormality, however, the possibility that the clinic pressure may overestimate the true pressure should be considered; this can be done either by self-monitoring or by ambulatory monitoring. A schema for the use of the different procedures for measuring blood pressure when evaluating a newly diagnosed hypertensive patient is shown in **Fig. 8.** If self-monitoring is chosen and reveals pressures comparable to the clinic value, treatment may be appropriate; but if the home readings are much lower than the clinic readings, it does not rule out the possibility that the blood pressure may be elevated at work: this is the advantage of ambulatory monitoring, which gives the best estimate of the full range of blood pressure experienced during everyday life.

Measurement of Blood Pressure in Special Populations and Circumstances

Infants and children

The Korotkoff sound technique is recommended as the standard for children older than 1 year; however, it may give systematic errors in infants, in whom the sounds are difficult to hear, and thus the true systolic pressure may be underestimated.[8] In infants the best indirect measurement technique is an ultrasonic flow detector.[86] A particular problem associated with blood pressure measurement in children of different ages is knowing which cuff size to choose. The BHS recommends choosing from 3 cuff sizes—4×13 cm, 8×18 cm, and 12×35 cm (adult cuff)—and putting on the widest cuff that will fit the arm.[87] The American Heart Association[26] and the National High Blood Pressure Education Program (NHBPEP)[88] have recommended that the cuff size be standardized to the circumference of the arm.

Pregnant women

In normal pregnancy there is a decrease in blood pressure, together with an increase of cardiac output and a large decrease of peripheral resistance. As a result of this hyperkinetic state, Korotkoff-like sounds occasionally may be heard over the brachial artery without any pressure being applied to the cuff. These sounds are most probably due to turbulent flow in the artery. Consequently, the use of phase 4 has frequently been recommended for registering diastolic pressure in pregnant women, which may be 12 mm Hg higher than phase 5.[89] The NHBPEP Working Group report recommends recording both phases 4 and 5 throughout pregnancy.[90] In one study of 85 pregnant women, however, phase 5 never approached zero, and phase 4 could be identified in only half, leading the investigators to recommend phase 5.[91]

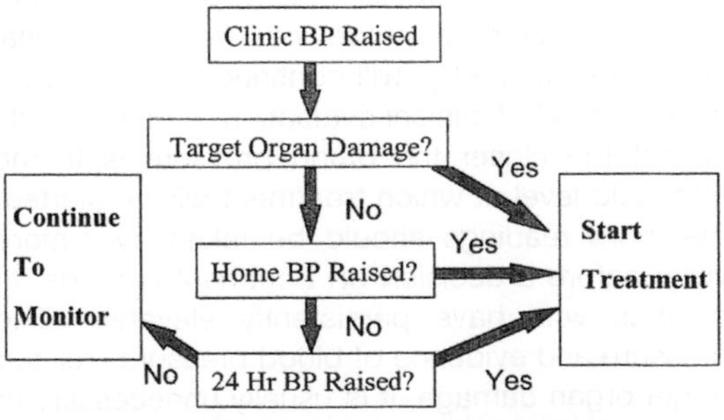

Fig. 8. Schema for combining different measures of blood pressure in the evaluation of patients with suspected hypertension.

Elderly patients

In some older people there is an increase of systolic pressure without a corresponding increase of diastolic pressure (systolic hypertension), which has been attributed to a diminished distensibility of the arteries with increasing age. In extreme cases this may result in a diminished compressibility of the artery by the sphygmomanometer cuff, so that falsely high readings may be recorded, often referred to as pseudohypertension of the elderly.[92] These patients represent the exception rather than the rule, however, because studies of healthy elderly subjects have not shown any greater discrepancy between direct and indirect measurements of pressure than in younger subjects.[93,94]

Obese patients

It is well known that the accurate estimation of blood pressure using the auscultatory method requires an appropriate match between cuff size and arm diameter. In obese subjects the regular adult cuff (12×23 cm) may seriously overestimate blood pressure.[95] The effect of arm circumference on the cuff method of measuring blood pressure was studied systematically by King.[3]

Exercise

During dynamic exercise the auscultatory method may underestimate systolic pressure by up to 15 mm Hg, whereas during recovery it may be overestimated by 30 mm Hg.[96,97] Errors in diastolic pressure are unlikely to be as large, except during the recovery period, when falsely low readings may be recorded.[96] This is the reason why the American Heart Association recommends taking the fourth phase of the Korotkoff sound after exercise.[26]

SUMMARY

Although the use of mercury sphygmomanometer is regarded as the gold standard for office blood pressure measurement, the widespread ban of use of mercury devices has diminished their role in hospital settings. Alternative methods such as automated electronic devices have gained increased popularity. The preferred location of measurement is the upper arm, but errors may occur because of changes in the position of the arm. Other technical sources of error include inappropriate cuff size and too rapid deflation of the cuff. Clinic readings may be unrepresentative of the patient's true blood pressure because of the white-coat effect, which is defined as the difference between the clinic readings and the average daytime blood pressure. Patients with elevated clinic pressure and normal daytime pressure are said to have white-coat hypertension, which is often explained by state anxiety or conditioned response. There are 3 commonly used methods for measuring blood pressure for clinical purposes: clinic readings, self-monitoring by the patient at home, and 24-hour ambulatory readings. Self-monitoring is generally performed using electronic devices that work on the oscillometric technique. Although standard validation protocols exist, many devices on the market have not been tested for accuracy. Such devices can record blood pressure from the upper arm, wrist, or finger, but the arm is preferred. Twenty-four-hour ambulatory monitoring is the best predictor of cardiovascular risk in the individual patient and is the only technique that can describe the diurnal rhythm of blood pressure accurately. Ambulatory monitoring is mainly used for diagnosing hypertension, whereas self-monitoring is used for following the response to treatment. Different techniques of blood pressure measurement may be preferred in certain situations. In infants the ultrasound technique is best, whereas in pregnancy and after exercise the diastolic pressure may be hard to measure using the conventional auscultatory method. In obese subjects it is important to use a cuff of the correct size.

REFERENCES

1. Pickering TG, Hall JE, Appel LJ, et al. Recommendations for blood pressure measurement in humans and experimental animals: part 1: blood pressure measurement in humans: a statement for professionals from the Subcommittee of Professional and Public education of the American Heart Association Council on high blood pressure research. Hypertension 2005;45:142.
2. Marey EJ. Pression et vitesse du sang. In: Masson G, editor. Physiologie experimentale, vol. 2. Paris; 1876. p. 307.
3. King GE. Errors in clinical measurement of blood pressure in obesity. Clin Sci 1967;32:223.
4. Mauck GW, Smith CR, Geddes LA, et al. The meaning of the point of maximum oscillations in cuff pressure in the indirect measurement of blood pressure—part II. J Biomech Eng 1980;102:28.
5. Yelderman M, Ream AK. Indirect measurement of mean blood pressure in the anesthetized patient. Anesthesiology 1979;50:253.
6. Borow KM, Newburger JW. Noninvasive estimation of central aortic pressure using the oscillometric method for analyzing systemic artery pulsatile blood flow: comparative study of indirect systolic, diastolic, and mean brachial artery pressure with simultaneous direct ascending aortic pressure measurements. Am Heart J 1982;103:879.
7. Santucci S, Cates EM, James GD, et al. A comparison of two ambulatory blood pressure monitors, the Del Mar Avionics Pressurometer IV and the Spacelabs 90202. Am J Hypertens 1989;2:797.
8. Elseed AM, Shinebourne EA, Joseph MC. Assessment of techniques for measurement of blood pressure in infants and children. Arch Dis Child 1973;48:932.
9. Penaz J. Photo-electric measurement of blood pressure, volume and flow in the finger. Dresden: digest of Tenth International Conference on Medical and Biological Engineering. Dresden (Germany), August 13–17, 1973.
10. Parati G, Casadei R, Groppelli A, et al. Comparison of finger and intra-arterial blood pressure monitoring at rest and during laboratory testing. Hypertension 1989;13:647.
11. van Egmond J, Hasenbos M, Crul JF. Invasive v. non-invasive measurement of arterial pressure. Comparison of two automatic methods and simultaneously measured direct intra-arterial pressure. Br J Anaesth 1985;57:434.
12. Imholz BP, Langewouters GJ, van Montfrans GA, et al. Feasibility of ambulatory, continuous 24-hour finger arterial pressure recording. Hypertension 1993;21:65.
13. Petrie JC, O'Brien ET, Littler WA, et al. Recommendations on blood pressure measurement. Br Med J (Clin Res Ed) 1986;293:611.
14. Netea RT, Smits P, Lenders JW, et al. Does it matter whether blood pressure measurements are taken with subjects sitting or supine? J Hypertens 1998;16:263.
15. Mitchell PL, Parlin RW, Blackburn H. Effect of vertical displacement of the arm on indirect blood-pressure measurement. N Engl J Med 1964;271:72.
16. Netea RT, Elving LD, Lutterman JA, et al. Body position and blood pressure measurement in patients with diabetes mellitus. J Intern Med 2002;251:393.

17. Netea RT, Lenders JW, Smits P, et al. Both body and arm position significantly influence blood pressure measurement. J Hum Hypertens 2003; 17:459.
18. Webster J, Newnham D, Petrie JC, et al. Influence of arm position on measurement of blood pressure. Br Med J (Clin Res Ed) 1984;288:1574.
19. Cushman WC, Cooper KM, Horne RA, et al. Effect of back support and stethoscope head on seated blood pressure determinations. Am J Hypertens 1990;3:240.
20. Parati G, Pomidossi G, Casadei R, et al. Lack of alerting reactions to intermittent cuff inflations during noninvasive blood pressure monitoring. Hypertension 1985;7:597.
21. Veerman DP, van Montfrans GA, Karemaker JM, et al. Inflating one's own cuff does not increase self-recorded blood pressure. J Hypertens Suppl 1988;6:S77.
22. Mejia AD, Egan BM, Schork NJ, et al. Artefacts in measurement of blood pressure and lack of target organ involvement in the assessment of patients with treatment-resistant hypertension. Ann Intern Med 1990;112:270.
23. King GE. Influence of rate of cuff inflation and deflation on observed blood pressure by sphygmomanometry. Am Heart J 1963;65:303.
24. Maxwell MH, Waks AU, Schroth PC, et al. Error in blood-pressure measurement due to incorrect cuff size in obese patients. Lancet 1982;2:33.
25. van Montfrans GA, van der Hoeven GM, Karemaker JM, et al. Accuracy of auscultatory blood pressure measurement with a long cuff. Br Med J (Clin Res Ed) 1987;295:354.
26. Perloff D, Grim C, Flack J, et al. Human blood pressure determination by sphygmomanometry. Circulation 1993;88:2460.
27. O'Brien E, Petrie J, Littler W, et al. The British Hypertension Society protocol for the evaluation of automated and semi-automated blood pressure measuring devices with special reference to ambulatory systems. J Hypertens 1990;8:607.
28. Association for the Advancement of Medical Instrumentation. Electronic of automated sphygmomanometer. Arlington (VA): American National Standard; 1992.
29. Gerin W, Schwartz AR, Schwartz JE, et al. Limitations of current validation protocols for home blood pressure monitors for individual patients. Blood Press Monit 2002;7:313.
30. Messelbeck J, Sutherland L. Applying environmental product design to biomedical products research. Environ Health Perspect 2000;108(Suppl 6): 997.
31. Canzanello VJ, Jensen PL, Schwartz GL. Are aneroid sphygmomanometers accurate in hospital and clinic settings? Arch Intern Med 2001;161:729.
32. Mion D, Pierin AM. How accurate are sphygmomanometers? J Hum Hypertens 1998;12:245.
33. Bailey RH, Knaus VL, Bauer JH. Aneroid sphygmomanometers. An assessment of accuracy at a university hospital and clinics. Arch Intern Med 1991;151: 1409.
34. Yarows SA, Qian K. Accuracy of aneroid sphygmomanometers in clinical usage: University of Michigan experience. Blood Press Monit 2001;6:101.
35. Ma Y, Temprosa M, Fowler S, et al. Evaluating the accuracy of an aneroid sphygmomanometer in a clinical trial setting. Am J Hypertens 2009;22:263.
36. Jhalani J, Goyal T, Clemow L, et al. Anxiety and outcome expectations predict the white-coat effect. Blood Press Monit 2005;10:317.
37. Ogedegbe G, Pickering TG, Clemow L, et al. The misdiagnosis of hypertension: the role of patient anxiety. Arch Intern Med 2008;168:2459.
38. Verdecchia P, Schillaci G, Borgioni C, et al. White coat hypertension and white coat effect. Similarities and differences. Am J Hypertens 1995;8:790.
39. Fagard RH, Staessen JA, Thijs L, et al. Response to antihypertensive therapy in older patients with sustained and nonsustained systolic hypertension. Systolic Hypertension in Europe (Syst-Eur) Trial Investigators. Circulation 2000;102:1139.
40. Padfield PL, Jyothinagaram SG, Watson DM, et al. Problems in the measurement of blood pressure. J Hum Hypertens 1990;4(Suppl 2):3.
41. Eilertsen E, Humerfelt S. The observer variation in the measurement of arterial blood pressure. Acta Med Scand 1968;184:145.
42. Ayman P, Goldshine AD. Blood pressure determinations by patients with essential hypertension I: the difference between clinic and home readings before treatment. Am J Med Sci 1940;200:465–74.
43. Mancia G, Bertinieri G, Grassi G, et al. Effects of blood-pressure measurement by the doctor on patient's blood pressure and heart rate. Lancet 1983;2:695.
44. Pickering TG, James GD, Boddie C, et al. How common is white coat hypertension? JAMA 1988; 259:225.
45. Comstock GW. An epidemiologic study of blood pressure levels in a biracial community in the Southern United States. Am J Hyg 1957;65:271.
46. McCubbin JA, Wilson JF, Bruehl S, et al. Gender effects on blood pressures obtained during an on-campus screening. Psychosom Med 1991;53:90.
47. Imai Y, Abe K, Sasaki S, et al. Clinical evaluation of semiautomatic and automatic devices for home blood pressure measurement: comparison between cuff-oscillometric and microphone methods. J Hypertens 1989;7:983.
48. Veerman DP, van Montfrans GA, Wieling W. Effects of cuff inflation on self-recorded blood pressure. Lancet 1990;335:451.

49. Cavallini MC, Roman MJ, Blank SG, et al. Association of the auscultatory gap with vascular disease in hypertensive patients. Ann Intern Med 1996;124:877.
50. Burke MJ, Towers HM, O'Malley K, et al. Sphygmomanometers in hospital and family practice: problems and recommendations. Br Med J (Clin Res Ed) 1982;285:469.
51. Kleinert HD, Harshfield GA, Pickering TG, et al. What is the value of home blood pressure measurement in patients with mild hypertension? Hypertension 1984;6:574.
52. Pickering TG, Miller NH, Ogedegbe G, et al. Call to action on use and reimbursement for home blood pressure monitoring: executive summary: a joint scientific statement from the American Heart Association, American Society Of Hypertension, and Preventive Cardiovascular Nurses Association. Hypertension 2008;52:1.
53. van Egmond J, Lenders JW, Weernink E, et al. Accuracy and reproducibility of 30 devices for self-measurement of arterial blood pressure. Am J Hypertens 1993;6:873.
54. Foster C, McKinlay S, Cruickshank JM, et al. Accuracy of the Omron HEM 706 portable monitor for home measurement of blood pressure. J Hum Hypertens 1994;8:661.
55. O'Brien E, Waeber B, Parati G, et al. Blood pressure measuring devices: recommendations of the European Society of Hypertension. BMJ 2001; 322:531.
56. Cooper R, Puras A, Tracy J, et al. Evaluation of an electronic blood pressure device for epidemiological studies. Blood Press Monit 1997;2:35.
57. Eckert S, Gleichmann S, Gleichmann U. Blood pressure self-measurement in upper arm and in wrist for treatment control of arterial hypertension compared to ABPM. Z Kardiol 1996;85(Suppl 3):109.
58. Wonka F, Thummler M, Schoppe A. Clinical test of a blood pressure measurement device with a wrist cuff. Blood Press Monit 1996;1:361.
59. Phillips RA, Diamond JA. Ambulatory blood pressure monitoring and echocardiography—noninvasive techniques for evaluation of the hypertensive patient. Prog Cardiovasc Dis 1991;41:397.
60. Pickering GW. High blood pressure. London: Churchill; 1968.
61. Villegas I, Arias IC, Botero A, et al. Evaluation of the technique used by health-care workers for taking blood pressure. Hypertension 1995;26:1204.
62. Bobrie G, Chatellier G, Genes N, et al. Cardiovascular prognosis of "masked hypertension" detected by blood pressure self-measurement in elderly treated hypertensive patients. JAMA 2004;291:1342.
63. Fagard RH, Van Den Broeke C, De Cort P. Prognostic significance of blood pressure measured in the office, at home and during ambulatory monitoring in older patients in general practice. J Hum Hypertens 2005;19:801.
64. Ohkubo T, Imai Y, Tsuji I, et al. Home blood pressure measurement has a stronger predictive power for mortality than does screening blood pressure measurement: a population-based observation in Ohasama, Japan. J Hypertens 1998;16:971.
65. Ohkubo T, Imai Y, Tsuji I, et al. Relation between nocturnal decline in blood pressure and mortality. The Ohasama Study. Am J Hypertens 1997;10: 1201.
66. Sega R, Facchetti R, Bombelli M, et al. Prognostic value of ambulatory and home blood pressures compared with office blood pressure in the general population: follow-up results from the Pressioni Arteriose Monitorate e Loro Associazioni (PAMELA) study. Circulation 2005;111:1777.
67. Niiranen TJ, Hanninen MR, Johansson J, et al. Home-measured blood pressure is a stronger predictor of cardiovascular risk than office blood pressure: the Finn-Home study. Hypertension 2010;55:1346.
68. Perloff D, Sokolow M. Ambulatory blood pressure: mortality and morbidity. J Hypertens Suppl 1991;9:S31.
69. Perloff D, Sokolow M, Cowan RM, et al. Prognostic value of ambulatory blood pressure measurements: further analyses. J Hypertens Suppl 1989;7:S3.
70. Verdecchia P, Schillaci G, Borgioni C, et al. Prognostic value of left ventricular mass and geometry in systemic hypertension with left ventricular hypertrophy. Am J Cardiol 1996;78:197.
71. Ohkubo T, Imai Y, Tsuji I, et al. Prediction of mortality by ambulatory blood pressure monitoring versus screening blood pressure measurements: a pilot study in Ohasama. J Hypertens 1997;15:357.
72. Redon J, Campos C, Narciso ML, et al. Prognostic value of ambulatory blood pressure monitoring in refractory hypertension: a prospective study. Hypertension 1998;31:712.
73. Khattar RS, Senior R, Lahiri A. Cardiovascular outcome in white-coat versus sustained mild hypertension: a 10-year follow-up study. Circulation 1892; 98:1998.
74. Staessen JA, Thijs L, Fagard R, et al. Predicting cardiovascular risk using conventional vs ambulatory blood pressure in older patients with systolic hypertension. Systolic Hypertension in Europe Trial Investigators. JAMA 1999;282:539.
75. Pickering TG. Blood pressure variability and ambulatory monitoring. Curr Opin Nephrol Hypertens 1993;2:380.
76. Pickering TG. The ninth Sir George Pickering memorial lecture ambulatory monitoring and the definition of hypertension. J Hypertens 1992;10:401.
77. Muller JE, Kaufmann PG, Luepker RV, et al. Mechanisms precipitating acute cardiac events: review

and recommendations of an NHLBI workshop. Circulation 1997;96:3233.
78. Clark LA, Denby L, Pregibon D, et al. A quantitative analysis of the effects of activity and time of day on the diurnal variations of blood pressure. J Chronic Dis 1987;40:671.
79. Ohkubo T, Hozawa A, Yamaguchi J, et al. Prognostic significance of the nocturnal decline in blood pressure in individuals with and without high 24-h blood pressure: the Ohasama study. J Hypertens 2002;20:2183.
80. Ingelsson E, Bjorklund-Bodegard K, Lind L, et al. Diurnal blood pressure pattern and risk of congestive heart failure. JAMA 2006;295:2859.
81. Chobanian AV, Bakris GL, Black HR, et al. The seventh report of the joint national committee on prevention, detection, evaluation, and treatment of high blood pressure: the JNC 7 report. JAMA 2003;289:2560.
82. Sander D, Kukla C, Klingelhofer J, et al. Relationship between circadian blood pressure patterns and progression of early carotid atherosclerosis: a 3-year follow-up study. Circulation 2000;102:1536.
83. Kikuya M, Hozawa A, Ohokubo T, et al. Prognostic significance of blood pressure and heart rate variabilities: the Ohasama study. Hypertension 2000;36:901.
84. Verdecchia P, Angeli F, Gattobigio R, et al. Impact of blood pressure variability on cardiac and cerebrovascular complications in hypertension. Am J Hypertens 2007;20:154.
85. Pringle E, Phillips C, Thijs L, et al. Systolic blood pressure variability as a risk factor for stroke and cardiovascular mortality in the elderly hypertensive population. J Hypertens 2003;21:2251.
86. Reder RF, Dimich I, Cohen ML, et al. Evaluating indirect blood pressure measurement techniques: a comparison of three systems in infants and children. Pediatrics 1978;62:326.
87. de Swiet M, Dillon MJ, Littler W, et al. Measurement of blood pressure in children. Recommendations of a working party of the British Hypertension Society. BMJ 1989;299:497.
88. Update on the 1987 Task Force Report on High Blood Pressure in Children and Adolescents: a working group report from the National High Blood Pressure Education Program. National High Blood Pressure Education Program Working Group on Hypertension Control in Children and Adolescents. Pediatrics 1996;98:649.
89. Villar J, Repke J, Markush L, et al. The measuring of blood pressure during pregnancy. Am J Obstet Gynecol 1989;161:1019.
90. Lenfant C. Working group report on high blood pressure in pregnancy. J Clin Hypertens (Greenwich) 2001;3:75.
91. Shennan A, Gupta M, Halligan A, et al. Lack of reproducibility in pregnancy of Korotkoff phase IV as measured by mercury sphygmomanometry. Lancet 1996;347:139.
92. Spence JD, Sibbald WJ, Cape RD. Direct, indirect and mean blood pressures in hypertensive patients: the problem of cuff artefact due to arterial wall stiffness, and a partial solution. Clin Invest Med 1979;2:165.
93. Finnegan TP, Spence JD, Wong DG, et al. Blood pressure measurement in the elderly: correlation of arterial stiffness with difference between intra-arterial and cuff pressures. J Hypertens 1985;3:231.
94. O'Callaghan WG, Fitzgerald DJ, O'Malley K, et al. Accuracy of indirect blood pressure measurement in the elderly. Br Med J (Clin Res Ed) 1983;286:1545.
95. Nielsen PE, Janniche H. The accuracy of auscultatory measurement of arm blood pressure in very obese subjects. Acta Med Scand 1974;195:403.
96. Gould BA, Hornung RS, Altman DG, et al. Indirect measurement of blood pressure during exercise testing can be misleading. Br Heart J 1985;53:611.
97. Henschel A, De La Vega F, Taylor HL. Simultaneous direct and indirect blood pressure measurements in man at rest and work. J Appl Phys 1954;6:506.

Initial Clinical Encounter with the Patient with Established Hypertension

Uchechukwu K.A. Sampson, MB, BS, MBA, MPH, MSc(Oxon)[a,b,*], George A. Mensah, MD, FACC, FACP, FACN[c]

KEYWORDS

• Hypertension • Patient • Treatment

Hypertension is a major risk factor for cardiovascular (CV) disease, implicated in the pathobiology of coronary artery disease (CAD), peripheral arterial disease (PAD), heart failure, and rhythm disorders, as well as renal, cerebrovascular, and ocular damage. Therefore, the initial clinical encounter with the patient with suspected or established hypertension can be a seminal teachable moment with clinical and public health importance. It provides the opportunity to set the tone for the provider-patient relationship, develop empathy, and assess the patient's literacy level and ability to self-manage. The initial encounter also presents the provider and patient with the opportunity to jointly set targets for blood pressure (BP) control, and assess the social, cultural, and environmental support systems available to the patient in self-management and care coordination. At the initial clinic visit, the provider and the patient agree on a multipronged treatment plan that includes, but is not limited to, an exercise program, evaluation by a dietician, smoking cessation or avoidance of second hand smoke exposure, social worker evaluation, and literacy level–appropriate education and self-management program.

This article addresses the comprehensive approach to patients with hypertension, with a focus on confirming or establishing the diagnosis of primary hypertension, looking for clues suggestive of secondary hypertension, and assessment for the presence and extent of target organ damage, as well as global CV risk evaluation. In addition, pragmatic approaches for assessing CV prognosis, BP control, patient health literacy (HL) and education, and patient self-management are discussed. Key recommendations are discussed that health providers should consider during the initial evaluation of the patient with hypertension. Although the importance of excluding secondary causes of hypertension is briefly mentioned, the strategies for evaluation and treatment are not discussed because they are addressed elsewhere in this issue.

UKAS is partially supported by the Harold Amos Medical Faculty Development Award of the Robert Wood Johnson Foundation and the Vanderbilt Clinical and Translational Scholars Award.
UKAS has nothing to disclose; GAM is a full-time employee of PepsiCo, although no conflicts of interest have been identified in his role.
[a] Division of Cardiovascular Medicine, Vanderbilt University Medical Center, 383 Preston Research Building, 2220 Pierce Avenue, Nashville, TN 37232, USA
[b] Department of Medicine, Meharry Medical College, Nashville, TN 37208, USA
[c] Heart Health and Global Health Policy, Global Research and Development, 700 Anderson Hill Road, PepsiCo, Inc, Building 6-2, Purchase, NY 10755, USA
* Corresponding author.
E-mail address: uchechukwu.sampson@vanderbilt.edu

Cardiol Clin 28 (2010) 587–595
doi:10.1016/j.ccl.2010.08.003

THE INITIAL COMPREHENSIVE EVALUATION

The initial encounter with the patient with hypertension should focus on a complete history and physical examination, with particular attention to the accurate determination of BP, assessment of hypertension-related target organ damage, and major identifiable causes of hypertension that may require specialist referral and intervention. During the clinical interview and the review of the past and present medical history, every effort should be made to determine the duration of hypertension and any previous actions or attempts at BP control. This information can inform the initial management strategy within the context of established guidelines. The foregoing should precede and guide ancillary investigation.

BP Measurement

Accurate measurement of BP is paramount for proper staging of hypertension. Furthermore, optimum follow-up schedule and application of treatment guidelines hinge on reliable and accurate BP measurements. Although there are many methods for BP measurement, the American Heart Association (AHA) recommends the use of a sphygmomanometer (a nonoscillometric method) by trained personnel for determination of ambulatory BP, with auscultation of the first and fifth phases of Korotkoff sounds using the bell side of the stethoscope.[1,2] Aneroid devices are becoming ubiquitous as a replacement for traditional mercury sphygmomanometers in the wake of concerns about mercury toxicity. A comprehensive discussion of the pros and cons of the different techniques for BP measurement has been provided by the AHA.[1] Regardless of the chosen technique, attention should be paid to patient preparation and position, and determination of midarm circumference for optimum cuff size selection and placement.

BP should not be measured if the patient is agitated or has engaged in recent (≤30 minutes) physical activity; the latter could include difficulties associated with the logistics of transportation to the clinic, and will require a period of relaxation and/or light-hearted conversation to elicit the appropriate patient mood. Similarly, a recent meal or the use of tobacco or caffeine up to 30 minutes before BP measurement is discouraged. For correct positioning, the patient should be seated with the back and legs supported and the feet resting on a firm surface. Determination of midarm circumference (midpoint between acromion and olecranon processes) should guide selection of appropriate cuff size (**Table 1**) to avoid overestimation or underestimation of BP measurement because of small or large cuff size, respectively. The landmark for cuff placement should be about 2 cm above the elbow crease, on bare arm, with the midline over the brachial artery. These recommendations are often ignored in the casual measurement of BP in the clinic or office.

BP measurement should proceed after determination of pulse obliteration pressure to avoid excessive inconvenience or discomfort to the patient and possible underestimation of the systolic blood pressure. Phase 1 and 5 Korotkoff sounds equate to systolic and diastolic BP respectively. Observer and parallax errors are common pitfalls that occur during BP measurement, which can be minimized by avoiding rounding or preference for a terminal digit in the case of observer error, or maintaining the observer's eyes at the level of the mercury in the case of parallax error. The classification of BP should be based on the average of 2 or more seated blood pressure measurements, properly measured with well-maintained and calibrated equipment, at each of 2 or more visits to the office or clinic.

BP CLASSIFICATION AND STAGING OF HYPERTENSION

Once accurate systolic and diastolic BP have been obtained, BP should be classified using the Joint National Committee (JNC) 7 scheme: normal (<120/80 mm Hg); prehypertension (120–139/80–89 mm Hg); and hypertension (>140/90 mm Hg: stage 1, 140–159/90–99 mm Hg; and stage 2, ≥160/100 mm Hg).[3] This classification has clinical implications and is not merely an academic exercise. Patients diagnosed with prehypertension

Table 1
Guide for blood pressure cuff sizing

Midarm Circumference (cm)	Cuff Dimensions (cm)	Cuff Size (cm)
22–26	12 × 22	Small adult arm
27–34	16 × 30	Adult arm
35–44	16 × 36	Large adult arm
45–52	16 × 42	Adult thigh

Data from Pickering TG, Hall JE, Appel LJ, et al. Recommendations for blood pressure measurement in humans and experimental animals: part 1: Blood pressure measurement in humans: a statement for professionals from the Subcommittee of Professional and Public Education of the American Heart Association Council on High Blood Pressure Research. Circulation 2005;111(5):697–716.

should be advised that they are at increased risk of developing hypertension, and therefore should actively embrace recommendations for therapeutic lifestyle modification in an effort to forestall progression to hypertension. It should be emphasized that the relationship between BP and CV risk is continuous and consistent, existing even at prehypertensive BP parameters, thus further justifying strict adherence to recommended lifestyle modification efforts. Persons with prehypertension do not require drug therapy unless there is associated history of diabetes or kidney disease. By contrast, all hypertensives (stages 1 and 2), regardless of the presence or absence of risk factors, require drug therapy in addition to lifestyle modification. In this regard, the cumulative CV risk of BP should also be communicated and factored into development of management strategy. The strategy should focus on timely BP control and assessment for existing target organ damage.

Assessment of Target Organ Damage

Ahead of ancillary investigations, the complete physical examination may provide pointers for the presence of hypertension-related target organ damage. The spectrum of target organ damage that can be precipitated by hypertension is shown in **Box 1**. An awareness of this spectrum should guide the clinician during the initial clinical encounter with, and physical examination of, the patient with hypertension. In addition, the presence of target organ damage provides objective insight on the duration and/or effectiveness of prior treatment efforts for hypertension. Delineation of the presence of any component in the spectrum of hypertension-related target organ damage has implications for patient management strategies. Physical signs such as displacement of apex beat or right parasternal heave suggest cardiomegaly or ventricular hypertrophy; however, evidence of changes in cardiac geometry are best delineated from noninvasive echocardiographic evaluation.

The experienced clinician can have a bedside insight on arterial stiffening or reduced distensibility, which signal the severity and/or duration of hypertension. The presence of carotid or abdominal bruit suggests the presence of carotid stenosis and abdominal aortic aneurysm, respectively. More importantly, ankle brachial index (ABI) is a simple bedside measurement that should be routinely incorporated into the initial clinic visit of the patient with hypertension. ABI has a 95% sensitivity and 99% specificity for the diagnosis of PAD,[4–6] which is highly prevalent[7–12] and associated with increased

Box 1
Spectrum of hypertensive damage to major target organs

Heart

- LV hypertrophy
- Impaired LV diastolic function
- Impaired LV systolic function
- Coronary microvascular disease
- Coronary atherosclerotic disease
- Chronic stable angina
- Unstable angina
- Coronary revascularization
- Myocardial infarction
- Chronic heart failure
- Sudden cardiac death
- Atrial fibrillation
- Ventricular arrhythmia

Blood vessels

- Reduced arterial distensibility
- Aortic dilatation
- Thoracic aortic aneurysms
- Abdominal aortic aneurysms
- Peripheral arterial aneurysms
- Aortic dissection
- PAD (including ABI <0.9; CIMT >0.9 mm)

Brain

- Acute and chronic hypertensive encephalopathy
- Lacunar infarction
- Intracerebral hemorrhage
- Intraparenchymal stroke
- Subarachnoid hemorrhage
- Transient ischemic attack

Eye

- Arteriolar narrowing
- Arteriovenous nicking
- Retinal microaneurysms
- Exudates and cotton-wool spots
- Hemorrhages
- Optic neuropathy

Kidney

- Nephropathy
- Nephrosclerosis
- Microalbuminuria
- Proteinuria
- Renal failure

Abbreviations: ABI, ankle brachial index; CIMT, carotid intima-media thickness; LV, left ventricle.

Data from The sixth report of the Joint National Committee on Prevention, Detection, Evaluation, and Treatment of High Blood Pressure. Arch Intern Med 1997;157(21):2413–46.

risk of CV and cerebrovascular events including death, myocardial infarction, and stroke.[13,14]

Hypertension is a major risk factor for PAD via its contribution to atherosclerosis, which is the usual underlying cause for PAD. Thus the presence of PAD in a patient with hypertension should be a cause for alarm akin to the presence of structural heart disease. Hypertensive retinopathy is amenable to bedside evaluation. The primary damages are noted in the retina, and have been well characterized; these include structural arterial and arteriolar changes, hemorrhage, exudates, and papilledema. A simplified bedside evaluation of hypertension-induced ocular damage has been made possible by Hyman's[15] user-friendly revision of the traditional Kate Wagner classification of hypertensive retinopathy. In many instances, hypertension-related organ damage can be suspected or inferred at bedside; however, ancillary investigation is usually necessary for further delineation and evaluation of other components of the spectrum for which bedside examination would not suffice.

Secondary Hypertension

A discussion of the evaluation and treatment of identifiable causes of hypertension is not within the scope of this article. However, it is an important part of the initial comprehensive evaluation of the patient with hypertension because many secondary causes of hypertension are curable and warrant specific investigations and therapeutic strategies. For example, the presence of renal artery bruit in a patient with hypertension suggests renovascular hypertension as a potential cause, as opposed to essential hypertension only. Similarly, the finding of abnormal pulses and brachial-femoral delay suggest aortic coarctation that warrants definitive evaluation. A list of recognized identifiable causes of hypertension and associated screening tests is provided in **Table 2**. Although these screening tests are not recommended in the routine evaluation of all patients with hypertension, they would be germane if the severity of hypertension, history, physical examination, and laboratory tests suggests any of these causes. These diagnostic tests are justified in the setting of poor response to drug therapy, an increase in BP of unknown cause after a period of optimal control, or sudden onset of hypertension in a young (<30 years) or older (>55 years) adult.

Table 2
Secondary hypertension: causes and screening tests

Diagnosis	Diagnostic Text
Chronic kidney disease	Estimated GFR
Coarctation of the aorta	CT angiography
Cushing syndrome and other glucocorticoid excess states including chronic steroid therapy	History; dexamethasone suppression test
Drug induced/related	History; drug screening
Pheochromocytoma	24-h urinary metanephrine and normetanephrine
Primary aldosteronism and other mineralocorticoid excess states	24-h urinary aldosterone level or specific measurements of other mineralocorticoids
Renovascular hypertension	Doppler flow study; magnetic resonance angiography
Sleep apnea	Sleep study with O_2 saturation
Thyroid/parathyroid disease	TSH; serum PTH

Abbreviations: CT, computed tomography; GFR, glomerular filtration rate; PTH, parathyroid hormone; TSH, thyroid-stimulating hormone.

INITIAL LABORATORY TESTS

Fundamental tests are required before the initiation of therapy. These include basic serum chemistry (potassium; sodium; creatinine or, preferably, estimated glomerular filtration rate [eGFR]; blood urea nitrogen; glucose), hematocrit, fasting lipid panel including high-density lipoprotein (HDL) and low-density lipoprotein (LDL) cholesterol and triglycerides, 12-lead electrocardiogram (ECG), and urinalysis. Testing for microalbuminuria is mandated for patients with diabetes or kidney disease, but otherwise is optional. Additional diagnostic testing is indicated in patients with a suspected identifiable cause of hypertension, as noted earlier (see **Table 2**).

Emerging biomarkers of CV risk can be evaluated in select populations to justify aggressive risk modulation. Such emerging risk markers include uric acid, high-sensitivity C-reactive protein (hsCRP), and homocysteine.[16,17] The presence of microalbuminuria or decreased eGFR is associated with increased CV risk[18–21]; similarly, increased hsCRP has been associated with increased CV risk even in patients classified as low risk by traditional measures.[22,23]

Although ECG can detect structural changes such as chamber enlargement and/or hypertrophy, it remains far less sensitive compared with echocardiography.[24] Such changes in cardiac structure and function elucidated by limited echocardiography may be essential in guiding therapeutic strategy and understanding the overall CV risk. However, in evaluating the patient with hypertension, a limited echocardiogram is recommended in the initial evaluation of patients who are untreated and at stage 1 or when the evidence of ventricular hypertrophy requires further clarification; notably, the probability of upgrading overall CV risk is highest when applied to patients older than 50 years.[25,26] Conceivably, our increasing understanding of the implications and treatment of diastolic dysfunction may justify the future use of limited echocardiography in the initial evaluation of subpopulations of patients with hypertension.

Ambulatory BP monitoring has an important role in optimization of therapy because 2 major confounding variables, white-coat effect and masked hypertension or isolated ambulatory hypertension, can reliably be resolved. The advent of automated devices makes ambulatory BP monitoring feasible and efficient. To the extent that this is true, ambulatory BP measurements recorded by patients constitute an important basis for adjustment of medications for optimal BP control. Although self-measurement of BP does not provide the 24-hour BP monitoring of which ambulatory BP devices are capable, it constitutes a practical method to assess differences between office and out-of-office measurements before deciding on the use of ambulatory BP monitoring.

In general, beyond the guideline-recommended fundamental tests, the decision to seek additional diagnostic information depends on the clinical context and the clinician's explicit and tacit perceptions of patient risk, as well as the likelihood that the test results will change patient management or prognosis.

ASSESSMENT OF GLOBAL CV RISK

Another objective that should be incorporated into the initial evaluation of the patient with hypertension is an assessment of the presence of additional CV risk factors and how they feature in the total or global CV risk. Although the established relationship between BP and risk of CV event is not dependent on these additional risk factors, they compound the risk of CV events from hypertension, thus contributing to the overall CV risk and prognosis of the individual. In this regard, it is important to control all additional CV risk factors according to their respective clinical practice guidelines. These risk factors include all components of target organ damage already delineated (see **Box 1**); family history of premature CAD; advanced age (older than 55 years for men and 65 years for women); microalbuminuria; sedentary lifestyle; the use of any tobacco product, especially cigarettes; and other components of metabolic syndrome, notably diabetes mellitus, increased LDL (or total) cholesterol or low HDL cholesterol, and obesity (body mass index $\geq$30 kg/m^2).

The JNC 7 BP stratification and treatment guidelines suggest that all patients with stage 1 or 2 hypertension require medications regardless of presence or absence of additional risk factors; however, a compelling indication should modulate the treatment target. That is, achieving a BP of less than 140/90 mm Hg is appropriate in patients without additional risk factors, but a lower target (<130/80 mm Hg) is required for patients with higher CV risk conferred by diabetes or renal disease. Herein, the application of risk algorithms is important in refining the management strategy. The use of established algorithms such as the Framingham Heart Study algorithm to assess short-term or 10-year CV risk can guide the urgency and intensity of treatment. Comprehensive risk stratification strategies should be encouraged in all persons, with careful attention to racial and ethnic populations who have a higher risk of CV death at younger ages compared with white people.[27] Screening carotid ultrasound should be considered, as appropriate, to determine carotid intima-media thickness (CIMT) values in patients, which adds to the assessment of long-term risk beyond the capability of traditional risk engines. The incidence of vascular outcomes correlates with increased CIMT (>0.9 mm), which increases with time and is associated with age.[28,29] Therefore, an increase in CIMT is evidence for vascular damage and should constitute a reason for a more stringent BP treatment goal when present in a patient with hypertension.

However, whether the rate of CIMT change might select younger patients for vascular risk, and its relation to traditional risk factors, is unknown. The relationship between CIMT accretion rate (CIMTar; ratio of maximum CIMT to age), a crude index of the rate of atherogenesis, and LDL cholesterol was recently evaluated in 564 subjects referred to a vascular medicine clinic.[30] At every level of baseline LDL cholesterol, there were individuals with CIMT and CIMTar greater than the median, suggesting that their carotid wall thickness was not entirely determined by the lipid concentration gradient between serum and the subendothelial space. Similar CIMTar values from a CV health study[31] and dissimilar LDL values suggest that factors other than the LDL gradient were also present in that cohort. The only baseline modifiable variable consistently associated with groups greater than the mean and median CIMT and CIMTar was systolic blood pressure.[30]

There are multiple mechanisms by which hypertension may increase CIMT: loss of smooth muscle architecture and subsequent lipid ingestion, an increase in lipid oxidation, increasing inflammation, and peptidergic signaling. Use of ultrasound techniques may also permit enhanced communication of future risk in examined subjects, and the visualization of atherosclerosis may be a means to increase potential adherence to programs of risk reduction including both lifestyle recommendations and medication(s). Rather than trying to communicate a value or number, CIMTar may enhance understanding of risk by showing apparent increased rate of lipid accumulation relative to age as opposed to a fixed cutoff value that fails to capture differential risk.

IMPORTANCE OF HL, SELF-MONITORING, AND LIFESTYLE CHANGES

The initial encounter with the patient with hypertension is a teachable moment that requires attention to multiple factors in the care delivery equation. A fundamental factor is patient HL, which affects health care costs and outcomes. HL is defined as the capacity to obtain, process, and understand basic health information and services needed to make appropriate health decisions.[32,33] The Institute of Medicine reports that 90 million people in the United States have difficulty understanding and using health information.[32] In addition to contributing to health care costs at the systemic and patient level,[34] limited HL is a stronger predictor of the health and outcome of patients than age, income, employment status, education level, and race.[35] Limited HL has been shown to foster nonadherence in CV disease, with attendant suboptimal risk factor control (eg, hypertension and hyperlipidemia)[3,36] and increased mortality.[37] Similar effects of limited HL on other adverse health outcomes, associated poorer intermediate disease phenotypes, and inefficient use of health services has been reported.[38,39]

Treatment of hypertension should involve the assessment of the HL level of the patient. There is increasing awareness of the poor attention to patient HL in health care delivery efforts despite readily available resources for this purpose (**Box 2**). These resources need to be used routinely in the initial encounter with the patient with hypertension. The awareness of HL should also prompt an evaluation of the readability and suitability of the patient education materials used in medical practices because there is evidence that many such materials in the CV arena are suboptimal.[40] Although the provider cannot reinvent the patient education materials on a whim, it is the collective responsibility of management and health care personnel to ensure that the readability and suitability of the materials used for patient education matches the HL of the population to which they cater. A prudent approach is to target the production of education materials that should not exceed the fifth grade readability level requirement; this will ensure broader use of such materials.

A major component of BP control is the contribution expected from the patient with hypertension. Commitment to self-monitoring of BP at home or at work may be vital to optimal management of hypertension. The advent of automated

Box 2
Selected resources for provider assessment of patient HL

http://www.pfizerhealthliteracy.com/physicians-providers/newest-vital-sign.html. Accessed June 13, 2010

http://www.ahrq.gov/populations/sahlsatool.htm. Accessed June 13, 2010

http://www.ama-assn.org/ama/pub/category/8035.html. Accessed June 13, 2010

Chew LD, Bradley KA, Boyko EJ. Brief questions to identify patients with inadequate health literacy. Fam Med 2004;36:588–94

Davis TC, Long SW, Jackson RH, et al. Rapid estimate of adult literacy in medicine: a shortened screening instrument. Fam Med 1993;25:391–95

Parker RM, Baker DW, Williams MV, et al. The test of functional health literacy in adults (TOFHLA): a new instrument for measuring patients' literacy skills. J Gen Intern Med 1995;10:537–42

Weiss BD, Mays MZ, Martz W, et al. Quick assessment of literacy in primary care: the newest vital sign . Ann Fam Med 2005;3(6):514–22 [published correction appears in Ann Fam Med 2006;4(1):83].

Lee SY, Bender DE, Ruiz RE, et al. Development of an easy-to-use Spanish health literacy test. Health Serv Res 2006;41(4 Pt 1):1392–412 oscillometric systems makes BP monitoring by the patient a practical approach to assess differences between office and out-of-office measurements. In some instances, this obviates the need for medication therapy or 24-hour monitoring to delineate masked hypertension or white-coat effect. Self-measurement encourages patient ownership in the management process. Self-measurement can also be used to make the patient with hypertension appreciate the consequences of poor habits, such as the acute effect of smoking on BP as well as the beneficial effects of therapeutic lifestyle changes.

Although the effects of therapeutic lifestyle changes are dose- and time-dependent and vary between individuals, they constitute a critical part of the algorithm for management of all stages of hypertension and prehypertension, and should be encouraged for the general well-being of everyone including normotensive individuals because these measures can prevent the development of hypertension. A fundamental and paramount action for overall CV risk reduction is smoking cessation. Other recommended modifications include weight reduction, adoption of dietary approaches to stop hypertension (DASH), reduction in dietary sodium intake, physical activity, and moderate consumption of alcohol. Weight reduction in overweight and obese individuals or maintenance of normal body weight (body mass index 18.5–24.9 kg/m^2) can result in 5 to 20 mm Hg drop in BP per 10 kg loss of weight[41,42]; the DASH eating plan entails a diet rich in fruits, vegetables, low-fat dairy products, and a reduced content of saturated and total fat, and can reduce BP by 8 to 14 mm Hg.[43,44] Dietary sodium reduction to no more than 100 mmol per day (2.4 g sodium or 6 g sodium chloride) can effect a 2 to 8 mm Hg BP reduction[43–45]; aerobic physical activity such as brisk walking for at least 30 minutes per day, more than 3 days a week, can result in a 4 to 9 mm Hg BP reduction[46,47]; and moderate alcohol consumption not exceeding 2 drinks (eg, 710 mL beer, 295 mL wine, or 89 mL 80-proof whiskey) per day in most men or 1 drink per day in women and lighter-weight persons can yield a 2 to 4 mm Hg BP reduction.[48]

Box 3
Key considerations during initial encounter with the patient with hypertension

- Confirm the diagnosis of hypertension and look for clues suggesting secondary, curable causes of hypertension
- Assess social, environmental, and lifestyle-related determinants of high blood pressure and CV risk
- Evaluate the need, and recommend appropriate referral, for social services, dietician care, and smoking-cessation services as indicated
- Assess patient health literacy
- Literacy level–appropriate education focused on lifestyle changes and CV risk
- Pursue patient ownership and empowerment through self-monitoring to encourage participation and adherence
- Discuss benchmarks, blood pressure targets, and timelines for success on lifestyle modification efforts
- Look for reasons to treat to the recommended target blood pressure levels especially in vulnerable populations in which an aggressive risk stratification strategy may be prudent

SUMMARY

The initial encounter with the patient with hypertension presents the opportunity to reprogram the trajectory of overall CV risk in the patient with suspected or established hypertension. Although the prescription of antihypertensive medications for the treatment and control of BP is important, the practicing clinician should strive to recognize other important considerations beyond drug prescription and treatment guidelines (**Box 3**). The initial clinical encounter with the patient with suspected or established hypertension is the prime opportunity to assess the patient's level of HL, social and economic implications of lifelong drug therapy and health care costs, and readiness for and effectiveness of patient self-management. This should be followed by delivery of patient education that is appropriate for literacy level. Major components of the education should be the importance of lifestyle modification and self-monitoring to track progress. Self-monitoring should be a tool to engage the patients in active participation, thus creating a sense of ownership and empowerment that might positively influence adherence. Comprehensive risk stratification should be encouraged in all patients, particularly those at risk for overall CV mortality and morbidity. Careful clinician adherence to established practice guidelines in overall risk assessment and treatment and control of BP to target levels remains crucial.

REFERENCES

1. Pickering TG, Hall JE, Appel LJ, et al. Recommendations for blood pressure measurement in humans and experimental animals. Part 1: blood pressure measurement in humans: a statement for professionals from the Subcommittee of Professional and

Public Education of the American Heart Association Council on High Blood Pressure Research. Hypertension 2005;45(1):142–61.
2. Beevers G, Lip GY, O'Brien E. ABC of hypertension: blood pressure measurement. Part II-conventional sphygmomanometry: technique of auscultatory blood pressure measurement. BMJ 2001; 322(7293):1043–7.
3. Chobanian AV, Bakris GL, Black HR, et al. The seventh report of the Joint National Committee on Prevention, Detection, Evaluation, and Treatment of High Blood Pressure: the JNC 7 report. JAMA 2003;289(19):2560–72.
4. Yao ST, Hobbs JT, Irvine WT. Ankle systolic pressure measurements in arterial disease affecting the lower extremities. Br J Surg 1969;56(9):676–9.
5. Ouriel K, Zarins CK. Doppler ankle pressure: an evaluation of three methods of expression. Arch Surg 1982;117(10):1297–300.
6. McDermott MM, Greenland P, Liu K, et al. The ankle brachial index is associated with leg function and physical activity: the walking and leg circulation study. Ann Intern Med 2002;136(12):873–83.
7. Selvin E, Erlinger TP. Prevalence of and risk factors for peripheral arterial disease in the United States: results from the national health and nutrition examination survey, 1999–2000. Circulation 2004;110(6): 738–43.
8. Criqui MH, Fronek A, Barrett-Connor E, et al. The prevalence of peripheral arterial disease in a defined population. Circulation 1985;71(3):510–5.
9. Lange S, Diehm C, Darius H, et al. High prevalence of peripheral arterial disease and low treatment rates in elderly primary care patients with diabetes. Exp Clin Endocrinol Diabetes 2004;112(10):566–73.
10. Diehm C, Schuster A, Allenberg JR, et al. High prevalence of peripheral arterial disease and co-morbidity in 6880 primary care patients: cross-sectional study. Atherosclerosis 2004;172(1):95–105.
11. Meijer WT, Hoes AW, Rutgers D, et al. Peripheral arterial disease in the elderly: the Rotterdam Study. Arterioscler Thromb Vasc Biol 1998;18(2): 185–92.
12. Hirsch AT, Criqui MH, Treat-Jacobson D, et al. Peripheral arterial disease detection, awareness, and treatment in primary care. JAMA 2001; 286(11):1317–24.
13. Criqui MH, Langer RD, Fronek A, et al. Mortality over a period of 10 years in patients with peripheral arterial disease. N Engl J Med 1992;326(6):381–6.
14. Weitz JI, Byrne J, Clagett GP, et al. Diagnosis and treatment of chronic arterial insufficiency of the lower extremities: a critical review. Circulation 1996; 94(11):3026–49.
15. Hyman BN. The eye as a target organ: an updated classification of hypertensive retinopathy. J Clin Hypertens (Greenwich) 2000;2(3):194–7.
16. Pearson TA, Mensah GA, Alexander RW, et al. Markers of inflammation and cardiovascular disease: application to clinical and public health practice: a statement for healthcare professionals from the Centers for Disease Control and Prevention and the American Heart Association. Circulation 2003;107(3):499–511.
17. Parsons DS, Reaveley DA, Pavitt DV, et al. Relationship of renal function to homocysteine and lipoprotein(a) levels: the frequency of the combination of both risk factors in chronic renal impairment. Am J Kidney Dis 2002;40(5):916–23.
18. Mann JF, Gerstein HC, Pogue J, et al. Renal insufficiency as a predictor of cardiovascular outcomes and the impact of ramipril: the HOPE randomized trial. Ann Intern Med 2001;134(8):629–36.
19. Beddhu S, Allen-Brady K, Cheung AK, et al. Impact of renal failure on the risk of myocardial infarction and death. Kidney Int 2002;62(5):1776–83.
20. Jensen JS, Feldt-Rasmussen B, Strandgaard S, et al. Arterial hypertension, microalbuminuria, and risk of ischemic heart disease. Hypertension 2000; 35(4):898–903.
21. Gerstein HC, Mann JF, Yi Q, et al. Albuminuria and risk of cardiovascular events, death, and heart failure in diabetic and nondiabetic individuals. JAMA 2001;286(4):421–6.
22. Ridker PM, Rifai N, Rose L, et al. Comparison of C-reactive protein and low-density lipoprotein cholesterol levels in the prediction of first cardiovascular events. N Engl J Med 2002;347(20): 1557–65.
23. Ridker PM, Hennekens CH, Buring JE, et al. C-reactive protein and other markers of inflammation in the prediction of cardiovascular disease in women. N Engl J Med 2000;342(12):836–43.
24. Liebson PR, Grandits G, Prineas R, et al. Echocardiographic correlates of left ventricular structure among 844 mildly hypertensive men and women in the treatment of mild hypertension study (TOMHS). Circulation 1993;87(2):476–86.
25. Sheps SG, Frohlich ED. Limited echocardiography for hypertensive left ventricular hypertrophy. Hypertension 1997;29(2):560–3.
26. Cuspidi C, Meani S, Valerio C, et al. Left ventricular hypertrophy and cardiovascular risk stratification: impact and cost-effectiveness of echocardiography in recently diagnosed essential hypertensives. J Hypertens 2006;24(8):1671–7.
27. Hurley LP, Dickinson LM, Estacio RO, et al. Prediction of cardiovascular death in racial/ethnic minorities using Framingham risk factors. Circ Cardiovasc Qual Outcomes 2010;3(2):181–7.
28. Bots ML, Hoes AW, Koudstaal PJ, et al. Common carotid intima-media thickness and risk of stroke and myocardial infarction: the Rotterdam Study. Circulation 1997;96(5):1432–7.

29. Chambless LE, Heiss G, Folsom AR, et al. Association of coronary heart disease incidence with carotid arterial wall thickness and major risk factors: the Atherosclerosis Risk in Communities (ARIC) Study, 1987–1993. Am J Epidemiol 1997;146(6): 483–94.
30. Sampson UK, Fazio F, Patton JW, et al. Carotid artery intima-media thickness accretion rate and the risk of atherogenesis in a primary prevention population [abstract]. J Am Coll Cardiol 2010;55. A156.E1461.
31. O'Leary DH, Polak JF, Kronmal RA, et al. Carotid-artery intima and media thickness as a risk factor for myocardial infarction and stroke in older adults. Cardiovascular Health Study Collaborative Research Group. N Engl J Med 1999;340(1):14–22.
32. Wilson JF. The crucial link between literacy and health. Ann Intern Med 2003;139(10):875–8.
33. Osborne H. Health literacy from A to Z: practical ways to communicate your health message. Sudbury (MA): Jones and Bartlett; 2005.
34. Eichler K, Wieser S, Brugger U. The costs of limited health literacy: a systematic review. Int J Public Health 2009;54(5):313–24.
35. Health literacy: report of the council on scientific affairs. ad hoc committee on health literacy for the Council on Scientific Affairs, American Medical Association. JAMA 1999;281(6):552–7.
36. Insull W. The problem of compliance to cholesterol altering therapy. J Intern Med 1997;241(4):317–25.
37. Influence of adherence to treatment and response of cholesterol on mortality in the coronary drug project. N Engl J Med 1980;303(18):1038–41.
38. Berkman ND, Dewalt DA, Pignone MP, et al. Literacy and health outcomes. Evid Rep Technol Assess (Summ) 2004;87:1–8.
39. Cho YI, Lee SY, Arozullah AM, et al. Effects of health literacy on health status and health service utilization amongst the elderly. Soc Sci Med 2008;66(8): 1809–16.
40. Murphy C, Keyes M, Taylor-Clarke K, et al. Potential impact of poor patient education materials on cardiovascular outcomes [abstract]. J Am Coll Cardiol 2010;55. A142.E1331.
41. Effects of weight loss and sodium reduction intervention on blood pressure and hypertension incidence in overweight people with high-normal blood pressure. The trials of Hypertension Prevention, phase II. The Trials of Hypertension Prevention Collaborative Research Group. Arch Intern Med 1997;157(6):657–67.
42. He J, Whelton PK, Appel LJ, et al. Long-term effects of weight loss and dietary sodium reduction on incidence of hypertension. Hypertension 2000;35(2): 544–9.
43. Vollmer WM, Sacks FM, Ard J, et al. Effects of diet and sodium intake on blood pressure: subgroup analysis of the DASH-sodium trial. Ann Intern Med 2001;135(12):1019–28.
44. Sacks FM, Svetkey LP, Vollmer WM, et al. Effects on blood pressure of reduced dietary sodium and the dietary approaches to stop hypertension (DASH) diet. DASH-sodium collaborative research group. N Engl J Med 2001;344(1):3–10.
45. Chobanian AV, Hill M. National heart, lung, and blood institute workshop on sodium and blood pressure: a critical review of current scientific evidence. Hypertension 2000;35(4):858–63.
46. Kelley GA, Kelley KS. Progressive resistance exercise and resting blood pressure: a meta-analysis of randomized controlled trials. Hypertension 2000; 35(3):838–43.
47. Whelton SP, Chin A, Xin X, et al. Effect of aerobic exercise on blood pressure: a meta-analysis of randomized, controlled trials. Ann Intern Med 2002;136(7):493–503.
48. Xin X, He J, Frontini MG, et al. Effects of alcohol reduction on blood pressure: a meta-analysis of randomized controlled trials. Hypertension 2001; 38(5):1112–7.

Management of High Blood Pressure in Children and Adolescents

Rae-Ellen W. Kavey, MD, MPH[a,*],
Stephen R. Daniels, MD, PhD[b,c], Joseph T. Flynn, MD, MS[d]

KEYWORDS

- High blood pressure • Hypertension • Children
- Adolescents • Management

Primary hypertension is an increasingly common diagnosis in children and adolescents.[1] In the past, hypertension in childhood was considered rare and usually secondary to an identifiable underlying cause, but epidemiologic studies have established reliable norms for blood pressures (BPs) measured in an outpatient setting, and BP screening, particularly in relation to the obesity epidemic, has identified increased BPs in 2% to 5% of American children and adolescents.[2–5] In the past, increased BPs in the medical setting were often attributed to anxiety but use of ambulatory monitoring with established norms has allowed assessment of BPs throughout the day in the home environment and therefore, confirmation of true hypertension even in young children.[6] Ultrasound applications have shown the presence of subclinical organ damage as evidence of the effect of hypertension in childhood.[7–9] At a prevalence as high as 5%, hypertension is one of the most common chronic diseases of childhood. Further, detection of hypertension in childhood identifies an individual at defined risk for hypertension as an adult and at increased risk for accelerated atherosclerosis and future premature cardiovascular disease.[10–12] By contrast, new information from epidemiologic studies and randomized trials indicates that healthy lifestyle choices in childhood are convincingly associated with lower BPs later in life.[13,14] A series of randomized trials summarized in the most recent pediatric BP Task Force report from the National Heart, Lung and Blood Institute (NHLBI) have shown the safety and efficacy of BP lowering drugs in children and adolescents.[2] This section describes an approach to diagnosis and management of the important and increasingly common problem of hypertension in childhood.

DIAGNOSIS OF HYPERTENSION

Because hypertension is a largely asymptomatic condition, it can be diagnosed only by routine measurement of BP. The Fourth Report on Childhood Blood Pressure from the NHLBI recommends that BP be measured routinely for all health care encounters in children aged 3 years and older.[2] This is not happening regularly for all children, and even when BP is measured, it may not be interpreted correctly.[15] Without appropriate measurement and interpretation, increased BP

[a] Department of Pediatrics, Division of Cardiology, Golisano Children's Hospital, University of Rochester Medical Center, 601 Elmwood Avenue, Rochester, NY 14642, USA
[b] Department of Pediatrics, University of Colorado, School of Medicine, 13123 East 16th Avenue, B065, Aurora, CO 80045, USA
[c] Department of Pediatrics, The Children's Hospital, 13123 East 16th Avenue, B065 Aurora, CO 80045, USA
[d] Division of Nephrology, Seattle Children's Hospital, 4800 Sandpoint Way North East, Seattle, WA 98105, USA
* Corresponding author. Division of Pediatric Cardiology, University of Rochester Medical Center, 601 Elmwood Avenue, Rochester, NY 14642.
E-mail address: Rae-ellen_kavey@urmc.rochester.edu

Cardiol Clin 28 (2010) 597–607
doi:10.1016/j.ccl.2010.07.004

cannot be recognized and necessary treatment strategies cannot be implemented.

There are several important issues to consider in the measurement of BP in children. Because children are growing and because of increasing obesity in childhood, appropriate cuff size can vary substantially among children of the same age. The cuff bladder should have a width that covers approximately two-thirds of the upper arm and a length that encircles at least 80% of the upper arm, preferably 100%. Ideally, BP should be measured by auscultation, using a mercury sphygmomanometer. Using an automated oscillometric device is acceptable for initial measurement, but elevated readings should be confirmed by auscultation. Once an accurate BP measurement is obtained, the interpretation of that BP is important. The definition of elevated BP for children is based on percentiles derived from population studies of healthy children. BP increase is defined as systolic or diastolic BP at or higher than the 95th percentile based on sex, age, and height percentile. Complete normative tables are available with these percentile values.[2] Hypertension is defined as BP persistently higher than that level on 3 or more occasions. If hypertension is present, it can be further classified as stage 1 if the BP is between the 95th percentile and the 99th percentile plus 5 mm Hg. Stage 2 hypertension is BP persistently higher than the 99th percentile plus 5 mm Hg. Prehypertension is defined as systolic or diastolic BP between 90th and 95th percentile for sex, age, and height. However, during puberty the 90th percentile is higher than the adult definition of prehypertension (120/80 mm Hg). So, in this age range, BPs higher than 120/80 mm Hg and lower than the 95th percentile should be considered prehypertension. The definitions for increased BP are presented in **Table 1**.

Table 1
Categorization of BP for pediatric patients

Category	Definition
Normal BP	Systolic or diastolic BP below the 90th percentile[a]
Prehypertension	Systolic or diastolic BP above the 90th percentile (or 120/80 mm Hg), but below the 95th percentile
Stage 1 hypertension	Systolic or diastolic BP higher than or equal to the 95th percentile, but lower than the 99th percentile plus 5 mm Hg
Stage 2 hypertension	Systolic or diastolic BP higher than or equal to the 99th percentile plus 5 mm Hg

[a] All BP percentiles are based on sex, age, and height percentiles.

The BP tables from the most recent NHLBI Task Force Report[2] are the most complete and accurate normative pediatric BP values available but they are lengthy and detailed, with knowledge of the patient's height percentile needed for interpretation of measured BP. Recently, a simplified table (**Table 2**) has been created based on age and gender using systolic and diastolic BP measurements higher than the 90th percentile norms for the lower limit of height from the NHLBI Task Force Report to identify children and adolescents in whom BP requires further evaluation.[16] This is a useful tool for screening BPs in children and adolescents.

White-coat hypertension is a concern in children and adolescents. This form of hypertension occurs when BPs are increased in a clinic or office setting, but are normal at home. White-coat hypertension can be evaluated in pediatric patients with established hypertension on clinic measurements by 24-hour ambulatory BP monitoring or home BP measurements. Standards have been established for pediatric ambulatory BPs.[6]

There may also be concerns about secondary forms of hypertension in children. Secondary hypertension can be caused by renal parenchymal disease, renal vascular disease, endocrine abnormalities, the use of certain medications, coarctation of the aorta, and certain neurologic conditions. Secondary hypertension probably represents about 5% of hypertension in children and adolescents and is more likely to be present in younger children, children with higher BP, and children who have little or no family history of hypertension. Most causes of secondary hypertension can be identified, or at least a strong suspicion developed, from a complete history and physical examination. Based on those results, confirmatory tests can be performed. When secondary hypertension is present, specific treatment can be initiated for the underlying abnormality. Another circumstance that raises concern about potential secondary hypertension occurs when pharmacologic treatment of hypertension is unsuccessful. The most common reason for this lack of success is poor adherence, but this difficulty in achieving successful treatment may also be a clue to an underlying secondary cause

Table 2
BP values requiring further evaluation, according to age and gender

	BP (mm Hg)			
	Male		Female	
Age (y)	Systolic	Diastolic	Systolic	Diastolic
3	100	59	100	61
4	102	62	101	64
5	104	65	103	66
6	105	68	104	68
7	106	70	106	69
8	107	71	108	71
9	109	72	110	72
10	111	73	112	73
11	113	74	114	74
12	115	74	116	75
13	117	75	117	76
14	120	75	119	77
15	120	76	120	78
16	120	78	120	78
17	120	80	120	78
18	120	80	120	80

These values represent the lower limits for abnormal BP ranges, according to age and gender. Any BP readings equal to or greater than these values represent BPs in the prehypertensive, stage 1 hypertensive or stage 2 hypertensive range and should be further evaluated by a physician.

Data from Kaelber DC, Pickett F. Simple table to identify children and adolescents needing further evaluation of blood pressure. Pediatrics 2009;123:e972–4.

of the BP increase. The initial standard laboratory evaluation for pediatric hypertension includes checking blood urea nitrogen and creatinine levels, urinalysis, and a complete blood count. These tests are particularly useful for excluding renal causes of hypertension.

Once a diagnosis of hypertension is made, it is also important to consider whether target-organ damage is present. The most useful way to evaluate target-organ damage is by assessing left ventricular (LV) mass using echocardiography. LV hypertrophy can result from prolonged exposure of the left ventricle to increased afterload caused by increased systemic BP. In this context, increased LV mass may be seen as adaptive, in adults LV hypertrophy is also a risk factor for adverse cardiovascular outcomes, including myocardial infarction, stroke, congestive heart failure, and sudden death. LV hypertrophy in the context of hypertension in children and adolescents may be as prevalent as 40%, with more severe LV hypertrophy present in approximately 10%.[9] Identification of LV hypertrophy may suggest the need for more urgent and more aggressive treatment of hypertension.

Hypertension should be easily recognizable during health maintenance visits in children and adolescents. The prevalence of hypertension of as high as 5% in the general childhood population indicates that this diagnosis should not be uncommon for pediatricians and family physicians. However, to accomplish this diagnosis, correct measurement of BP is necessary. The observed BP must be compared with percentile values to determine if it is increased. This process often does not occur routinely in pediatric primary care.

OBESITY-RELATED HYPERTENSION

As described earlier, secondary hypertension is rare in childhood and presents most frequently in children less than 10 years of age with severe BP elevation. By contrast, hypertension associated with obesity is now the most common presentation in children and adolescents, with prevalence increasing as both age and the degree of obesity increase. Analysis of pooled data from 8 large epidemiologic studies involving more than 47,000 children revealed that regardless of race, gender, and age, the risk of increased BP was significantly higher for children in the upper compared with lower decile of body mass index (BMI, calculated as weight in kilograms divided by the square of height in meters).[17] Among obese children with BMI higher than the 90th percentile for age/sex in an obesity treatment program, the prevalence of hypertension averaged 30%.[18] However, in the most severely obese group with BMI higher than the 99.5th percentile, obesity prevalence was reported to be 45%. In a school-based survey in the United States published in 2004, the overall prevalence of hypertension among adolescents was 4.5%.[19] However, in the group with BMI higher than the 95th percentile, hypertension was reported in 34% of subjects. From epidemiologic studies, a serial analysis of combined National Health Examination Survey and National Health and Nutrition Examination Survey (NHANES) data showed that the prevalence of hypertension in children trended downward on each survey obtained between 1976 until 1988, after which prevalence progressively increased, coincident with the onset and progression of the obesity epidemic.[1] Between 1988 and 2002, prehypertension increased significantly by 2.3% and hypertension by 1%. In 1999 to 2002, hypertension prevalence was 4.2% for blacks, 3.3% for whites, and 4.6% for Mexican-Americans. Higher BMI and waist circumference both significantly increased the likelihood of hypertension. This trend continues into young adult life, with NHANES data from 1999 to 2004 showing that in individuals aged 18 to 39 years, the prevalence of both isolated systolic hypertension and combined systolic and diastolic hypertension has increased compared with results from 1988 to 1994 and that hypertension correlates significantly with obesity, smoking, and low socioeconomic status.[20] Hypertension is common among obese children and adolescents, involving at least one-third of all subjects when findings from epidemiologic and specific population studies are considered.

Mechanisms for Obesity-Related Hypertension

The mechanisms by which obesity contributes to the development of hypertension are multiple, complex, and, as yet, incompletely understood. As in adults, an upper body fat distribution has been shown to correlate with the development of hypertension in children.[21] Sodium retention is believed by many to be the common pathway leading to obesity-related hypertension. Hyperinsulinemia and/or insulin resistance, often seen with abdominal obesity, can result in chronic sodium retention by direct effects on the renal tubules and indirectly through stimulation of the sympathetic nervous system (SNS) and augmentation of aldosterone secretion.[22–24] Insulin is also believed to be the signal that links dietary intake and nutritional status to SNS activity, with increased SNS activity reported in obese individuals in multiple studies.[25,26] Hypertension is commonly seen in association with hyperuricemia, and this may also be related to hyperinsulinemia. However, recent studies in adults have shown that hyperuricemia independently predicts development of hypertension, suggesting that increased uric acid may play a causative role.[27] In adolescents with essential hypertension, almost 90% were reported to have increased uric acid levels compared with only 30% of adolescents with secondary hypertension and no normotensive controls.[28] A recent randomized, double-blind, placebo-controlled, crossover trial of allopurinol in children with newly diagnosed essential hypertension showed a significant reduction in BP associated with reduction of uric acid levels.[29] Alterations in vascular structure and function have been described in obese children and adolescents; these may be primary and therefore contributory to pressure increase or secondary to established hypertension. Findings include increased carotid artery intimal-medial thickness (cIMT) and reduced forearm blood flow response to ischemia with increased minimum vascular resistance.[30,31] Increased cIMT has been shown to occur with obesity alone and to a greater extent with obesity and hypertension. Increased vascular resistance has been shown to correlate directly with fasting insulin levels and to improve with weight loss. Stimulation of the renin-angiotensin-aldosterone system (RAAS) is also believed to contribute to the development of hypertension in obese individuals. The RAAS is an important modulator of efferent glomerular arteriolar tone and of tubular reabsorption of sodium. Plasma renin activity and aldosterone levels both decrease with weight loss in obese adults.[32] In obese adolescents, Rocchini and colleagues[33] reported significantly higher supine and upright aldosterone levels with no difference in plasma renin levels. However, a given increment in plasma renin activity produced a greater change in aldosterone levels in obese than in nonobese patients. In this study, weight loss resulted in a significant decrease in plasma aldosterone in the obese adolescent patients. Weight loss has been consistently shown to lower BP in multiple studies in obese adults and children.[23,34,35] The BP change has been shown to be independent of sodium restriction.

Diagnosis of Hypertension in Obese Children and Adolescents

The principles of BP measurement and interpretation outlined in the preceding section apply equally to obese children. Care must be taken to select an appropriate cuff size, which can be challenging for patients with large arms. White-coat hypertension is at least as common among obese children as it is in nonobese children, so ambulatory BP monitoring is an important way to confirm the diagnosis of hypertension, especially if drug treatment is being considered.[30,36]

Assessment for evidence of LV hypertrophy should be performed if a diagnosis of hypertension is made. Echocardiographic determination of LV mass is based on standard measurements indexed for body size using height to the 2.7 power. This method has been shown to most closely account for lean body mass, excluding the effects of obesity. Increased LV mass has been reported in obese children and in 34% to 38% of children with untreated hypertension. Outcome-based standards are not available for children. A conservative cut point for the presence of increased LV mass is 51 g/m^2;[7] this is higher than the 99th percentile throughout childhood and adolescence, and in adults with hypertension has been shown to be associated with increased morbidity.[9]

Treatment of Hypertension in Obese Children and Adolescents

Weight loss is the cornerstone of hypertensive management in obese children and adolescents. Several recent studies have addressed the role of diet specifically as it relates to BP. A meta-analysis of the effect of reducing salt intake on BP in children and adolescents found that a modest reduction in salt intake did decrease BP, with a significant effect size of −1.17 mm of mercury (mm Hg) for systolic BP and −2.47 mm Hg for diastolic BP in normotensive children aged 8 to 16 years; in infants, salt reduction decreased systolic BP by 2.47 mm Hg.[37] In the Dietary Approaches to Stop Hypertension (DASH) intervention trial in adults, a diet rich in fruits and vegetables, low-fat or fat-free dairy products, whole grains, fish, poultry, beans, seeds, and nuts and lower in salt and sodium, sweets and added sugars, fats, and red meat than the typical US diet substantially reduced both systolic and diastolic BP among hypertensive and normotensive individuals.[38] Sustained adherence to a DASH-style diet has been shown to be associated with lower risk of coronary heart disease and stroke on long-term follow-up.[39] A randomized controlled trial of the DASH diet was assessed in 57 adolescents with prehypertension or hypertension. At 3-month follow-up, the DASH group had a significantly greater decrease in systolic BP associated with higher intake of fruits, low-fat dairy products, potassium, and magnesium and a lower intake of total fat than did the usual care group.[40] Maximal decreases in BP have been achieved when a weight loss program combines diet change with physical conditioning.

When diet, exercise, and behavior counseling are not effective in reducing weight and controlling BP, drug therapy to support weight loss can be considered. Drug treatment of obesity to manage hypertension has not been specifically studied but pharmacologic treatment of obesity has been investigated in a series of randomized controlled trials in adolescents. For male and female adolescents with severe increase of BMI and insulin resistance, including females with polycystic ovarian syndrome, the addition of metformin to a comprehensive multidisciplinary weight loss program significantly reduced weight and BMI and improved insulin resistance and lipid levels at 4- to 6-month follow-up[41–43] For adolescents older than 12 years, the addition of orlistat, which causes fat malabsorption through inhibition of enteric lipase, to a comprehensive multidisciplinary weight loss program improved weight loss and BMI at 6- to 12-month follow-up in 3 of 4 studies.[44–46] However, orlistat therapy was associated with a high reported rate of gastrointestinal symptoms. In 12- to 16-year-old adolescents with severe elevation of BMI (32–44 kg/m^2), the addition of sibutramine, a serotonin reuptake inhibitor, to a comprehensive multidisciplinary weight loss program improved weight loss, BMI, and measures of metabolic risk at 12-month follow-up.[47,48] A large multicenter randomized controlled trial of sibutramine versus placebo in obese adolescents specifically addressed the cardiovascular effects of sibutramine.[49] At the 12-month end point, the sibutramine group had a significantly greater decrease in BMI and both groups had small mean decreases in heart rate and BP. However, tachycardia was reported as an adverse event in significantly more patients treated with sibutramine. Discontinuation of treatment did not differ between the 2 groups and no patient treated with sibutramine required discontinuation of treatment because of hypertension. Recent small case series of adolescents with a BMI higher than the 95th percentile with significant comorbidities and adolescents with a BMI 35 kg/m^2 or greater, at or above the 97th percentile, who had failed a weight loss program indicate that bariatric surgery in conjunction with a comprehensive multidisciplinary weight loss program can improve weight loss, BMI, insulin resistance, glucose tolerance, and BP.[50,51] Drug therapy to control hypertension is described in the next section.

PHARMACOLOGIC TREATMENT OF CHILDHOOD HYPERTENSION

Nonpharmacologic measures (dietary changes, exercise, and weight loss) have long been recommended as primary therapy for childhood hypertension,[2] especially in those with primary hypertension or obesity-related hypertension (see preceding section). The efficacy of these measures has been subject to question, however, primarily because of high rates of nonadherence with prescribed lifestyle changes. Thus, some hypertensive children and adolescents, including those with secondary hypertension, require pharmacologic treatment.

Medications Available for Use in Children

A major issue related to use of antihypertensive medications in young people is the availability of safety and efficacy data. Historically, few drug trials were conducted in children, with the consequence that many drugs had to be used empirically, without the benefit of specific pediatric efficacy, safety, or dosing information. Given the low incidence of hypertension in childhood, it is not surprising that this situation was especially true for antihypertensive medications.[52] The passing of the US Food and Drug Administration Modernization Act (FDAMA) in 1997, which contained a provision that granted 6 additional months of patent protection to drug manufacturers if they conducted pediatric trials, has had an enormous effect on pediatric drug development.[53] Subsequent legislation (Best Pharmaceuticals for Children Act, Pediatric Research Equity Act, FDA Amendments Act of 2007) has extended this provision and has led to other initiatives, including public posting of internal FDA pharmacology and efficacy reviews on the Internet, and mechanisms to promote studies of medications with lapsed patent protection. These initiatives have led to many pediatric clinical trials of antihypertensive medications and have also increased the number of such medications with specific pediatric labeling (**Table 3**), correcting a significant deficiency for antihypertensive medications and increasing the amount of clinically useful information for practitioners. More recently, the European Medicines Agency has enacted the so-called pediatric rule, which requires manufacturers to study medications in children to be able to market them in Europe.[54]

Because many children cannot swallow standard pills and capsules, drug formulation is another important issue for pediatricians and others who care for hypertensive children. The FDAMA and related legislation do not contain provisions to mandate marketing of liquid preparations of medications studied in children, leaving this need unfulfilled. However, several of the recent pediatric drug trials have incorporated an extemporaneous suspension into the study design, and the suspensions used have subsequently been incorporated into the FDA-approved label information for these compounds. Although this does provide some useful information for these medications, there are many unresolved questions with respect to stability of extemporaneously prepared suspensions that highlight the problems faced in prescribing most antihypertensive medications to children.[55]

Indications for Use of Antihypertensive Medications in Children

Because there has never been a natural history study of untreated primary hypertension in the pediatric age group, the long-term consequences of untreated hypertension in an asymptomatic, otherwise healthy child or adolescent remain unknown.[2] In addition, aside from one recent study of an angiotensin-receptor blocker (ARB),[56] there is an almost complete lack of data on the long-term effects of antihypertensive medications on the growth and development of children. Therefore, consensus organizations have recommended that use of pharmacologic therapy be limited

Table 3
Pediatric labeling of antihypertensive medications: effect of the FDAMA and successor legislation

Had Pediatric Labeling Before FDAMA	New Pediatric Labeling Since FDAMA[a]	Under Study, Awaiting Labeling, or Anticipated Future Study
Captopril[b]	Amlodipine	Aliskiren
Chlorothiazide	Benazepril	Candesartan
Diazoxide[b]	Enalapril	Olmesartan
Furosemide	Eplerenone[c]	Ramipril
Hydralazine	Fenoldopam	Sodium nitroprusside
Hydrochlorothiazide	Fosinopril	Telmisartan
Methyldopa	Irbesartan[c]	
Minoxidil	Losartan	
Propranolol	Lisinopril	
Spironolactone	Metoprolol Valsartan	

[a] Does not include medications studied and granted exclusivity but not pediatric labeling.
[b] No specific dose recommendations included in label.
[c] Label specifically states drug not effective in hypertensive children.

to children and adolescents with one of the following indications[2]:

- Symptomatic hypertension
- Secondary hypertension
- Hypertensive target-organ damage
- Diabetes (types 1 and 2)
- Persistent hypertension despite nonpharmacologic measures.

There are some subpopulations of children in which the benefits of pharmacologic treatment are reasonably clearly established, making the decision to prescribe more likely to produce a clinical benefit. Chief among these are children with chronic kidney disease (CKD), in whom it has recently been shown that lower BP reduces the rate of CKD progression.[57] In addition, one recent small study has shown that pharmacologic treatment can reduce LV mass index and urinary microalbumin excretion in a group of mostly obese children and adolescents with primary hypertension.[58] However, in other groups of children a conservative approach still seems warranted given the lack of evidence of benefit and the concern over possible adverse medication effects unique to the pediatric age group.

Approach to Prescribing Antihypertensive Medications in the Pediatric Patient

The approach to prescribing antihypertensive medications in the hypertensive child or adolescent has several differences from the approach usually followed in adults. The first of these differences relates to choice of initial medication. Although many individual antihypertensive compounds have now been studied in the pediatric age group, no pediatric studies comparing different agents have been conducted. Therefore, it is unknown whether one class of agent is better than another in children and adolescents. This situation leaves the prescriber without evidence-based guidance for choice of drug. This is reflected in the most recent consensus guidelines, which state that any class of agent is acceptable for use in children and adolescents.[2] Given this state of affairs, various approaches for choice of initial medication have been proposed, including tailoring drug choice to the patient's underlying pathophysiology and presence of concurrent conditions.[59]

The second difference from drug prescribing in adults is that most medications in children are dosed based on body weight; the one-size-fits-all approach used in adults is not followed in pediatrics. Ideally, such prescribing is based on the results of appropriately conducted clinical trials designed to establish a dose response for the compound under study. Many of the recent pediatric trials of antihypertensive medications have failed to show a dose response because of design flaws.[60] Nevertheless, as illustrated in **Table 4**, most antihypertensive medications used in children and adolescents do have accepted dose ranges based on body weight. This finding forms the basis for the stepped-care approach to drug treatment outlined in **Fig. 1**. Stepped care allows for the individualization of therapy according to the needs of the patient and also facilitates detection of adverse effects when drug doses are increased or new agents added. It has been endorsed by the last 3 pediatric working groups of the National High Blood Pressure Education Program as an appropriate approach to the use of antihypertensive drugs in children and adolescents.[2]

Another difference related to prescribing of antihypertensive medications in the pediatric age group is that ideally, drugs prescribed for use in children and adolescents should have FDA-approved pediatric labeling and should be indicated for pediatric use. As discussed earlier, many agents do not have such labeling, despite the recent legislative efforts that have been made to address this issue.[52,53,56] Given this situation, and given that essentially all classes of antihypertensive agents have now been studied in children (with the exception of commonly used diuretics), it is reasonable to limit prescribing to those agents that are labeled for use in children and adolescents.

Long-term Considerations for Use of Antihypertensive Medications in Children and Adolescents

As in adults, antihypertensive therapy in children and adolescents must be monitored closely both for efficacy and for potential adverse effects. BP should be measured in the office every 2 to 4 weeks until good control is achieved. For children with uncomplicated primary hypertension and no hypertensive target-organ damage, goal BP should be less than the 95th percentile for age, gender, and height, whereas for children with secondary hypertension, diabetes, or hypertensive target-organ damage, goal BP should be less than the 90th percentile for age, gender, and height.[2] These goals are consistent with current recommendations for therapy for hypertension in adults and also parallel the prescribing practices of many pediatric nephrologists. Once control is achieved, then office BP measurement every 3 to 4 months is appropriate. Home BP

Table 4
Doses for selected antihypertensive agents for use in hypertensive children and adolescents

Class	Drug	Starting Dose	Interval	Maximum Dose[a]
Aldosterone receptor antagonists	Eplerenone	25 mg/d	QD-BID	100 mg/d
	Spironolactone[b]	1 mg/kg/d	QD-BID	3.3 mg/kg/d up to 100 mg/d
ACE inhibitors	Benazepril[b]	0.2 mg/kg/d up to 10 mg/d	QD	0.6 mg/kg/d up to 40 mg/d
	Captopril[b]	0.3–0.5 mg/kg/dose	BID-TID	6 mg/kg/d up to 450 mg/d
	Enalapril[b]	0.08 mg/kg/d	QD	0.6 mg/kg/d up to 40 mg/d
	Fosinopril	0.1 mg/kg/d up to 10 mg/d	QD	0.6 mg/kg/d up to 40 mg/d
	Lisinopril[b]	0.07 mg/kg/d up to 5 mg/d	QD	0.6 mg/kg/d up to 40 mg/d
	Quinapril	5–10 mg/d	QD	80 mg/d
ARBs	Candesartan	2–4 mg/d	QD	32 mg/d
	Losartan[b]	0.75 mg/kg/d up to 50 mg/d	QD	1.4 mg/kg/d up to 100 mg/d
	Olmesartan	2.5 mg/d	QD	40 mg/d
	Valsartan[b]	1.3 mg/kg/d up to 40 mg/d <6 y: 5–10 mg/d	QD	2.7 mg/kg/d up to 160 mg/d <6 y: 80 mg/d
α and β-adrenergic antagonists	Labetalol[b]	2–3 mg/kg/d	BID	10–12 mg/kg/d up to 1.2 g/d
	Carvedilol	0.1 mg/kg/dose up to 12.5 mg BID	BID	0.5 mg/kg/dose up to 25 mg BID
β-adrenergic antagonists	Atenolol[b]	0.5–1 mg/kg/d	QD-BID	2 mg/kg/d up to 100 mg/d
	Bisoprolol/ HCTZ	0.04 mg/kg/d up to 2.5/6.25 mg/d	QD	10/6.25 mg/d
	Metoprolol	1–2 mg/kg/d	BID	6 mg/kg/d up to 200 mg/d
	Propranolol	1 mg/kg/d	BID-TID	16 mg/kg/d up to 640 mg/d
Calcium channel blockers	Amlodipine[b]	0.06 mg/kg/d	QD	0.3 mg/kg/d up to 10 mg/d
	Felodipine	2.5 mg/d	QD	10 mg/d
	Isradipine[b]	0.05–0.15 mg/kg/dose	TID-QID	0.8 mg/kg/d up to 20 mg/d
	Extended-release nifedipine	0.25–0.5 mg/kg/d	QD-BID	3 mg/kg/d up to 120 mg/d
Central α-agonist	Clonidine[b]	5–10 μg/kg/d	BID-TID	25 μg/kg/d up to 0.9 mg/d
Diuretics	Amiloride	5–10 mg/d	QD	20 mg/d
	Chlorthalidone	0.3 mg/kg/d	QD	2 mg/kg/d up to 50 mg/d
	Furosemide	0.5–2.0 mg/kg/dose	QD-BID	6 mg/kg/d
	HCTZ	0.5–1 mg/kg/d	QD	3 mg/kg/d up to 50 mg/d
Vasodilators	Hydralazine	0.25 mg/kg/dose	TID-QID	7.5 mg/kg/d up to 200 mg/d
	Minoxidil	0.1–0.2 mg/kg/d	BID-TID	1 mg/kg/d up to 50 mg/d

Abbreviations: BID, twice daily; HCTZ, hydrochlorothiazide; QD, once daily; QID, 4 times daily; TID, 3 times daily.
[a] The maximum recommended adult dose should never be exceeded.
[b] Information on preparation of a stable extemporaneous suspension is available for these agents.

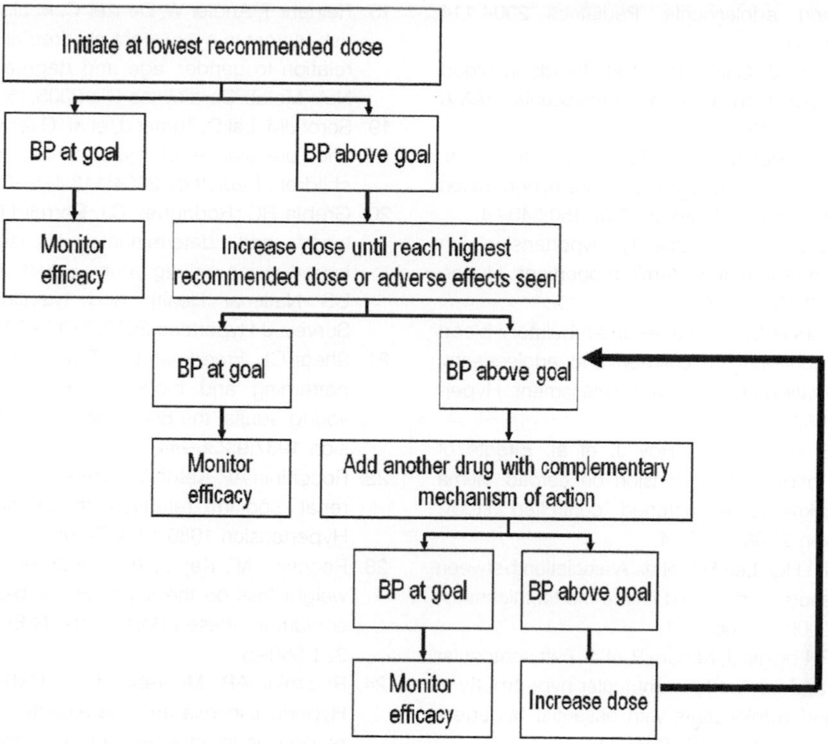

Fig. 1. Stepped-care approach to antihypertensive drug therapy in children and adolescents.

measurement should also be incorporated into the treatment plan, as this may help improve compliance with treatment, as well as achievement of goal BP. Periodic laboratory monitoring may also be required, particularly if a diuretic or agent affecting the renin-angiotensin system is prescribed, or if the hypertensive child or adolescent has underlying renal disease as the cause of their hypertension. Women of childbearing potential should be counseled regarding the need to use an effective method of contraception if treatment with an angiotensin-converting enzyme (ACE) inhibitor or ARB is indicated.

Adherence to treatment is an important long-term issue in the treatment of hypertension in children and adolescents because most patients have so few symptoms. In adolescents, this situation is particularly difficult because they often do not like to take their medications and do not like to be perceived as different from their peers. If BP control can be achieved with a single drug that is taken once a day, this improves the likelihood of compliance and this should be taken into consideration when the initial agent is chosen. The adverse effect profile of the medication may also affect adherence; newer agents such as long-acting calcium channel blockers and agents affecting the renin-angiotensin system have lower rates of adverse effects than older agents such as β-adrenergic blockers, and may therefore be preferable in the pediatric age group.

A few hypertensive children and adolescents, specifically those obese patients who make significant progress with lifestyle modification, may be candidates for withdrawal of therapy after a period of sustained BP control. Parents may be especially interested in attempting this goal to avoid an indefinite period of drug therapy beginning at a young age. Home BP monitoring and monitoring for resolution of hypertensive target-organ damage are especially important if withdrawal of medications is contemplated.

Antihypertensive medications lower BP in hypertensive children and adolescents. What remains for future study is whether use of antihypertensive drugs in the young results in prevention or amelioration of the long-term cardiovascular sequelae of hypertension.

REFERENCES

1. Din-Dzietham R, Liu Y, Bielo MV, et al. High blood pressure trends in children and adolescents in National Surveys, 1963 to 2003. Circulation 2007;116:1488–96.
2. National High Blood Pressure Education Program Working Group on High Blood Pressure in Children and Adolescents. The fourth report on the diagnosis, evaluation and treatment of high blood pressure in

children and adolescents. Pediatrics 2004;114 (Suppl):555–76.

3. Muntner P, He J, Cutler JA, et al. Trends in blood pressure among children and adolescents. JAMA 2004;291:2107–13.
4. McNiece KL, Poffenbarger TS, Turner JL, et al. Prevalence of hypertension and pre-hypertension among adolescents. J Pediatr 2007;150:640–4.
5. Sorof J, Daniels SR. Obesity hypertension inn children: a problem of epidemic proportions. Hypertension 2002;40:441–7.
6. Urbina E, Alpert B, Flynn J, et al. Ambulatory blood pressure monitoring in children and adolescents: recommendations for standard assessment. Hypertension 2008;552:433–51.
7. Lande MB, Carson NL, Roy J, et al. Effects of childhood primary hypertension on carotid intima media thickness. A matched controlled study. Hypertension 2006;48:40–4.
8. Lim SM, Kim HC, Lee HS, et al. Association between blood pressure and carotid intima-media thickness. J Pediatr 2009;154:667–71.
9. Daniels SR, Loggie J, Khoury P, et al. Left ventricular geometry and severe left ventricular hypertrophy in children and adolescents with essential hypertension. Circulation 1998;97:1907–11.
10. Chen X, Wang Y. Tracking of blood pressure from childhood to adulthood: a systematic review and meta-analysis. Circulation 2008;117:3171–80.
11. Raitakari OT, Juonola M, Kahonen M, et al. Cardiovascular risk factors in childhood and carotid artery intima-media thickness in adulthood: the Cardiovascular Risk in Young Finns Study. JAMA 2003;290: 2277–83.
12. Li S, Chen W, Srinivasan SR, et al. Childhood cardiovascular risk factors and carotid vascular changes in adulthood: the Bogalusa Heart Study. JAMA 2003;290:2271–6.
13. Gidding SS, Barton BA, Dorgan JA. Higher self-reported activity is associated with lower systolic blood pressure: the Dietary Intervention Study in Childhood (DISC). Pediatrics 2006;118:2388–93.
14. Niinikoski H, Jula A, Viikari J, et al. Blood pressure is lower in children and adolescents with low-saturated-fat diet since infancy: the Special Turku Coronary Risk Factor Intervention Project. Hypertension 2009;53:918–24.
15. Hansen ML, Gunn PW, Kaelber DC. Underdiagnosis of hypertension in children and adolescents. JAMA 2007;298(8):874–9.
16. Kaelber DC, Pickett F. Simple table to identify children and adolescents needing further evaluation of blood pressure. Pediatrics 2009;123:e972–4.
17. Rosner B, Prineas R, Daniels SR, et al. Blood pressure differences between blacks and whites in relation to body size among US children and adolescents. Am J Epidemiol 2000;151:1007–19.
18. Reinehr T, Andler W, Denzer C, et al. Cardiovascular risk factors in overweight children and adolescents: relation to gender, age and degree of overweight. Nutr Metab Cardiovasc Dis 2005;15:181–7.
19. Sorof JM, Lai D, Turner J, et al. Overweight, ethnicity and prevalence of hypertension in school-aged children. Pediatrics 2004;113:475–82.
20. Grebla RC, Rodriguez CJ, Borrell LN, et al. Prevalence and determinants of isolated systolic hypertension among young adults: the 1999–2004 US National Health and Nutrition Examination Survey. J Hypertens 2010;28:15–23.
21. Shear CL, Freedman DS, Burke GL, et al. Body fat patterning and blood pressure in children and young adults: the Bogalusa Heart Study. Hypertension 1987;9:236–44.
22. Rocchinin AP, Katch V, Kveselis D, et al. Insulin and renal sodium retention in obese adolescents. Hypertension 1989;14:367–74.
23. Rocchini AP, Key J, Bondie D, et al. The effect of weight loss on the sensitivity of blood pressure to sodium in obese adolescents. N Engl J Med 1989; 321:580–5.
24. Rocchini AP, Moorehead C, DeRemer S, et al. Hyperinsulinemia and the aldosterone and pressor responses to angiotensin II. Hypertension 1990;15: 861–6.
25. Jiang X, Srinivasan SR, Urbina E, et al. Hyperdynamic circulation and cardiovascular risk in children and adolescents: the Bogalusa Heart Study. Circulation 1995;91:1101–6.
26. Sorof JM, Poffenbarger T, Franco K, et al. Isolated systolic hypertension, obesity and hyperkinetic hemodynamic states in children. J Pediatr 2002; 140:660–6.
27. Feig DI, Kang D-H, Johnson RJ. Uric acid and cardiovascular risk. N Engl J Med 2008;359: 1811–21.
28. Feig DI, Johnson RJ. Hyperuricemia in childhood primary hypertension. Hypertension 2003;42: 247–52.
29. Feig DI, Soletsky B, Johnson RJ. Effect of allopurinol on blood pressure of adolescents with newly diagnosed essential hypertension: a randomized trial. JAMA 2008;300:924–32.
30. Stabouli S, Kotsis V, Papamichael C, et al. Adolescent obesity is associated with high ambulatory blood pressure and increased carotid intimal-medial thickness. J Pediatr 2005;147:651–6.
31. Rocchini AP, Moorehead C, Katch V, et al. Forearm resistance vessel abnormalities and insulin resistance in obese adolescents. Hypertension 1992;19:615–20.
32. Tuck MI, Sowers J, Dornfield L, et al. The effect of weight reduction on blood pressure plasma renin activity and plasma aldosterone level in obese patients. N Engl J Med 1981;304:930–3.

33. Rocchini AP, Katch VL, Grekin R, et al. Role for aldosterone in blood pressure regulation of obese adolescents. Am J Cardiol 1986;57:613–8.
34. Sjostrom CD, Lissner L, Wedel H, et al. Differential long-term effects of intentional weight loss on diabetes and hypertension. Hypertension 2000;36:20–5.
35. Rocchini AP, Katch V, Anderson J, et al. Blood pressure in obese adolescents: effect of weight loss. Pediatrics 1988;82:116–23.
36. Kavey REW, Kveselis DA, Atallah N, et al. White coat hypertension in childhood: evidence for end-organ effect. J Pediatr 2007;150:491–7.
37. He FJ, Graham AM. Importance of salt in determining blood pressure in children. Meta-analysis of controlled trials. Hypertension 2006;48:861–9.
38. Appel LJ, Moore TJ, Obarzanek E, et al. A clinical trial of the effects of dietary patterns on blood pressure. DASH Collaborative Research Group. N Engl J Med 1997;336(16):1117–24.
39. Folsom AR, Parker ED, Harnack LJ. Degree of concordance with DASH diet guidelines and incidence of hypertension and fatal cardiovascular disease. Am J Hypertens 2007;20(3):225–32.
40. Couch SC, Saelens BE, Levin L, et al. The efficacy of a clinic-based behavioral nutrition intervention emphasizing a DASH-type diet for adolescents with elevated blood pressure. J Pediatr 2008;152(4):494–501.
41. Kay JP, Alemzadeh R, Langley G, et al. Beneficial effects of metformin in normoglycemic morbidly obese adolescents. Metabolism 2001;50(12):1457–61.
42. Srinivasan S, Ambler GR, Baur LA, et al. Randomized, controlled trial of metformin for obesity and insulin resistance in children and adolescents: improvement in body composition and fasting insulin. J Clin Endocrinol Metab 2006;91(6):2074–80.
43. Freemark M, Bursey D. The effects of metformin on body mass index and glucose tolerance in obese adolescents with fasting hyperinsulinemia and a family history of type 2 diabetes. Pediatrics 2001;107(4):E55.
44. Maahs D, de Serna DG, Kolotkin RL, et al. Randomized, double-blind, placebo-controlled trial of orlistat for weight loss in adolescents. Endocr Pract 2006;12(1):18–28.
45. Chanoine JP, Hampl S, Jensen C, et al. Effect of orlistat on weight and body composition in obese adolescents: a randomized controlled trial. JAMA 2005;293(23):2873–83.
46. Ozkan B, Bereket A, Turan S, et al. Addition of orlistat to conventional treatment in adolescents with severe obesity. Eur J Pediatr 2004;163(12):738–41.
47. Berkowitz RI, Wadden TA, Tershakovec AM, et al. Behavior therapy and sibutramine for the treatment of adolescent obesity: a randomized controlled trial. JAMA 2003;289(14):1805–12.
48. García-Morales LM, Berber A, Macias-Lara CC, et al. Use of sibutramine in obese Mexican adolescents: a 6-month, randomized, double-blind, placebo-controlled, parallel-group trial. Clin Ther 2006;28(5):770–82.
49. Daniels SR, Long B, Crow S, et al. Sibutramine Adolescent Study Group. Cardiovascular effects of sibutramine in the treatment of obese adolescents: results of a randomized, double-blind, placebo-controlled study. Pediatrics 2007;120(1):e147–57.
50. Tsai WS, Inge TH, Burd RS. Bariatric surgery in adolescents: recent national trends in use and in-hospital outcome. Arch Pediatr Adolesc Med 2007;161(3):217–21.
51. Ippisch HM, Inge TH, Daniels SR, et al. Reversibility of cardiac abnormalities in morbidly obese adolescents. J Am Coll Cardiol 2008;51:1342–8.
52. Flynn JT. Pediatric use of antihypertensive medications: much more to learn. Curr Ther Res Clin Exp 2001;62:314–28.
53. Roberts R, Rodriguez W, Murphy D, et al. Pediatric drug labeling: improving the safety and efficacy of pediatric therapies. JAMA 2003;290:905–11.
54. Dunne J. The European Regulation on medicines for paediatric use. Paediatr Respir Rev 2007;8:177–83.
55. Ghulam A, Keen K, Tuleu C, et al. Poor preservation efficacy versus quality and safety of pediatric extemporaneous liquids. Ann Pharmacother 2007;41:857–60.
56. Flynn JT, Meyers KC, Neto JP, et al. Pediatric Valsartan Study Group. Efficacy and safety of the angiotensin receptor blocker valsartan in children with hypertension aged one to five years. Hypertension 2008;52:222–8.
57. Wühl E, Trivelli A, Picca S, et al. for the ESCAPE Trial Group. Strict blood-pressure control and progression of renal failure in children. N Engl J Med 2009;361:1639–50.
58. Assadi F. Effect of microalbuminuria lowering on regression of left ventricular hypertrophy in children and adolescents with essential hypertension. Pediatr Cardiol 2007;28:27–33.
59. Flynn JT, Daniels SR. Pharmacologic treatment of hypertension in children and adolescents. J Pediatr 2006;149:746–54.
60. Benjamin DK Jr, Smith PB, Jadhav P, et al. Pediatric antihypertensive trial failures: analysis of end points and dose range. Hypertension 2008;51:834–40.

Treatment and Control of High Blood Pressure in Adults

George A. Mensah, MD, FACC, FACP, FAHA[a,*],
George Bakris, MD, FASH, FASN, FAHA[b]

KEYWORDS

- Hypertension • Prehypertension
- Antihypertensive medications • Lifestyle modification

In patients with established hypertension, the treatment and control of systolic and diastolic blood pressure (BP) to target levels remain the primary objectives. However, the overall goal of treatment is the reduction of cardiovascular, cerebrovascular, renal, and all-cause mortality and morbidity. These goals and objectives require accurate measurements of baseline and follow-up BP and a comprehensive assessment using the clinical history, physical examination, and laboratory tests to establish the presence or absence of target organ damage, coexistent risk factors, and global (or total) cardiovascular risk. This assessment is crucial in informing the initial choice of drugs, urgency and intensity of treatment, and frequency of follow-up visits as recommended in established clinical guidelines.

To ensure patient adherence to provider recommendations for hypertension treatment, it is also important to assess the patient's health literacy level, ability to self-manage, and readiness to adopt behavioral and lifestyle changes, as well as the social, environmental, cultural, and financial sources of support in care. Although all of these are important in the treatment and control of hypertension in adults and the elderly, this article focuses only on the classification and staging of hypertension and the strategies for pharmacologic management as recommended in the Seventh Report of the Joint National Committee on Prevention, Detection, Evaluation, and Treatment of High BP (JNC 7).[1]

Whenever appropriate, changes in clinical practice that represent deviations from recommendations in JNC 7 are discussed when indicated by compelling clinical trial results available since publication of the JNC 7 report or suggested by more recent evidence-based recommendations from published national, international, or professional society guidelines for the prevention, treatment, and control of hypertension in adults and the elderly.[2–6] In addition, these guidelines are supplemented with updated guidelines and position papers by other societies such as the European Society of Hypertension/European Society of Cardiology[7] and the American Society of Hypertension and the American Heart Association/American College of Cardiology.

CLASSIFICATION OF BP LEVELS AND STAGING OF HYPERTENSION IN ADULTS

The JNC 7 report recommends that all patients should be classified as normal, prehypertensive, or hypertensive based on the level of the systolic and/or diastolic BP. As shown in **Table 1**, the classification of normal BP requires a systolic BP less than 120 mm Hg and a diastolic BP less than 90 mm Hg. Prehypertension, a term first formally introduced in the series of hypertension guidelines

[a] Heart Health and Global Health Policy, Global Research and Development, 700 Anderson Hill Road, PepsiCo, Inc, Building 6-2, Purchase, NY 10755, USA
[b] University of Chicago Pritzker School of Medicine, 5841 South Maryland Avenue, MC 1027, Chicago, IL 60637, USA
* Corresponding author.
E-mail address: george.mensah@pepsico.com

Cardiol Clin 28 (2010) 609–622
doi:10.1016/j.ccl.2010.08.002

by the Joint National Committee in the JNC 7 report, is defined as BP levels higher than normal, with systolic BP of 120 to 139 mm Hg or diastolic BP of 80 to 89 mm Hg. Patients classified in this way as prehypertensive should not be labeled as having a disease but should be informed of an increased risk of developing hypertension. Although they are not candidates for drug therapy unless they also have preexisting diabetes, kidney disease, or cardiovascular disease, they should be firmly and unambiguously advised to begin or continue therapeutic lifestyle changes because this intervention clearly aids in delaying the onset of hypertension.[1]

Hypertension is defined as systolic or diastolic BP of at least 140 mm Hg or 90 mm Hg, respectively. Hypertension must be further classified as stage 1 or stage 2 according to the level of systolic and diastolic BP, as shown in **Table 1**. It is important that the BP values used in this classification be based on the average of 2 or more properly measured, seated BP readings on each of 2 or more office visits.[1] Lifestyle modification, with emphasis on sodium intake, fruit and vegetable consumption, regular physical activity, and maintenance of ideal body weight, must be encouraged in persons with normal BP and recommended for persons with hypertension or prehypertension.[1] The beneficial effect of these lifestyle changes on BP levels have been well documented and can be as little as a reduction of 2 to 4 mm Hg (for moderation of alcohol intake in those who use alcohol) or as much as 5 to 20 mm Hg (in overweight or obese persons who are able to lose 10 kg of body weight), as shown in **Table 2**. These benefits were reaffirmed in the recent evidence review for the 2009 Canadian Hypertension Education Program recommendations.[2]

DEFINITION AND RISK ASSESSMENT FOR TREATMENT PLANNING IN HYPERTENSION

Since the publication of the JNC 7 report, several investigators have expressed the need for redefining hypertension.[8–12] The American Society of Hypertension Writing Group has proposed refinements in the definition of hypertension, and suggested that BP be recognized as a biomarker for hypertension and that a distinction be made between the various stages of hypertension and global cardiovascular risk.[9] Inherent in this evolving definition and risk assessment of hypertension are several crucial practical questions. For example, at what level of BP should drug treatment of hypertension begin, and should the definition and levels for starting treatment change based on the comorbid conditions?[8] What evidence supports aggressive control of BP to goals of less than 130/80 mm Hg? At present, it is uncertain whether all of these questions will be addressed in the JNC 8 guideline update.

LIFESTYLE MODIFICATIONS FOR THE PREVENTION AND CONTROL OF HIGH BP

Behavioral and lifestyle modifications are fundamental to successful prevention and control of high BP.[13–16] As shown in **Table 2**, the JNC 7 report recommended these modifications in persons with hypertension and prehypertension. They must even be strongly encouraged in persons with normal BP levels. The major modifications recommended are in the 5 areas of weight reduction or maintenance of ideal body weight, adoption of a Dietary Approaches to Stop Hypertension (DASH) eating plan, reduction of dietary sodium intake, engagement in regular aerobic physical activity, and moderation of alcohol consumption.

It has been estimated that a 1600 mg sodium DASH eating plan can reduce BP levels to the same extent as single-drug therapy.[17] Although such a diet may not be palatable to some persons, similar reductions in BP can be seen with a 2400 mg sodium plan. The magnitude of expected BP reductions is shown in **Table 2**. Combining several of these changes, for example dietary sodium reduction, moderation of alcohol intake, and increased physical activity, can have an even greater effect on BP levels. From a population perspective, these changes can have a major effect on the reduction of cardiovascular risk. For example, more than half of Americans aged 18 years and older have hypertension or prehypertension[18,19] and are candidates for these behavioral and lifestyle changes. In persons with prehypertension or stage 1 hypertension, a combination of 2 or more of these behavioral and lifestyle interventions has been shown to significantly reduce the estimated 10-year coronary heart disease risk by 12% and 14%, respectively.[20]

SPECTRUM OF ORAL ANTIHYPERTENSIVE DRUGS AND CHOICE OF INITIAL THERAPY

One of the greatest clinical and public health accomplishments of the last half century is the wide spectrum of safe and effective oral medications available for the treatment and control of hypertension. **Table 3** shows more than a dozen classes of oral antihypertensive drugs available for clinical use in the United States. Despite this plethora of safe and effective medications, hypertension treatment and control in the United States

Table 1
Classification and staging of BP and considerations of initial drug therapy

BP Classification	SBP[a] (mm Hg)	DBP[a] (mm Hg)	Lifestyle Modification	Initial Drug Therapy: Without Compelling Indications	Initial Drug Therapy: With Compelling Indications
Normal	<120	<80	Encourage	No antihypertensive drug indicated	Drug(s) for compelling indications[b]
Prehypertension	120–139	or 80–89	Yes		
Stage 1 hypertension	140–159	90–99	Yes	Thiazide-type diuretics for most. May consider ACEI, ARB, BB, CCB, or combination	Drug(s) for the compelling indications.[b] Other antihypertensive drugs (diuretics, ACEI, ARB, BB, CCB) as needed
Stage 2 hypertension	≥160	≥100	Yes	Two-drug combination for most[c] (usually thiazide-type diuretic and ACEI or ARB or BB or CCB)	

Abbreviations: ACEI, angiotensin-converting enzyme inhibitor; ARB, angiotensin receptor blocker; BB, β-blocker; CCB, calcium channel blocker; DBP, diastolic blood pressure; SBP, systolic blood pressure.

[a] Treatment determined by highest BP category.

[b] Initial combined therapy should be used cautiously in those at risk for orthostatic hypotension.

[c] Treat patients with chronic kidney disease or diabetes to BP goal of less than 130/80 mmHg.

Reproduced from National High Blood Pressure Education Program. JNC 7 Express: The Seventh Report of the Joint National Committee on Prevention, Detection, Evaluation, and Treatment of High Blood Pressure. Bethesda, MD: US Department of Health and Human Services; 2003.

Table 2
Therapeutic lifestyle modifications for the prevention and control of high BP

Modification	Recommendation	Approximate SBP Reduction (Range in mm Hg)
Weight reduction	Maintain normal body weight (body mass index 18.5–24.9 kg/m^2)	5–20 10 kg weight loss
Adopt DASH eating plan	Consume a diet rich in fruits, vegetables, and low-fat dairy products with a reduced content of saturated and total fat	8–14
Dietary sodium reduction	Reduce dietary sodium intake to no more than 100 mmol per day (2.4 g sodium or 6 g sodium chloride)	2–8
Physical activity	Engage in regular aerobic physical activity such as brisk walking (at least 30 min per day on most days	4–9
Moderation of alcohol consumption	Limit to no more than 2 drinks (30 mL ethanol; eg, 710 mL beer, 300 mL wine, or 90 mL 80-proof whiskey) per day in most men, and no more than 1 drink per day in women and lighter-weight persons	2–4

Reproduced from National High Blood Pressure Education Program. JNC 7 Express: The Seventh Report of the Joint National Committee on Prevention, Detection, Evaluation, and Treatment of High Blood Pressure. Bethesda, MD: US Department of Health and Human Services; 2003.

and throughout the world has generally been suboptimal,[21,22] leading to several calls for renewed action to prevent, treat, and control hypertension.[23–28] The recent analysis of the 2007 to 2008 National Health and Nutrition Survey (NHANES) data provides evidence that hypertension treatment and control rates in the United States improved during the period since the 1999 to 2004 survey.[19] For the first time in the United States, hypertension control rates exceeded 50%, with most of the improvement since 1988 occurring after 1999 to 2000.[19] Hypertension treatment increased from 61% to 73%, and BP control (defined by systolic level of <140 mm Hg and diastolic BP level of <90 mm Hg) increased from 35% to 50%.[19] As Chobanian[22] pointed out, this 50% control rate is particularly impressive and meets the Healthy People 2010 national objective.

These antihypertensive medications are indicated for patients with stage 1 or 2 established hypertension. For these patients, the choice of which medication to use for initial drug therapy, including the decision to use a single-drug monotherapy, fixed-dose combination therapy, or 2 drugs in combination, should be made based on the hypertension stage, baseline risk factors, target organ damage, and any compelling indications. For persons with stage 2 hypertension who have more than a 20 mm Hg (systolic) and 10 mm Hg difference between their starting BP level and the goal BP, JNC 7 recommends initiating combination therapy with 2 drugs from different antihypertensive drug classes. **Table 4** shows examples of drug combinations available in fixed-dose preparations. For individuals with prehypertension who have no compelling indications, the goal is to lower BP to the normal range using only therapeutic lifestyle changes. Antihypertensive drugs are not indicated in this setting.

By definition, a compelling indication is a specific high-risk condition for which compelling clinical trial data exist showing that the use of a particular class of antihypertensive treatment has benefit in terms of mortality or morbidity reduction. If a patient with hypertension also has one of these specific high-risk conditions, then the initial drug choice must be from the antihypertensive drug class indicated by the clinical trial results. These high-risk conditions include heart failure, postmyocardial infarction status, high coronary disease risk, diabetes, chronic kidney disease, and recurrent stroke prevention. **Table 5** shows which drug classes are indicated for the specific compelling indications. In diabetes, **Fig. 1** shows a suggested approach for achieving goal BP. The treatment of hypertensive crises is addressed elsewhere in this issue.

Table 3
Oral antihypertensive drugs available in the United States

Class	Drug (Trade Name)	Usual Dose Range in mg/d (Daily Frequency)
Thiazide diuretics	Chlorothiazide (Diuril)	125–500 (1)
	Chlorthalidone (generic)	12.5–25 (1)
	Hydrochlorothiazide (Microzide, HydroDIURIL[a])	12.5–50 (1)
	Polythiazide (Renese)	2–4 (1)
	Indapamide (Lozol[a])	1.25–2.5 (1)
	Metolazone (Mykrox)	0.5–1.0 (1)
	Metolazone (Zaroxolyn)	2.5–5 (1)
Loop diuretics	Bumetanide (Bumex[a])	0.5–2 (2)
	Furosemide (Lasix[a])	20–80 (2)
	Torsemide (Demadex[a])	2.5–10 (1)
Potassium-sparing diuretics	Amiloride (Midamor[a])	5–10 (1–2)
	Triamterene (Dyrenium)	50–100 (1–2)
Aldosterone receptor blockers	Eplerenone (Inspra)	50–100 (1–2)
	Spironolactone (Aldactone[a])	25–50 (1–2)
β-Blockers	Atenolol (Tenormin[a])	25–100 (1)
	Betaxolol (Kerlone[a])	5–20 (1)
	Bisoprolol (Zebeta[a])	2.5–10 (1)
	Metoprolol (Lopressor[a])	50–100 (1–2)
	Metoprolol extended release (Toprol XL)	50–100 (1)
	Nadolol (Corgard[a])	40–120 (1)
	Propranolol (Inderal[a])	40–160 (2)
	Propranolol long acting (Inderal LA[a])	60–180 (1)
	Timolol (Blocadren[a])	20–40 (2)
β-Blockers with intrinsic sympathomimetic activity	Acebutolol (Sectral[a])	200–800 (2)
	Penbutolol (Levatol)	10–40 (1)
	Pindolol (generic)	10–40 (2)
Combined α- and β-blockers	Carvedilol (Coreg)	12.5–50 (2)
	Labetalol (Normodyne, Trandate[a])	200–800 (2)
ACE inhibitors	Benazepril (Lotensin[a])	10–40 (1–2)
	Captopril (Capoten[a])	25–100 (2)
	Enalapril (Vasotec[a])	2.5–40 (1–2)
	Fosinopril (Monopril)	10–40 (1)
	Lisinopril (Prinivil, Zestril[a])	10–40 (1)
	Moexipril (Univasc)	7.5–30 (1)
	Perindopril (Aceon)	4–8 (1–2)
	Quinapril (Accupril)	10–40 (1)
	Ramipril (Altace)	2.5–20 (1)
	Trandolapril (Mavik)	1–4 (1)
Angiotensin II antagonists	Candesartan (Atacand)	8–32 (1)
	Eprosartan (Tevetan)	400–800 (1–2)
	Irbesartan (Avapro)	150–300 (1)
	Losartan (Cozaar)	25–100 (1–2)
	Olmesartan (Benicar)	20–40 (1)
	Tilmisartin (Micardis)	20–80 (1)
	Valsartan (Diovan)	80–320 (1)

(continued on next page)

Table 3
(continued)

Class	Drug (Trade Name)	Usual Dose Range in mg/d (Daily Frequency)
Calcium channel blockers: non-dihydropyridines	Diltiazem extended release (Cardizem CD, Dilacor XR, Tiazac[a])	180–420 (1)
	Diltiazem extended release (Cardizem LA)	120–540 (1)
	Verapamil immediate release (Calan, Isoptinf)	80–320 (2)
	Verapamil long acting (Calan SR, Isoptin SR[a])	120–360 (1–2)
	Verapamil: Coer (Covera HS, Verelan PM)	120–360 (1)
Calcium channel blockers: dihydropyridines	Amlodipine (Norvasc)	2.5–10 (1)
	Felodipine (Plendil)	2.5–20 (1)
	Isradipine (Dynacirc CR)	2.5–10 (2)
	Nicardipine sustained release (Cardene SR)	60–120 (2)
	Nifedipine long acting (Adalat CC, Procardia XL)	30–60 (1)
	Nisoldipine (Sular)	10–40 (1)
α_1-Blockers	Doxazosin (Cardura)	1–16 (1)
	Prazosin (Minipress[a])	2–20 (2–3)
	Terazosin (Hytrin)	1–20 (1–2)
Central α_2-agonists and other centrally acting drugs	Clonidine (Catapres[a])	0.1–0.8 (2)
	Clonidine patch (Catapres-TTS)	0.1–0.3 (1 weekly)
	Methyldopa (Aldomet[a])	250-1000 (2)
	Reserpine (generic)	0.05[b]–0.25 (1)
	Guanfacine (generic)	0.5–2 (1)
Direct vasodilators	Hydralazine (Apresoline[a])	25–100 (2)
	Minoxidil (Loniten[a])	2.5–80 (1–2)

Abbreviation: ACE, angiotensin-converting enzyme.
[a] These dosages may vary from those listed in the Physicians' Desk Reference; are now or will soon become available in generic preparations.
[b] A 0.1 mg dose may be given every other day to achieve this dosage.
Reproduced from National High Blood Pressure Education Program. JNC 7 Express: The Seventh Report of the Joint National Committee on Prevention, Detection, Evaluation, and Treatment of High Blood Pressure. Bethesda, MD: US Department of Health and Human Services; 2003.

THE ALGORITHM FOR HYPERTENSION TREATMENT AND FOLLOW-UP

Fig. 2 shows the algorithm for hypertension treatment recommended by the National High Blood Pressure education Program[29] and in the JNC 7 report.[1] In this algorithm, lifestyle changes and initial drug selection are based on hypertension stage, comorbid conditions, global cardiovascular risk, and the presence or absence of compelling indications.[1] For most patients with uncomplicated hypertension, the JNC 7 report recommended that a thiazide-type diuretic should be the preferred initial drug treatment, either alone or in combination with drugs from other classes.[1] Chobanian,[22] chair of committee for the JNC 7 report, admitted in his Shattuck lecture of 2009 that several important clinical trials[30–32] now indicate a need for a more flexible approach. These studies show that several drug classes with reasonable side effect profiles can reduce cardiovascular complications to a degree similar to that associated with diuretics. In addition, generic preparations of these drug classes are, or will soon become, available, thus making the low-cost advantage of thiazide diuretics less important.[22]

Fig. 3 shows the refinement in the algorithm for hypertension treatment based on the more flexible approach suggested by clinical trial results

Table 4
Combination drugs for treatment of hypertension

Combination Type	Fixed-dose Combination (mg)[a]	Trade Name
ACEIs and CCBs	Amlodipine/benazepril hydrochloride (2.5/10, 5/10, 5/10, 10/20)	Lotrel
	Enalapril maleate/felodipine (5/5)	Lexxel
	Trandolapril/verapamil (2/180, 1/240, 2/240, 4/240)	Tarka
ACEIs and diuretics	Benazepril/hydrochlorothiazide (5/6.25, 10/12.5, 20/12.5, 20/25)	Lotensin HCT
	Captopril/hydrochlorothiazide (25/15, 25/25, 50/15, 50/25)	Capozide
	Enalapril maleate/hydrochlorothiazide (5/12.5, 10/25)	Vaseretic
	Lisinopril/hydrochlorothiazide (10/12.5, 20/12.5, 20/25)	Prinzide
	Moexipril HCl/hydrochlorothiazide (7.5/12.5, 15/25)	Uniretic
	Quinapril HCl/hydrochlorothiazide (10/12.5, 20/12.5, 20/25)	Accuretic
ARBs and diuretics	Candesartan cilexetil/hydrochlorothiazide (16/12.5, 32/12.5)	Atacand HCT
	Eprosartan mesylate/hydrochlorothiazide (600/12.5, 600/25)	Teveten/HCT
	Irbesartan/hydrochlorothiazide (150/12.5, 300/12.5)	Avalide
	Losartan potassium/hydrochlorothiazide (50/12.5, 100/25)	Hyzaar
	Telmisartan/hydrochlorothiazide (40/12.5, 80/12.5)	Micardis/HCT
	Valsartan/hydrochlorothiazide (80/12.5, 160/12.5)	Diovan/HCT
BBs and diuretics	Atenolol/chlorthalidone (50/25, 100/25)	Tenoret FC
	Bisoprolol fumarate/hydrochlorothiazide (2.5/6.25, 5/6.25, 10/6.25)	Ziac
	Propranolol LA/hydrochlorothiazide (40/25, 80/25)	Inderide
	Metoprolol tartrate/hydrochlorothiazide (50/25, 100/25)	Lopressor HCT
	Nadolol/bendrofluthiazide (40/5, 80/5)	Corzide
	Timolol maleate/hydrochlorothiazide (10/25)	Timolide
Centrally acting drug and diuretic	Methyldopa/hydrochlorothiazide (250/15, 250/25, 500/30, 500/50)	Aldoril
	Reserpine/chlorothiazide (0.125/250, 0.25/500)	Diupres
	Reserpine/hydrochlorothiazide (0.125/25, 0.125/50)	Hydropres
Diuretic and diuretic	Amiloride HCl/hydrochlorothiazide (5/50)	Moduretic
	Spironolactone/hydrochlorothiazide (25/25, 50/50)	Aldactone
	Triamterene/hydrochlorothiazide (37.5/25, 50/25, 75/50)	Dyazide, Maxzide

Drug abbreviations: ACEI, angiotensin-converting enzyme inhibitor; ARB, angiotensin receptor blocker; BB, β-blocker; CCB, calcium channel blocker.

[a] Some drug combinations are available in multiple fixed doses. Each drug dose is reported in milligrams.

Reproduced from National High Blood Pressure Education Program. JNC 7 Express: The Seventh Report of the Joint National Committee on Prevention, Detection, Evaluation, and Treatment of High Blood Pressure. Bethesda, MD: US Department of Health and Human Services; 2003.

published since the JNC 7 report.[22] In patients with stage 2 hypertension, a stepped-care strategy, beginning with lifestyle changes alone, is inappropriate. Ideally, lifestyle changes and a starting dose of a 2-drug combination should be initiated in most patients. More recent guidelines, based on the results of the Avoiding Cardiovascular Events Through Combination Therapy in Patients Living with Systolic Hypertension (ACCOMPLISH) trial, recommend initiating therapy with a renin-angiotensin-aldosterone system blocker plus calcium antagonist instead of a thiazide diuretic.[33] Moreover, recent data of the 24-hour ambulatory blood pressure monitoring from this trial showed no difference in BP with an additional 20% CV risk reduction in a cohort of more than 11,000 patients with a mean age of 69 years when amlodipine was used with an angiotensin-converting enzyme (ACE) inhibitor compared with a diuretic.[30]

Specific recommendations from position papers of the American Society of Hypertension state that, in the initial stages of managing hypertension, there should be frequent visits in the first 2 to 4 months until BP approaches goal. Most modern treatments take 2 to 4 weeks to achieve maximum effect and should be titrated after this time period. The physician should always ask about sodium intake at every visit because this is one of the most common causes of failure to

Table 5
Compelling indications and the corresponding recommended drug class

	Recommended Drugs					
Compelling Indication[a]	**Diuretic**	**BB**	**ACEI**	**ARB**	**CCB**	**Aldo ANT**
Heart failure	•	•	•	•		•
After myocardial infarction		•	•			•
High coronary disease risk	•	•	•		•	
Diabetes	•	•	•	•	•	
Chronic kidney disease			•	•		
Recurrent stroke prevention	•		•			

Drug abbreviations: ACEI, angiotensin-converting enzyme inhibitor; ARB, angiotensin receptor blocker; Aldo ANT, aldosterone antagonist; BB, β-blocker; CCB, calcium channel blocker.

[a] Compelling indications for antihypertensive drugs are based on benefits from outcome studies or existing clinical guidelines; the compelling indication is managed in parallel with the BP.

Reproduced from National High Blood Pressure Education Program. JNC 7 Express: The Seventh Report of the Joint National Committee on Prevention, Detection, Evaluation, and Treatment of High Blood Pressure. Bethesda, MD: US Department of Health and Human Services; 2003.

achieve BP goal. It should be noted that all patients should be reviewed in the context of their own genotype and phenotype after lifestyle modifications are implemented and are being adhered to; health care providers must appreciate that the initial therapy is not as important as the combination of antihypertensive medications that will achieve BP goals.

STRATEGIES FOR DRUG SELECTION BEYOND THE INITIAL THERAPY

Sequential Monotherapy

This approach to lower BP was popularized in the Joint National Committee's fifth report. It is a strategy that is not considered to be effective, in particular because it leaves the patient unprotected for periods of time and can potentially

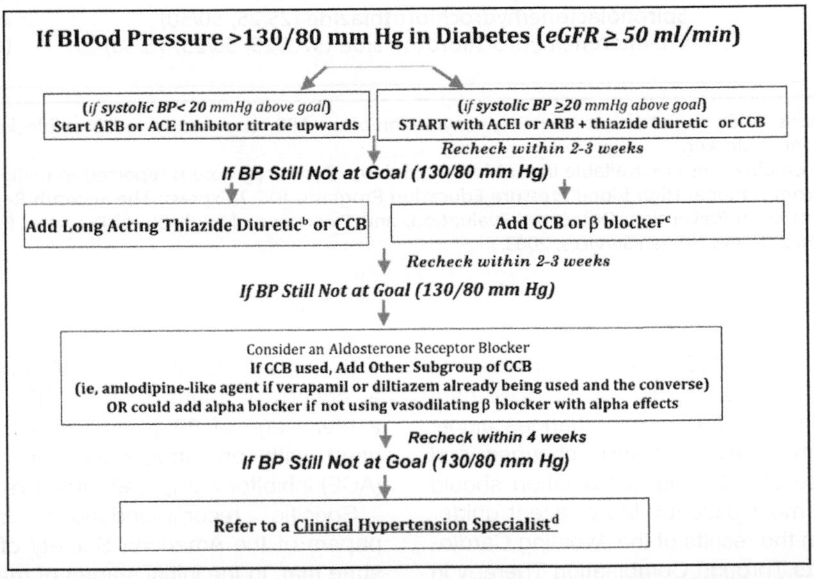

Fig. 1. A suggested approach to achieve BP goal in patients with diabetes. [a]Kidney function (estimated glomerular filtration rate [eGFR]), which generally responds well to thiazide diuretics. [b]Chlorthalidone is the suggested thiazidelike diuretic because it is used in clinical trials and forms the bases for the cardiovascular outcome data. [c]Vasodilating β-blockers have a better tolerability profile and less metabolic consequences compared with older agents such as atenolol. [d]Specialists can be found at http://www.ash-us.org/specialist_program/directory.htm#. (*Adapted from* Ruilope L, Kjeldsen SE, de la Sierra, A et al. The kidney and cardiovascular risk–implications for management: a consensus statement from the European Society of Hypertension. Blood Press 2007;16(2):74; with permission.)

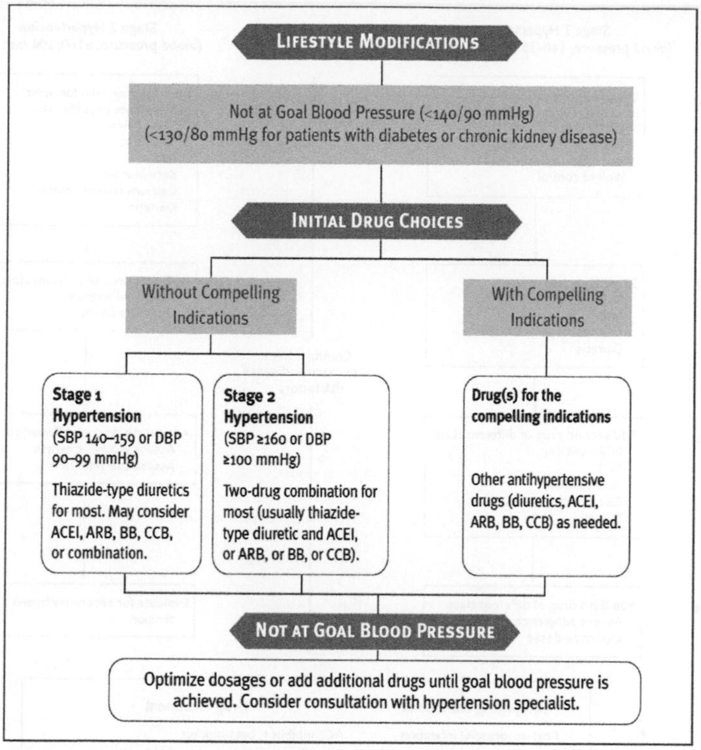

Fig. 2. The algorithm for hypertension treatment. ACEI, angiotensin-converting enzyme inhibitor; ARB, angiotensin receptor blocker; BB, β-blocker; CCB, calcium channel blocker; DBP, diastolic blood pressure; SBP, systolic blood pressure. (*Reproduced from* National High Blood Pressure Education Program. JNC 7 Express: The Seventh Report of the Joint National Committee on Prevention, Detection, Evaluation, and Treatment of High Blood Pressure. Bethesda, MD: US Department of Health and Human Services; 2003.)

cause patients to lose faith in the health care provider unless the physician is lucky enough to find the best single therapy for the patient. In the absence of a perfect method to predict the single best therapy for each individual patient, understanding the physiology of the disease process and selecting an appropriate drug based on the pharmacologic properties of the antihypertensive medications seems optimal.

Combination Therapy with 2 or More Medications

More than 75% of patients with hypertension require 2 or more medications to achieve BP goal. Thus, early combination therapy is preferred to sequential monotherapy. When the initial monotherapy fails to control BP to target levels, the current recommendation is to start with low-dose combination therapy, ideally using a different, but complimentary, drug class. Alternatively, the second medication added could be a low dose of a fixed-dose combination, yielding a 3-drug combination therapy.

IMPORTANCE OF ADDRESSING ADVERSE DRUG EVENTS

Currently available antihypertensive medications are generally safe. In particular, their associated risk of adverse effects is far less than the risk of cardiovascular, renal, and cerebrovascular complications in untreated and uncontrolled hypertension. However, every effort should be made to assure the patient that all adverse effects should be reported and that these adverse effects will be addressed and, if necessary, changes in medication dosage or drug class will be made. The spectrum of adverse effects is broad and can range from potassium loss (typically with loop and thiazide diuretics) to constipation (with calcium channel blockers and central α agonists). Most of these are not life threatening and are well tolerated when recognized and addressed early.

Angioedema is among the most serious and life-threatening adverse effects. It is most commonly seen in ACE inhibitor treatment but has been reported in all renin-angiotensin-system blockers. It

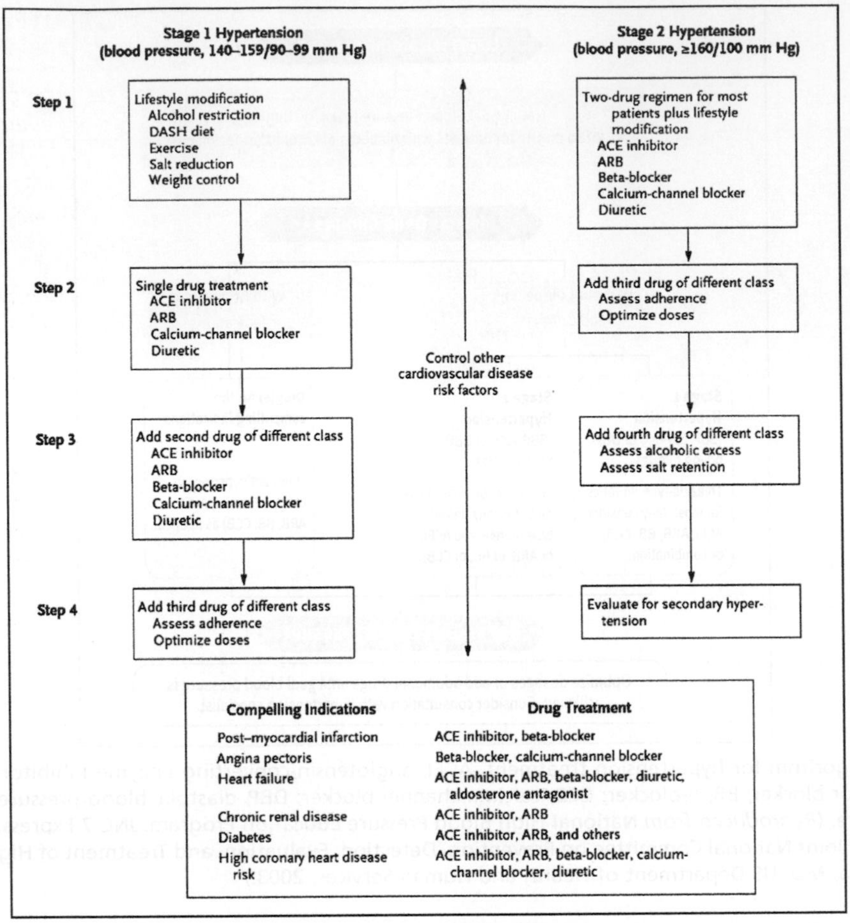

Fig. 3. A further refinement in the algorithm for the management of hypertension. ACE, angiotensin-converting enzyme; ARB, angiotensin receptor blocker; DASH, Dietary Approaches to Stop Hypertension. (*Reproduced from* Chobanian AV. Shattuck Lecture. The hypertension paradox—more uncontrolled disease despite improved therapy. N Engl J Med 2009;361(9):882; with permission.)

is more commonly seen in black patients in whom a sixfold higher risk has been noted. It typically presents as a transient swelling of the face, lips, tongue, and upper respiratory tract.[34] If unrecognized early, angioedema can be life threatening. Prompt recognition, discontinuation of the culprit medication, and conservative management with antihistamine and, if necessary, epinephrine and/or steroid therapy as warranted.[35] A prior history of ACE inhibitor–related angioedema is a contraindication to the use of ACE inhibitors, and, in general, angiotensin receptor blockers should not be used unless there is a compelling indication, in which case they should be used cautiously.[35]

Sexual dysfunction, although not life threatening, can be an important reason for patient nonadherence to medication regimens. It can occur with all agents that reduce BP, and it is especially prevalent in patients whose BP has been poorly controlled and now is at goal. Although older agents such as β-blockers, and adrenergic agents are offenders by direct mechanisms, all agents that help achieve control have this effect transiently. Patience needs to be exercised and tone will return except when complicated by the presence of diabetic neuropathy, in which case appropriate referral for evaluation and treatment should be made.

ANTIHYPERTENSIVE THERAPY IN SPECIFIC POPULATIONS

Patients with hypertension and specific comorbid conditions require special attention and follow-up. These conditions include ischemic heart disease, chronic heart failure, diabetes, chronic kidney disease, stroke, peripheral arterial disease, left ventricular hypertrophy, obesity, and the metabolic syndrome.[1] The JNC 7 report has provided useful guidance on the management of these patients, with emphasis on the compelling indications for the use of specific drugs in these settings. In addition, attention should be paid to the goal BP, especially in the setting of diabetes and/or proteinuric kidney disease, for which the treatment goal should be less than 120 (systolic) and less than 80 mm Hg (diastolic), typically requiring 2 or more antihypertensive medications. Similarly, in patients with ischemic heart disease, a goal BP should be 130/80 mm Hg or lower. Other sections of this issue discuss key concepts in the management of other population groups, including patients who have undergone organ transplantation, pregnant women, patients with autonomic dysfunction and baroreceptor dysfunction, and African Americans.

In addition to these populations, the elderly represent another group in whom the treatment and control of hypertension require additional considerations. Hypertension is common in older adults, especially those aged 60 years and older, in whom hypertension prevalence may be as high as 60 to 80%. Although hypertension awareness and treatment are high in these older adults, the proportion of those treated and controlled is lower compared with adults aged 18 to 39years ($P<.001$) and those 40 to 59 years ($P = .008$).[19] In these patients, a normal diastolic BP should not be construed as representing an absence of hypertension, because isolated systolic hypertension (ISH), defined as systolic BP more than 160 mm Hg and a diastolic BP less than 90 mm Hg, is common. There is some debate as to the optimal threshold (systolic BP >150 mm Hg vs 160 mm Hg) for initiating antihypertensive drug therapy. Regardless of the threshold used, treatment should be started at lower doses and titrated up slowly to avoid hypotension and/or hypoperfusion with associated symptoms of confusion and lethargy. In general, 2 or more drugs in combination therapy are needed, when BP is greater than 20/10 mm Hg more than the goal. The goal BP for patients older than 70 years who have ISH should be less than 150/90 mm Hg. Goal BP for patients younger than 70 years who typically have primary hypertension, but not ISH, should be less than 140 mm Hg (systolic). The general recommended BP goal in uncomplicated hypertension in the elderly is less than 140/90 mm Hg. However, as emphasized in the ACC/AHA Expert Consensus Document on Hypertension in the Elderly, this target is based on expert opinion rather than on data from randomized controlled trials.[36] It remains unclear whether the goal systolic BP should be the same in 65 to 79 year olds as in patients older than 80 years.[37]

EMERGING TREATMENT OF HYPERTENSION

Emerging Drug Therapies

Although a vast array of safe and effective treatments for hypertension is now available, there is continued research for new therapies. The endothelin receptor type A antagonist darusentan is likely to be approved for the management of resistant hypertension. In a recent randomized, double-blind, placebo-controlled trial, Weber and colleagues showed that darusentan provided additional BP reduction in patients with established resistant hypertension.[37] The main adverse effects were related to fluid accumulation. Edema, or fluid retention, occurred in nearly twice as many patients on darusentan compared with those on placebo (27% vs 14%). Other drug therapies in the research and development stages include cannabinoid-1 receptor antagonists[38] and advanced glycation end product cross-link breakers.[39,40]

Vaccine Therapy

Advances in the last decade have some promise in the use of vaccines against targets in the renin-angiotensin-aldosterone system such as angiotensin I, angiotensin II, and angiotensin II type 1 receptors in the management of hypertension.[41] Although effective BP control is the desired outcome of these studies, demonstrated safety is a major concern, especially because early vaccines against renin had the undesired adverse effect of autoimmune disease in animal studies.[41] Several vaccines that target either angiotensin II or its receptors remain experimental but show significant promise.[42–44]

Baroreceptor Stimulation

Several recent advances in the baroreceptor control of long-term sympathetic output and renal fluid volume regulation led to successful development and testing of an animal model of BP control using electrical stimulation of the carotid sinus.[45] Human trials to evaluate the clinical application of electrical carotid sinus manipulation in the treatment of systemic hypertension are underway with encouraging initial results.[45]

Renal Sympathetic Denervation

The crucial role of renal sympathetic nerve activity in the pathogenesis and maintenance of hypertension is well established.[46] Recent development of safe, effective, minimally invasive, percutaneous radiofrequency renal denervation from within the renal artery has provided an emerging approach for hypertension treatment.[47] One multicenter proof-of-principle trial of this approach in 50 patients with resistant hypertension showed that BP was reduced by 27/17 mm Hg at 12 months, without impairment of the estimated glomerular filtration rate.[48]

SUMMARY

As the leading risk factor cause of death worldwide, hypertension remains a major clinical and public health challenge. Prevention and control of prehypertension through behavioral and lifestyle changes and the treatment of hypertension to goal BP remain important objectives. Antihypertensive medications now available for clinical practice are generally safe and effective and should be used with lifestyle modification to attain goal BP in all patients with stage 1 or stage 2 hypertension. In the presence of diabetes or proteinuric chronic renal failure, goal BP should be less than 120/80 mm Hg. In patients with cardiovascular disease, goal BP should be 120 mm Hg or lower. The goal BP for patients older than 70 years who have ISH should be less than 150/90 mm Hg. The generally recommended BP goal in uncomplicated primary hypertension in the elderly is less than 140/90 mm Hg.

In most of these patients, 2 or more medications with complementary mechanisms of action should be used in combination. When patients fail to attain goal BP while adherent on 3 or more appropriately dosed antihypertensive medications, including a diuretic, they should be referred to a hypertension specialist for evaluation of resistant hypertension. Although a stepped-care approach (beginning with lifestyle changes and then only adding drug treatment when goal BP is not attained) may be appropriate in persons with stage 1 hypertension, it should not be used in stage 2 hypertension or in patients in whom the initial BP is greater than 20/10 mm Hg more than goal. In patients with underlying ischemic heart disease, chronic heart failure, diabetes, chronic kidney disease, stroke, peripheral arterial disease, left ventricular hypertrophy, obesity, and the metabolic syndrome, attention should be paid to the compelling indications for the use of specific drugs in these settings.

Adverse drug effects such as angioedema, electrolyte abnormalities, and sexual dysfunction should be identified early and managed promptly to address both patient safety and treatment adherence. Similarly, other factors that can affect adherence, including cost of medications and the patient's health literacy level and ability to self-manage, as well as the social, environmental, cultural, and financial sources of support in care, must be addressed to achieve the full benefits in the treatment and control of hypertension and prehypertension.

REFERENCES

1. Chobanian AV, Bakris GL, Black HR, et al. The Seventh Report of the Joint National Committee on Prevention, detection, evaluation, and treatment of high blood pressure: the JNC 7 report. JAMA 2003;289(19):2560–72.
2. Khan NA, Hemmelgarn B, Herman RJ, et al. The 2009 Canadian hypertension education program recommendations for the management of hypertension: part 2–therapy. Can J Cardiol 2009;25(5):287–98.
3. Padwal RS, Hemmelgarn BR, Khan NA, et al. The 2009 Canadian hypertension education program recommendations for the management of hypertension: part 1–blood pressure measurement, diagnosis and assessment of risk. Can J Cardiol 2009;25(5):279–86.
4. Sanchez RA, Ayala M, Baglivo H, et al. Latin American guidelines on hypertension. Latin American Expert Group. J Hypertens 2009;27(5):905–22.
5. Mancia G, de BG, Dominiczak A, et al. 2007 ESH-ESC practice guidelines for the management of arterial hypertension: ESH-ESC Task Force on the Management of Arterial Hypertension. J Hypertens 2007;25(9):1751–62.
6. Japanese Society of Hypertension. Japanese Society of Hypertension guidelines for the management of hypertension (JSH 2004). Hypertens Res 2006;29(Suppl):S1–105:S1–105.
7. Mancia G, de Backer G, Dominiczak A, et al. 2007 Guidelines for the management of arterial hypertension: the Task Force for the Management of Arterial Hypertension of the European Society of Hypertension (ESH) and of the European Society of Cardiology (ESC). J Hypertens 2007;25(6):1105–87.
8. Ram CV, Giles TD. The evolving definition of systemic arterial hypertension. Curr Atheroscler Rep 2010;12(3):155–8.
9. Giles TD, Materson BJ, Cohn JN, et al. Definition and classification of hypertension: an update. J Clin Hypertens (Greenwich) 2009;11(11):611–4.
10. Giles TD. Should we redefine hypertension? Curr Cardiol Rep 2006;8(6):395–8.
11. Giles TD, Berk BC, Black HR, et al. Expanding the definition and classification of hypertension. J Clin Hypertens (Greenwich) 2005;7(9):505–12.
12. Kostis JB, Messerli F, Giles TD. Hypertension: definitions and guidelines. J Clin Hypertens (Greenwich) 2005;7(9):538–9.
13. Khan NA, Hemmelgarn B, Herman RJ, et al. The 2008 Canadian Hypertension Education Program recommendations for the management of

hypertension: part 2-therapy. Can J Cardiol 2008; 24(6):465–75.
14. Moore TJ, Alsabeeh N, Apovian CM, et al. Weight, blood pressure, and dietary benefits after 12 months of a Web-based Nutrition Education Program (DASH for health): longitudinal observational study. J Med Internet Res 2008;10(4):e52.
15. Whelton PK, He J, Appel LJ, et al. Primary prevention of hypertension: clinical and public health advisory from the National High Blood Pressure Education Program. JAMA 2002;288(15):1882–8.
16. Appel LJ. The role of diet in the prevention and treatment of hypertension. Curr Atheroscler Rep 2000; 2(6):521–8.
17. Sacks FM, Svetkey LP, Vollmer WM, et al. Effects on blood pressure of reduced dietary sodium and the Dietary Approaches to Stop Hypertension (DASH) diet. DASH-Sodium Collaborative Research Group. N Engl J Med 2001;344(1):3–10.
18. Ostchega Y, Yoon SS, Hughes J, et al. Hypertension awareness, treatment, and control–continued disparities in adults: United States, 2005–2006. NCHS Data Brief 2008;(3):1–8.
19. Egan BM, Zhao Y, Axon RN. US trends in prevalence, awareness, treatment, and control of hypertension, 1988–2008. JAMA 2010;303(20):2043–50.
20. Maruthur NM, Wang NY, Appel LJ. Lifestyle interventions reduce coronary heart disease risk: results from the PREMIER Trial. Circulation 2009;119(15):2026–31.
21. Mensah GA. The global burden of hypertension: good news and bad news. Cardiol Clin 2002;20(2): 181–5, v.
22. Chobanian AV. Shattuck lecture. The hypertension paradox–more uncontrolled disease despite improved therapy. N Engl J Med 2009;361(9):878–87.
23. Rubinstein A, Alcocer L, Chagas A. High blood pressure in Latin America: a call to action. Ther Adv Cardiovasc Dis 2009;3(4):259–85.
24. Campbell NR, Leiter LA, Larochelle P, et al. Hypertension in diabetes: a call to action. Can J Cardiol 2009;25(5):299–302.
25. Bakris G, Hill M, Mancia G, et al. Achieving blood pressure goals globally: five core actions for health-care professionals. A worldwide call to action. J Hum Hypertens 2008;22(1):63–70.
26. Lackland DT. Hypertension control among African Americans: an urgent call for action. J Clin Hypertens (Greenwich) 2004;6(6):333–4.
27. Carter BL, Elliott WJ. The role of pharmacists in the detection, management, and control of hypertension: a national call to action. Pharmacotherapy 2000;20(2):119–22.
28. Lenfant C, Roccella EJ. A call to action for more aggressive treatment of hypertension. J Hypertens Suppl 1999;17(1):S3–7.
29. National High Blood Pressure Education Program. JNC 7 express: the seventh report of the Joint National Committee on Prevention, Detection, Evaluation, and Treatment of High Blood Pressure. Bethesda (MD): US Department of Health and Human Services; 2003.
30. Jamerson K, Weber MA, Bakris GL, et al. Benazepril plus amlodipine or hydrochlorothiazide for hypertension in high-risk patients. N Engl J Med 2008; 359(23):2417–28.
31. Wing LM, Reid CM, Ryan P, et al. A comparison of outcomes with angiotensin-converting–enzyme inhibitors and diuretics for hypertension in the elderly. N Engl J Med 2003;348(7):583–92.
32. Dahlof B, Devereux RB, Kjeldsen SE, et al. Cardiovascular morbidity and mortality in the Losartan Intervention for Endpoint Reduction in Hypertension study (LIFE): a randomised trial against atenolol. Lancet 2002;359(9311):995–1003.
33. Bakris GL, Sarafidis PA, Weir MR, et al. Renal outcomes with different fixed-dose combination therapies in patients with hypertension at high risk for cardiovascular events (ACCOMPLISH): a prespecified secondary analysis of a randomised controlled trial. Lancet 2010;375(9721):1173–81.
34. Greaves M, Lawlor F. Angioedema: manifestations and management. J Am Acad Dermatol 1991;25(1 Pt 2):155–61.
35. Sica DA, Black HR. Current concepts of pharmacotherapy in hypertension: ACE inhibitor-related angioedema: can angiotensin-receptor blockers be safely used? J Clin Hypertens (Greenwich) 2002;4(5):375–80.
36. Aronow WS, Fleg JL, Pepine CJ, et al. ACCF/AHA/NHLBI 2010 Expert consensus document on hypertension in the elderly: a report of the American College of Cardiology foundation task force on expert consensus documents. J Am Coll Cardiol, in press.
37. Weber MA, Black H, Bakris G, et al. A selective endothelin-receptor antagonist to reduce blood pressure in patients with treatment-resistant hypertension: a randomised, double-blind, placebo-controlled trial. Lancet 2009;374(9699):1423–31.
38. Batkai S, Pacher P, Osei-Hyiaman D, et al. Endocannabinoids acting at cannabinoid-1 receptors regulate cardiovascular function in hypertension. Circulation 2004;110(14):1996–2002.
39. Zieman SJ, Melenovsky V, Clattenburg L, et al. Advanced glycation endproduct crosslink breaker (alagebrium) improves endothelial function in patients with isolated systolic hypertension. J Hypertens 2007;25(3):577–83.
40. Bakris GL, Bank AJ, Kass DA, et al. Advanced glycation end-product cross-link breakers. A novel approach to cardiovascular pathologies related to the aging process. Am J Hypertens 2004;17(12 Pt 2): 23S–30S.
41. Do TH, Chen Y, Nguyen VT, et al. Vaccines in the management of hypertension. Expert Opin Biol Ther 2010;10(7):1077–87.

42. Ruilope LM, Dukat A, Bohm M, et al. Blood-pressure reduction with LCZ696, a novel dual-acting inhibitor of the angiotensin II receptor and neprilysin: a randomised, double-blind, placebo-controlled, active comparator study. Lancet 2010;375(9722): 1255–66.
43. Maurer P, Bachmann MF. Immunization against angiotensins for the treatment of hypertension. Clin Immunol 2010;134(1):89–95.
44. Tissot AC, Maurer P, Nussberger J, et al. Effect of immunisation against angiotensin II with CYT006-AngQb on ambulatory blood pressure: a double-blind, randomised, placebo-controlled phase IIa study. Lancet 2008;371(9615):821–7.
45. Kougias P, Weakley SM, Yao Q, et al. Arterial baroreceptors in the management of systemic hypertension. Med Sci Monit 2010;16(1):RA1–8.
46. Oparil S. The sympathetic nervous system in clinical and experimental hypertension. Kidney Int 1986; 30(3):437–52.
47. Schlaich MP, Krum H, Sobotka PA. Renal sympathetic nerve ablation: the new frontier in the treatment of hypertension. Curr Hypertens Rep 2010; 12(1):39–46.
48. Krum H, Schlaich M, Whitbourn R, et al. Catheter-based renal sympathetic denervation for resistant hypertension: a multicentre safety and proof-of-principle cohort study. Lancet 2009;373(9671):1275–81.

Hypertension in Special Populations: Chronic Kidney Disease, Organ Transplant Recipients, Pregnancy, Autonomic Dysfunction, Racial and Ethnic Populations

John M. Flack, MD, MPH[a,*], Keith C. Ferdinand, MD[b], Samar A. Nasser, PA-C, MPH[a], Noreen F. Rossi, MD[c]

KEYWORDS

• Hypertension • Pregnancy • Baroreceptor reflex
• African American • Organ transplant • Kidney disease

HYPERTENSION AND CHRONIC KIDNEY DISEASE

Hypertension, after diabetes mellitus (DM), is the second leading cause of end-stage renal disease (ESRD) and together these entities account for over 60% of ESRD cases. Moreover, the deleterious impact of elevated blood pressure (BP), particularly systolic BP (SBP), on cardiovascular-renal disease manifests well below conventional BP threshold for hypertension (≥140/90 mm Hg).[1–3]

Renal excretory function (glomerular filtration rate [GFR]) declines 1 to 2 mL/min/y beginning in the third to fourth decade of life. Obesity, a common contributor to both hypertension and DM, plausibly causes and contributes to kidney injury and the decline in renal function. Estimates of chronic kidney disease (CKD) in the United States using the continuous National Health and Nutrition Examination Survey (NHANES) dataset 1999 to 2004 demonstrate that 13% of the population (26.3 million people) had CKD stages 1 to 4.[4] In the NHANES III data, approximately 3% of United States adults (5.6 million people) have elevated levels of serum creatinine, and 70% of this group has concomitant hypertension.[5] Although 75% of persons with CKD receive antihypertensive treatment, only 11% have BP controlled to less than 130/85 mm Hg and only 27% less than 140/90 mm Hg.[5]

Similar to GFR, increased urinary albumin excretion has diagnostic and prognostic value.[6] Random spot urine samples for determination of the albumin/creatinine ratio instead of timed urine collections are now recommended. Microalbuminuria (spot urine albumin/creatinine ratio is between 30 and 200 mg albumin/g creatinine and albumin/creatinine ratio values >200 mg albumin/g creatinine), even if estimated GFR is above 60 mL/min/1.73 m^2, represents CKD. Albuminuria, even within the range of microalbuminuria, is highly informative in individuals with hypertension. Accordingly, albuminuria is a marker for BP, particularly SBP, elevations[7] and similar

[a] Division of Translational Research and Clinical Epidemiology, Department of Medicine, Wayne State University and the Detroit Medical Center, 4201 St Antoine, Suite 2E, Detroit, MI 48201, USA
[b] Cardiology Division, Department of Medicine, Morehouse School of Medicine, Emory University, 1364 Clifton Road North East, Suite F414, Atlanta, GA 30322, USA
[c] Division of Nephrology, Department of Medicine, Wayne State University and the Detroit Medical Center, 4160 John R Street, Suite 908, Detroit, MI 48201, USA
* Corresponding author.
E-mail address: jflack@med.wayne.edu

Cardiol Clin 28 (2010) 623–638
doi:10.1016/j.ccl.2010.07.007
0733-8651/10/$ – see front matter

levels of albuminuria predict pharmacologic resistance to antihypertensive drug therapy.[8] That is, hypertensive patients with albuminuria require more intense antihypertensive therapy to achieve goal BP levels, take longer to attain goal BP levels, and less frequently ever attain goal BP.

The kidney is important in the genesis of hypertension and declining renal function predicts an elevated risk for cardiovascular disease (CVD). The primacy of the kidney in the pathogenesis of essential hypertension has been demonstrated by the cure of hypertension in patients with ESRD after receipt of kidney transplants from normotensive donors.[9]

BP Reduction and CKD

The benefits of appropriate BP control include reductions in proteinuria and a slowing of the progressive loss of kidney function. In individuals with CKD and albuminuria, evidence confirms lowering SBP (110–129 mm Hg) and decreasing urinary albumin excretion ratio (<1 g/d) with angiotensin-converting enzyme inhibitor (ACEI) or angiotensin converting inhibitor–containing regimens protects against ESRD.[10–16] Despite lesser BP lowering efficacy of ACEI as monotherapy in African Americans, the African American Study of Kidney disease and hypertension proved the effectiveness of renin-angiotensin system (RAS) blockade of ramipril in slowing the progressive loss of kidney function in nondiabetic hypertensive nephropathy in blacks.[17] Nevertheless, African Americans with hypertensive CKD achieving a mean BP of 128/78 mm Hg had similar reduction in renal function as those achieving 141/85 mm Hg[18]; possible explanations for lower BP not slowing the progressive loss of kidney function were (1) the cohort had relatively low prevalence of significant proteinuria; (2) the follow-up period was short (<3 years); and (3) BP lowering was of insufficient magnitude. In patients with CKD, necessary hypertension treatment, even if ACEI and angiotensin receptor blocker (ARB) are not used, may lead to a transient rise in serum creatinine. The magnitude of the initial decrease in GFR with ACEI or ARB has actually been linked directly to the subsequently slowing of the loss of renal function.[1] Over-diuresis can potentiate the rise in serum creatinine occurring when RAS blockers are used in patients with CKD.[1] Also, simply lowering BP in patients with CKD contributes to the rise in serum creatinine levels because of disordered autoregulation of glomerular pressure in the setting of reduced nephron mass.

Optimal Antihypertensive Regimens and CKD

Multiple guidelines, including those issued by the American Society of Nephrology and the National Kidney Foundation, along with Joint National Committee-7, recommend for all patients with CKD a goal of less than 130/80 mm Hg.[1,19] In most cases, multiple medications, including an ACEI or ARB, and diuretics are required and with GFR below 30 to 40 mL/min/1.73 m^2, a loop diuretic rather than a thiazide-type diuretic is usually necessary to adequately reach BP goals.

Nevertheless, the necessity of combining a diuretic with an ACEI and ARB to decrease cardiovascular and renal outcomes has been challenged by recent data from 11,506 high-risk patients with hypertension at high risk for cardiovascular events in the Avoiding Cardiovascular Events in Combination Therapy in Patients Living with Systolic Hypertension trial.[20] In addition to a reported 20% decrease in cardiovascular events with benazepril plus amlodipine versus benazepril plus hydrochlorothiazide, there were fewer CKD events (113 [2%] vs 215 [3.7%]) in the benazepril plus hydrochlorothiazide group (hazard ratio [HR] 0.52; 0.41–0.65; P<.0001).[20] The authors concluded that initial antihypertensive treatment, benazepril plus amlodipine, should be considered in preference to benazepril plus hydrochlorothiazide. In the Telmisartan Randomized Assessment Study in ACE Intolerant Subjects With Cardiovascular Disease trial, 5926 ACEI-intolerant adults with CVD or diabetes, but without macroalbuminuria or heart failure, were treated for 4 to 5 years with telmisartan.[21] Telmisartan-treated patients compared with placebo had less proteinuria, but more often experienced doubling of serum creatinine and slight reductions in estimated GFR. Symptomatic hypotension (1% vs 0.5%) and hyperkalemia greater than 5.5 mmol/L (3.8% vs 1.4%) were more common with telmisartan. With few patients developing ESRD that required dialysis, telmisartan did not prevent severe kidney disease more than placebo.

In the Ongoing Telmisartan Alone and in Combination with Ramipril Global Endpoint Trial (ONTARGET), 85% of participants had CVD, 69% had hypertension, and 38% had DM.[22] This trial was the first study to demonstrate comparable renoprotective and cardioprotective effects between an ARB (telmisartan) and ramipril in a large cohort of 25,260 at-risk patients, on top of usual standard care.[22] The primary renal outcome of a composite of dialysis, doubling of serum creatinine, and death was similar for telmisartan (N = 1147 [13.4%]) and ramipril (N = 1150 [13.5%]; HR 1.00; 95% confidence interval [CI], 0.92–1.09), but was higher in the combination therapy group (1233 [14.5%]; HR 1.09; 95% CI, 1.01–1.18; $P = .037$).[22] Although combination therapy reduced proteinuria to a greater extent than monotherapy, there were more adverse renal outcomes and more participant discontinuations because of hypotension.[22]

Nevertheless, for patients with ESRD, preliminary recent data have suggested a unique benefit of ACEI-ARB combination for peritoneal dialysis patients, based on inhibiting the local tissue RAS, and potentially less development of peritoneal fibrosis and a longer life for the peritoneal membrane.[23]

Management of hypertension in the dialysis population should focus on ambulatory measurements of BP and the use of longer-acting antihypertensive drugs, with their dosage and timing adjusted according to their dialytic clearances. Unless contraindicated, ACEIs are indicated for hypertension in patients with autosomal-dominant polycystic kidney disease, in whom diastolic cardiac dysfunction is a prominent feature.

Future Considerations: Hypertension Therapy and CKD

A newer antihypertensive agent, aliskiren, an oral direct renin inhibitor, may contribute to decreasing proteinuria and deterioration of renal function when added to conventional therapy. Aliskiren in the Evaluation of Proteinuria in Diabetes trial studied 599 patients with diabetic nephropathy and proteinuria and a baseline estimated GFR of approximately 68 mL/min/1.73 m^2 and a baseline albumin/creatinine ratio of approximately 500.[24] After losartan, 100 mg daily, in addition to other BP-lowering medications and an average baseline BP of approximately 135/78 mm Hg, patients were randomly assigned to the addition of aliskiren, 300 mg daily, or placebo.[24] The primary outcome of the reduction in the albumin/creatinine ratio in the aliskiren-based treatment was significant. Moreover, when comparing treatment groups, there were minimal differences in BP (−2/1 mm Hg in favor of aliskiren) and no significant differences in adverse event rates.[24] Nonsteroidal anti-inflammatory drugs are widely used for osteoarthritis, a leading cause of physical disability. Both cyclooxygenase-2 inhibitors and traditional nonsteroidal anti-inflammatory drugs can exacerbate, if not cause, hypertension, particularly in patients with CKD. The use of nonsteroidal anti-inflammatory drugs can further reduce glomerular filtration, increase salt and water retention, and augment the likelihood of hyperkalemia, particularly when used with concomitant medications that impair potassium excretion, such as ACEI, heparin, potassium-sparing diuretics, and to a somewhat lesser degree ARBs. Naproxcinod, an investigational cyclooxygenase-inhibiting nitric oxide donator, may lower SBP more so than rofecoxib.[25]

HYPERTENSION AND ORGAN TRANSPLANTATION

The number of new kidney transplants per 1 million people increased 31% between 1997 and 2006 (15.6 per 1 million in 1997 vs 22.2 in 2006).[26] Hypertension is also common among kidney transplant recipients and contributes to graft loss and premature death.

Elevated BP with levels consistent with hypertension is common in patients who have received organ transplants, specifically cardiac and kidney allografts, exceeding 65% of these patients. In kidney transplant recipients, the prevalence of hypertension is 60% to 80%, and despite polytherapy, optimal BP control is not achieved in most patients.[27] Not only is hypertension common, but many individuals posttransplant have nocturnal hypertension with blunted or reversed diurnal BP rhythms. As a result, they may need more specific evaluation including ambulatory BP monitoring.[27]

The cause of increased BP and hypertension in patients with transplantation is of multiple origins including, but not limited to, vasoconstriction, vascular remodeling caused by immunosuppressive drugs, and corticosteroids. To avoid organ rejection, the mandated use of immunosuppressive drugs exposes patients to calcineurin inhibitors. After calcineurin inhibitors, the two drugs used are cyclosporine and tacrolimus, which is the newer agent with an improved profile with respect to hypertension, dyslipidemia, and long-term renal function. In patients with cardiac transplantation and in those who have undergone successful renal transplantation, drug-induced decreases in kidney function and sodium and water retention are important concerns. In some cases, transplant renal artery stenosis may be another contributing factor to hypertension.

Appropriate BP control in patients with cardiac transplantation is necessary to decrease cardiovascular complications and deterioration of graft function in patients with renal transplantation.[27] Large-scale, randomized, controlled trials confirming the renal and cardiovascular benefit of BP control in patients posttransplantation are, however, not available. Nevertheless, considering the risk for cardiovascular events and graft occlusion with renal transplantation, there may be a benefit from lowering BP to less than 130/80 mm Hg. Despite the importance of dietary salt as a contributor to hypertension in the general population, its role in cyclosporine-induced hypertension is minimal, and in tacrolimus-based immunosuppression, no appreciable influence of dietary salt intake on BP has been demonstrated. With measured 24-hour urine sodium excretion as an estimate of intake in a group of stable renal transplant recipients on tacrolimus (N = 143), there was no correlation between urine sodium excretion and either SBP or diastolic BP (DBP) ($R = 0.13$; $R = 0.11$; $P =$ NS).[28] In general, restricting dietary salt intake in these patients is not recommended. The target BP in transplant recipients is the same as in the CKD population, although in this case there is no preference for one class of antihypertensive agents over the other. However, multiple drugs in combination are needed to control BP in almost all patients. Similar to patients with intrinsic renal disease, patients treated with ACEIs or ARBs require close monitoring of serum creatinine and potassium. A greater than 1 dL increase in serum creatinine may indicate the need to investigate for the presence of renal artery stenosis.

Cardiac transplantation is an established intervention for end-stage heart disease and clinical outcomes in older cardiac transplant patients have improved over the last decade, similar to those in younger patients. Nevertheless, there remains significant morbidity and mortality because of infections, cancer, and chronic allograft vasculopathy. Perhaps as many as 95% of the patients with cardiac transplantation have hypertension.[29] A recent study of 253 cardiac transplant patients showed 109 (43%) developed new-onset hypertension, with associated variables including male recipient or donor, idiopathic dilated cardiomyopathy as the indication for transplant, and renal deterioration.[29]

Individualized immunosuppression is now available, modified based on the patient's requirements and problems, including new antibodies for induction therapy; a choice between cyclosporine and tacrolimus; and the advent of mycophenolate mofetil and proliferation signal inhibitors (everolimus, sirolimus).[30] However, compared with cyclosporine, tacrolimus seems to reduce the adverse effect profile for hypertriglyceridemia and renal dysfunction and the need for hypertensive medications.[31] In particular, the lesser propensity of tacrolimus to raise BP and adversely affect lipids may influence the choice between tacrolimus and cyclosporine.[31–34] The weaning of corticosteroids should have a positive impact on BP, osteoporosis, and diabetes. Progression of CKD post–cardiac transplantation can be ameliorated with calcineurin inhibitor–free immunosuppression, including mycophenolate mofetil and proliferation signal inhibitors.[30] Hypertension after pediatric cardiac transplantation is also common and primarily associated with the immunosuppressive regimen. In a study of 51 children 1 year posttransplant, the incidence of hypertension was present in 49%; associated factors included taking significantly more immunosuppressive agents, higher tacrolimus levels, maintenance prednisone therapy, or regimens including sirolimus.[35]

HYPERTENSION IN PREGNANCY

Epidemiology

Hypertension is the most common medical problem encountered during pregnancy, occurring in 6% to 10% of all pregnancies in the United States, of which 70% are first-time pregnancies.[36] Hypertensive disorders in pregnancy are among the leading causes of maternal mortality, along with thromboembolism, hemorrhage, and nonobstetric injuries. Between 1991 and 1999, pregnancy-induced hypertension caused 15.7% of maternal deaths in the United Staes.[37] Although maternal DBP greater than 110 mm Hg is associated with an increased risk for placental abruption and fetal growth restriction, two studies suggest that DBP greater than 85 mm Hg or mean arterial pressures of greater than or equal to 90 mm Hg at any stage of gestation are associated with significantly higher fetal mortality.[38,39] Pressure-related fetal complications include abruptio placentae, intrauterine growth restriction, premature delivery, and intrauterine fetal death. Additionally, hypertension before pregnancy or during early pregnancy is associated with a twofold greater risk of gestational DM.[40]

Physiology of the Pregnant State

During pregnancy there is an increase of plasma-extracellular fluid volume, cardiac output, GFR, renal blood flow, and overall vascular compliance and a marked fall in peripheral vascular resistance. The net effect of these physiologic changes is that BP falls beginning in the first trimester, peaking mid-second trimester (5–10 mm Hg systolic, 10–15 mm Hg diastolic), with a subsequent return to baseline levels by late third trimester.

BP is the product of cardiac output and systemic vascular resistance (SVR; BP = cardiac output × SVR). Despite the large increase in cardiac output, the maternal BP is decreased until later in pregnancy as a result of the relatively greater decrease in SVR that nadirs mid-pregnancy followed by a gradual rise until term.

Nevertheless, even at full term, SVR remains 21% lower than prepregnancy values in pregnancies unaffected by gestational hypertension or preeclampsia.[41] Plausible contributors to the decreased SVR are progesterone-mediated smooth muscle relaxation and raised nitric oxide, which blunts vascular responsiveness to potent vasoconstrictors, such as angiotensin II and norepinephrine.

BP Measurement

Accurate measurement of BP is required to determine the true level of BP and to correctly diagnose hypertension. In pregnant women BP should be measured after several minutes of rest in the seated position with the legs uncrossed with the arm being used for measurement stationary heart level. The fifth-phase Korotkoff sound should be used to determine the DBP. The definition of hypertension is SBP greater than or equal to 140 or DBP greater than or equal to 90 mm Hg that is confirmed over two readings separated by at least 4 to 6 hours.[36,42] Even though the change in BP from prepregnancy levels is no longer in the definition of hypertension in pregnancy, women experiencing a rise in SBP greater than 30 mm Hg or DBP greater than 15 mm Hg, despite absolute BP levels less than 140/90 mm Hg, should be considered high-risk patients.[36]

Chronic Hypertension

Chronic hypertension antedating the onset of gestation increases the risk of fetal, neonatal, and maternal morbidity. During pregnancy BP normally falls starting early in the first trimester reaching a nadir around 20 weeks gestation. The early fall in BP can mask the detection of chronic or pre-existing hypertension during the first half of pregnancy. The prevalence of hypertension in premenopausal women is close to 25% in whites and 30% in blacks and increases over time with age. Approximately 2% to 5% of pregnancies are complicated by chronic hypertension.[43]

Chronic hypertension is defined as BP greater than or equal to 140/90 mm Hg before pregnancy or before 20 weeks gestation or persisting longer than 12 weeks postpartum. When hypertension is first identified at less than 20 weeks gestation, the BP elevations usually represent chronic hypertension. In contrast, new onset of elevated BP after 20 weeks gestation mandates the consideration and exclusion of preeclampsia.

Preeclampsia and Ecclampsia

Preeclampsia is the new onset of hypertension and proteinuria after 20 weeks gestation, with SBP greater than or equal to 140/90 mm Hg, and proteinuria of 0.3 g or greater in a 24-hour urine specimen or a spot urine protein:creatinine ratio greater than 0.3. The appearance of proteinuria of this magnitude may, however, be a late occurrence. Thus, preeclampsia should be suspected when late-onset hypertension is accompanied by such symptoms as headache; abdominal pain; or abnormal laboratory tests, such as low platelets or abnormal liver function tests. Preeclampsia occurs in up to 5% of all pregnancies, in 10% of first pregnancies, and in 20% to 25% of women with a history of chronic hypertension and tends to occur near the time of delivery with a predilection for nulliparas. Preeclampsia is more common at the extremes of maternal age (<18 years and >35 years). The increased prevalence of preeclampsia in older women is much more striking than in younger women. This observation, in all likelihood, is attributable to the higher prevalence of chronic hypertension and other comorbid medical illnesses (eg, diabetes) that significantly augment the risk for preeclampsia.

There are several classifications of preeclampsia: (1) mild preeclampsia; (2) severe preeclampsia; and (3) eclampsia (occurrence of generalized convulsion or coma in the setting of preeclampsia, with no other neurologic condition). Severe preeclampsia must have one of the following manifestations listed in **Box 1**. Preeclampsia at less than 34 weeks gestation also has worse outcomes than when its onset is nearer the time of delivery.[44] Nevertheless, preeclampsia can rapidly progress to the onset of convulsions even in women without "severe" preeclampsia or in preeclampsia that appears near the time of delivery. Therefore, the stratification of preeclampsia by severity and time of onset can be somewhat misleading. Observations from the Women in Child Health Development Studies in Pregnancy cohort show that women with preeclampsia have significantly increased long-term CVD risk.[45] In this study median follow-up was 37 years. Observed preeclampsia was independently associated with CVD death (HR = 2.14; 95% CI, 2.14–3.57); however, if preeclampsia occurred by 34 weeks gestation, the risk for CVD death was strikingly higher (HR = 9.54; 95% CI, 9.54–20.26).

There is some understanding of the pathophysiologic mechanisms involved in preeclampsia. Preeclampsia is primarily a disorder of placental dysfunction leading to a syndrome of endothelial dysfunction with associated vasospasm. Pathologic examination of the placenta has shown multiple placental abnormalities: (1) diffuse placental thrombosis, (2) an inflammatory placental endometrium vasculopathy, or (3) abnormal

Box 1
Characteristics of severe preeclampsia

Symptoms of central nervous system dysfunction: blurred vision, scotomata, altered mental status, severe headache

Symptoms of liver capsule distention: right upper quadrant or epigastric pain

Nausea, vomiting

Hepatocellular injury: serum transaminase concentration at least twice normal

Severe BP elevation: systolic BP $\geq$160 mm Hg or diastolic $\geq$110 mm Hg on two occasions at least 6 hours apart

Thrombocytopenia: <100,000 platelets per cubic millimeter

Proteinuria: $\geq$5 g in 24 hours

Oliguria: <500 mL in 24 hours

Severe fetal growth restriction

Pulmonary edema or cyanosis

Cerebrovascular accident

trophoblastic invasion of the endometrium. There is also evidence supporting an altered maternal immune response to fetal and placental tissue as contributing to the development of preeclampsia. Thus, preeclampsia is a multidimensional disease affecting both the placenta and the maternal circulation.[46,47] Preeclampsia involves dysfunction of multiple organ systems, including the central nervous, hepatic, pulmonary, renal, and hematologic systems. Endothelial damage leads to a pathologic capillary leak that can cause the pregnant woman with preeclampsia to manifest rapid weight gain; nondependent edema (face or hands); pulmonary edema; or hemoconcentration. The diseased placenta can also negatively impact the fetus by decreased uteroplacental blood flow. Progression to eclamptic seizures is typically, although not invariably, preceded by warning signs (eg, headache, visual disturbances, epigastric pain, hyperreflexia) and tend to occur near the time of delivery or immediately postpartum (within 48 hours of delivery).

The hypertension occurring in preeclampsia occurs with arterial constriction and relatively lower intravascular volume compared with normal pregnancy. The vasculature of normal pregnant women typically demonstrates decreased responsiveness to vasoactive peptides, such as angiotensin II and epinephrine. In contrast, women with preeclampsia actually manifest hyperresponsiveness to these hormones, an alteration that may precede BP elevations and other systemic manifestations of preeclampsia. In addition, BP in preeclampsia is labile and normal circadian BP rhythms may be either blunted or reversed. One study found increased arterial stiffness in women with preeclampsia, and in those with gestational hypertension, compared with normotensive controls; treatment with methyldopa significantly improved but did not normalize the vascular stiffness in preeclampsia.[48]

Appropriate management of preeclampsia is critically important for both the health of the mother and the baby. Confirmed or suspected preeclampsia necessitates hospitalization because this condition can rapidly progress and deteriorate. The only known definitive cure for preeclampsia is delivery. However, it is reasonable to continue the gestation in women with preeclampsia as BP is controlled and there are no worrisome signs, such as declining kidney function; clotting or liver abnormalities; or signs of imminent convulsions (headache, epigastric pain, hyperreflexia).[44]

Preeclampsia Superimposed on Chronic Hypertension

Approximately 15% to 25% of women with chronic hypertension in pregnancy develop superimposed preeclampsia.[43] Superimposed preeclampsia is a major contributor to the excess maternal and fetal risk that has been observed in women with chronic hypertension. Superimposed preeclampsia is most often diagnosed late in gestation.

Gestational Hypertension

Gestational hypertension is the onset of hypertension after 20 weeks gestation without proteinuria. BP elevations attributable to gestational hypertension should, however, normalize within 12 weeks of delivery. Approximately one third of women initially diagnosed with gestational hypertension (or transient hypertension of pregnancy) eventually satisfy the diagnostic criteria for preeclampsia. This ominous evolution more often occurs when hypertension develops before 30 weeks gestation. Maternal and fetal outcomes are usually normal in pregnancies complicated by gestational hypertension. Nevertheless, gestational hypertension may also indicate a higher risk for chronic hypertension later in life. Risk factors for the occurrence of hypertension in pregnancy are displayed in **Box 2**.

Hypertension Treatment During Pregnancy

In cases of mild, low-risk hypertension, there are no definitive data to support a benefit from the short-term use of antihypertensive drugs.[49,50] There is very clear benefit, however, in reducing the progression to severe hypertension with antihypertensive

Box 2
Factors impacting the occurrence of hypertension in pregnancy

- Nulliparity
- Preeclampsia in a previous pregnancy
- Age >40 years or <8 years
- Family history of pregnancy-induced hypertension
- Chronic hypertension
- Chronic renal disease
- Antiphospholipid antibody syndrome or inherited thrombophilia
- Vascular or connective tissue disease
- DM (pregestational and gestational)
- Multifetal gestation
- High body mass index
- Male partner whose previous partner had preeclampsia
- Hydrops fetalis
- Unexplained fetal growth restriction

drug therapy; there is a 50% reduction in the incidence of severe hypertension.[51] Severe, uncontrolled hypertension during pregnancy may worsen end-organ damage in those with preexisting conditions, such as renal disease, cardiac dysfunction (ie, left ventricular hypertrophy), or DM complicated by vascular disease.[52,53] There is, however, no convincing evidence that antihypertensive therapy reduces the risk of superimposed preeclampsia or placental abruption.[54] There is also no evidence that antihypertensive drug therapy improves fetal outcomes. Thus, the most important considerations when instituting antihypertensive drug therapy is maternal safety balanced against drug exposure risks to the fetus.

Both the American College of Gynecology and the National High Blood Pressure Education Program recommend initiating antihypertensive therapy when the systolic pressures reach levels of 150 to 160 mm Hg or higher or diastolic pressures 100 to 110 mm Hg or when there is elevated BP (above conventional BP thresholds) in the presence of pressure-related target-organ injury (eg, left ventricular hypertrophy, CKD).[36,42,44] The normal decline in BP though mid-trimester may allow some women with chronic hypertension to be safely withdrawn from pharmacologic antihypertensive therapy during pregnancy. In this situation, the BP must, however, be continuously monitored.

Although uncommonly used in the nonpregnant population, methyldopa, a centrally acting agent that reduces sympathetic outflow from the central nervous system, is first-line antihypertensive therapy in pregnant patients.[36,42] The wide use of this drug in pregnancy is based on the well-documented maternal and fetal safety record and the favorable long-term pediatric follow-up data.[55] Importantly, methyldopa does not alter maternal cardiac output or blood flow to the uterus or kidneys.[55] There are, however, several caveats to consider when using methyldopa. First, methyldopa is relatively short-acting necessitating that it be dosed three to four times daily. Second, long-term methyldopa use may cause salt and water retention that can attenuate the BP lowering effect, which can be restored by simultaneous use of diuretics.[56] Finally, uptitration to higher doses may lead to an increase in central nervous system–related side effects.

Labetalol, a combined α- and β-blocker, is a good alternative to methyldopa as a first-line antihypertensive agent.[57,58] In women with mild chronic hypertension, data from studies demonstrated no deleterious effects from the use of either methyldopa or labetalol.[59] In a randomized comparative trial of 263 pregnant women between 6 and 13 weeks gestation with mild to moderate hypertension, treatment with either labetalol or methyldopa achieved significantly lower maternal BPs throughout gestation compared with no medication, although there were no differences among the three groups with respect to various clinical outcomes (eg, gestational age at delivery, birth weight, fetal growth retardation).[60] However, because the safety record of labetalol in pregnancy is not as well established as that of methyldopa, it is considered a second-line antihypertensive agent. Use of the cardioselective β-blocker atenolol early in pregnancy in women with chronic hypertension has been shown to result in significantly lower birthweights compared with placebo and other antihypertensive agents.[61] The results of these and other studies indicate that treatment with atenolol is associated with fetal growth impairment and that this effect is related to duration of therapy.[61,62] Thus, atenolol should be avoided in early pregnancy and used only with caution in later pregnancy.

Nifedipine (a calcium-channel blocker) is another antihypertensive medication commonly used during pregnancy. When administered in late pregnancy, oral calcium antagonists have been shown to reduce maternal BP in pregnant women with mild to moderate hypertension, including those with preeclampsia, without apparent adverse fetal or perinatal effects.[55] However, little is known about the effects of long-term administration of these drugs in pregnant women, particularly in the first trimester. Among the calcium antagonists, nifedipine has been the most studied agent in pregnancy, although most of its use has been in the later stages of gestation. Hydralazine, a vasodilator often used intravenously to acutely control hypertension, can also be used orally for maintenance therapy as a second- or third-line agent. Possible side effects include a lupus-like syndrome, headache, palpitations, and tachycardia. Oral hydralazine is effective as monotherapy or as add-on therapy to methyldopa in the long-term management of chronic hypertension in pregnancy. Hydralazine seems to be reasonably safe for the fetus, although a few cases of fetal thrombocytopenia have been reported. In general, effective long-term antihypertensive therapy with hydralazine (ie, for chronic hypertension in pregnancy) often requires combination therapy (typically with a sympatholytic agent, such as methyldopa or a β-blocker) and such combinations also help attenuate reflex sympathetic activation associated with this agent.

The use of diuretics during pregnancy has been somewhat controversial.[58] Often used to treat chronic mild hypertension in nongravid women, these drugs are frequently discontinued during pregnancy.[19] Diuretics can attenuate the normal plasma volume expansion occurring during pregnancy. Diuretics should be regarded as a second- or third-line option. In the setting of fetal growth restriction or superimposed preeclampsia, diuretics should be discontinued immediately because of their ability to lower plasma volume and uteroplacental perfusion.[63] Edema in patients with nephropathy may sometimes be treated throughout pregnancy with diuretics, provided volume status is monitored. With regard to teratogenicity, hypospadias has been linked to first-trimester furosemide exposure, and neonatal thrombocytopenia may be associated with third-trimester use of thiazides. Overall, the data do not suggest an increased risk of congenital anomalies or adverse perinatal outcomes associated with first-trimester diuretic use.[58,59]

ACEIs and ARBs have teratogenic potential in both the first and second trimesters, and should be discontinued immediately once pregnancy is confirmed. Moreover, these drugs (and direct renin inhibitors) should be avoided in women of childbearing potential who are not using effective contraception. One study demonstrated a possible association between first-trimester ACEI use and congenital anomalies, specifically cardiac and central nervous system malformations.[64] In the second trimester, ACEIs are associated with renal failure, which can result in oligohydramnios, limb contractures, and lung hypoplasia. As a general rule, if a patient becomes pregnant and is already using an antihypertensive drug that provides adequate BP control, it is reasonable to continue this medication during the pregnancy, with the exception of ACEIs, ARBs, atenolol, and direct renin inhibitors.

There is no clear consensus on the management of mild to moderate hypertension in pregnancy to optimize pregnancy outcomes. Overall, medication therapy to lower BP during pregnancy should be used mainly for maternal safety because of the lack of data to support an improvement in fetal outcome. Nevertheless, national hypertension guidelines list methyldopa, labetalol, and long-acting nifedipine as acceptable oral antihypertensive agents if drug therapy is required in pregnant women with mild to moderate hypertension.[36]

BARORECEPTOR DYSFUNCTION AND FAILURE AND HYPERTENSION

Autonomic failure and baroreceptor failure are distinctly different entities, although they have sometimes been discussed as if they were synonymous. The focus here is almost exclusively on baroreceptor failure, the more common of the two conditions.

In normal individuals the baroreceptor reflex arc responds to increases in BP that stretch baroreceptors in the aortic arch, carotid sinuses, and the great vessels of the thorax. The afferents from these stretch-sensitive baroreceptors join the afferent (glossopharyngeal and vagus) nerves and along with cortical input by other afferent nerves send signals to the nucleus tractus solitarii in the dorsal medullary brainstem resulting in decreased sympathetic and greater parasympathetic efferent nervous system outflow to the vasculature and heart. The net result is a decrease in heart rate, contractility, and vascular resistance resulting in lower BP. A drop in BP resulting in less distention of the baroreceptors has the opposite effect. Nonselective baroreceptor failure occurs as a consequence of damage to either the afferent or efferent nerves in the baroreceptor reflex arc.

The acute and chronic clinical presentations of baroreceptor failure are displayed in **Box 3**. Common causes of baroreceptor failure include neck trauma or surgery, carotid endartectomy, and neck irradiation. Moreover, brainstem infarction or other pathology affecting the nucleus tractus solitarii can also result in baroreceptor failure.[65,66] Patients with acute baroreceptor failure after neck surgery may experience abrupt and severe rises in BP, extreme BP lability, and apneic spells attributable to loss of carotid body

Box 3
Clinical presentations in baroreceptor failure

Acute
- Strikingly high BP elevations
- Tachycardia
- Headache

Subacute and chronic
- Volatile hypertension
  - Severe BP elevations after physical/emotional stress, pain, or exercise
  - Low early morning BP
  - BP–pulse dissociation
- Intermittent tachycardia
- Decreased respiratory sinus arrhythmia
- Intermittent episodes of
  - Diaphoresis
  - Irritability
  - Headache
  - Anxiety
- BP is exquisitely volume sensitive
- BP is highly sensitive to vasoactive drugs

input.[66] Tachycardia, paroxysms of severe arterial hypertension, flushing, headache, diaphoresis, and emotional lability that resemble the clinical presentation of pheochromocytoma may also occur.[65] Over the long-term, however, BP tends to decline in acute baroreceptor failure patients. The onset of baroceptor failure tends to be more insidious, however, in those who have undergone neck irradiation occurring over months to years. Nevertheless, extremely labile hypertension is a common presentation of subacute to chronic nonselective (involves sympathetic and parasympathetic nerve fibers) baroreceptor failure.[66]

Pathophysiology of Extreme BP Readings

In baroreceptor failure the reflex arc through the dorsal medullary brainstem that modulates sympathetic and parasympathetic nervous system tone in response to vascular baroreceptor input has been functionally isolated from such input. Nevertheless, the cortical inputs remain intact explaining how emotional upset, physical exertion, or pain can lead to strikingly high BP elevations. These BP spikes are dependent on high synaptic concentrations of norepinephrine in the periphery. Catecholamine levels may be elevated to levels similar to those observed in pheochromocytoma.[67] Conversely, in the early morning when cortical inputs are minimal, BP can fall to very low levels.

Medication Sensitivity in Baroreceptor Failure

The norepinephrine transporter is responsible for approximately 80% to 90% of the norepinephrine removal from the synapse.[68] Tricyclic antidepressants, commonly used antidepressants that inhibit this transporter, may impressively raise BP in individuals with baroreceptor failure, as can cocaine and amphetamines.[69] For obvious reasons, monoamine oxidase inhibitors should also be avoided in patients with baroreceptor failure. Over-the-counter medications, dietary supplements, and tyramine-containing foods and beverages can also raise BP significantly in patients with baroreceptor failure.[69]

Patients with baroreceptor failure are exquisitely volume sensitive in both directions. For example, when treated with diuretics individuals may develop orthostatic hypotension, which is not a common clinical finding in baroreceptor failure. BP may rise dramatically during intravascular volume expansion. Additionally, arterial (eg, calcium antagonists) and mixed arterial-venous dilators (eg, nitrates, ACEIs) may precipitate dizziness, orthostatic hypotension, and prominent drops in BP.

Suspecting Baroreceptor Failure on Clinical Grounds

The clinician can have a very high index of suspicion of baroreceptor failure in patients with prior neck surgery or irradiation who present with widely fluctuating BP readings that are very low in the early morning. In addition, prominent BP elevations during or after emotional upset or excitement are also consistent with the diagnosis of baroreceptor failure. On 24-hour ambulatory BP monitoring there is a lesser correlation between the BP and pulse than is typically observed; also, BP variability (standard deviation) is significantly higher than normal. Clues may also be obtained from serial home BP readings taking in the early morning hours and throughout the day and during or after emotional upset. The pattern of readings is very low in the early morning and highly variable, similar to the pattern observed during 24-hour ambulatory BP monitoring. Although orthostatic hypotension is not a common clinical feature of baroreceptor failure, some patients may show a paradoxic rise in BP when assuming upright posture.[70] Beat-to-beat BP variability is reduced during deep breathing and Valsalva maneuver. The rise in heart rate and BP during isometric hand grip or cold pressor testing is usually normal to increased, however, because the sympathetic efferent fibers to the heart and vasculature are intact.[65,71]

Pharmacologic Diagnosis of Baroreceptor Failure

In general, the absence of a bradycardic response to pressor agents or the absence of a tachycardic response to vasodilators is highly consistent with, but not sufficient for, the diagnosis of baroreceptor failure.[65] It must be remembered that patients with baroreceptor failure are very sensitive to vasoactive agents. A dose of phenylephrine (12.5 μg) sufficient to increase BP by 20 mm Hg should lead to a 7 to 21 beats per minute reduction in heart rate. A dose of nitroprusside (0.1 μg/kg/min) that lowers BP by 20 mm Hg should increase heart rate by 9 to 28 beats per minute.[65] Patients with baroreceptor failure tend to show pulse changes of less than 4 beats per minute of directionally appropriate pulse change during these provocative tests.

Treatment of Hypertension in Baroreceptor Failure

The nonpharmacologic and pharmacologic treatment of hypertension or BP elevations in patients with baroreceptor failure is not entirely straightforward or intuitive. For example, dietary sodium restriction, a staple of nonpharmacologic treatment in most hypertensive patients, often needs to be avoided; it may be necessary for patients to upwardly adjust their intake of dietary sodium. Also, two of the most effective antihypertensive drug types (diuretics and vasodilators) are potentially problematic when prescribed to the patient with baroreceptor failure. Accordingly, these agents must be prescribed at very low doses with diligent patient monitoring for iatrogenic side effects if they are to be used at all. Again, the major goal of hypertension treatment is to avoid the precipitous, severe BP elevations that can occur during emotional stimulation. Two centrally acting sympatholytic drugs, clonidine and α-methyldopa, may be useful for this purpose. The sedative effect of these drugs is also a plus given the potential of this effect to modulate emotion-driven severe elevations in BP. Heusser and colleagues[72] have, however, speculated that the clonidine patch may be less effective than oral clonidine in these patients because of cutaneous vasoconstriction attributable to sympathetic activation. Other antiadrenergic drugs may also be useful including α-blockers, β-blockers, and α-β blockers. Anxiolytic agents, such as benzodiazepines, may also be useful, especially during the acute phase of baroreceptor failure, because BP elevations are significantly driven by cortical influences.

HYPERTENSION IN AFRICAN AMERICANS

Hypertension in African Americans is a major clinical and public health problem that contributes significantly to premature morbidity and mortality and to the shorter lifespan in African Americans compared with whites. Higher BP readings in African Americans than in whites have been documented early in life beginning in childhood.[73] Non-Hispanic black men (44.4%) and women (43.9%) have the highest age-adjusted prevalence of hypertension among the three major race-ethnicity groups in the United States.[74] Although African Americans have often been labeled as having the highest hypertension rates in the world, they do not, because adults in Spain, Finland, and Germany all have higher age-adjusted hypertension prevalence.[75]

Hypertension awareness rates are higher in African American women (81.8%) than in any of the major race-gender groups in the United States; they are roughly equivalent in African American (67.8%) and white men (70.4%).[76] Hypertension treatment rates are again higher in African American women (71.4%) than white women; African American men, however, have slightly lower treatment rates than white men (56.4% vs 60%). BP control rates (<140/90 mm Hg) remain too low in populations, and are lowest in African American men (29.9%). Nevertheless, control rates have improved most dramatically in African American men over the last several decades. Finally, still fewer than 50% of drug-treated African American hypertensives have controlled BP.[77]

Ambulatory BP Patterns

Twenty-four–hour ambulatory BP recordings can be highly informative because they more accurately predict CVD risk than office cuff BP determinations. Nighttime BP levels that are 10% to 20% lower than daytime levels reflect normal diurnal variation in BP. It is certainly plausible that this normal nocturnal decline or dipping in BP is "healthy" for the vasculature and pressure-sensitive target organs. African Americans more often than whites manifest a nondipping ambulatory BP pattern,[78] which may contribute to the inordinate amounts of injury to pressure-sensitive target-organs that has been repeatedly documented in African Americans. Although it is intuitively appealing to postulate that nondipping causes target-organ injury, there are also data supporting the thesis that nondipping of ambulatory BP may also be a consequence of pressure-sensitive target injury.

Nondipping ambulatory BP is not invariably linked to African American race because obesity, salt sensitivity, low dietary potassium intake, high dietary sodium intake, CKD, and sleep-disordered breathing, most of which are excessively prevalent in African Americans, have all been linked to a blunted nocturnal decline in BP.[79]

Salt Sensitivity

Salt sensitivity can be conceptualized as a rise in BP occurring during sodium loading or a fall in BP during sodium restriction that exceeds directionally appropriate random fluctuations in BP. Salt sensitivity is a very practical concern given the nearly ubiquitous intake of dietary sodium by African Americans that is far in excess of any known physiologic need. Even those African Americans with BP in the normal range have typically been found to manifest more salt sensitivity than whites.[80] The observations of greater salt sensitivity in African Americans fueled much speculation, with scant empiric evidence, that African Americans had an expansion of the intravascular fluid compartment. More recent observations suggest that salt sensitivity represents a complex manifestation of the interplay between dietary intake of sodium and potassium, baroreceptor responses or lack thereof to the transient volume expansion occurring during high sodium intake, the peripheral vasculature, and renal sodium excretory capacity. An aberrant vascular response (vasoconstriction) to dietary sodium loading and transient volume expansion in both the renal[81] and peripheral vasculature[82] is present in African Americans manifesting salt sensitivity. Importantly, it is imperative to appreciate that African Americans are not invariably salt sensitive. Moreover, factors linked to salt sensitivity include obesity, low dietary potassium intake, CKD, diabetes, and older age. High levels of dietary potassium intake have been shown to abolish salt sensitivity.[81]

Subclinical Vascular Dysfunction

African Americans (even those with "normal" BP levels) have more evidence of subclinical microvascular and macrovascular dysfunction and anatomic abnormalities than their white counterparts.[83–88] Normotensive, healthy young African Americans have higher carotid and central aortic BP and more stiffness of these vessels than whites.[83] Moreover, these abnormalities are not reflected in the peripheral brachial arteries, the anatomic site of most clinic BP determinations. The functional vascular abnormalities in African Americans are both endothelium-dependent and independent[85,86] and correlate with lesser ability of the resistance

Table 1
Treatment goals according to risk category or stratum

Risk Category	Recommended Treatment	Goal BP, mm Hg
Primary prevention BP ≥135/85 mm Hg without target-organ damage,[b] preclinical CVD,[c] or CVD[d]	Lifestyle modification[a] (up to 3 months without drugs) + drug therapy	<135/85
Secondary prevention/ target-organ damage[b,c,d] BP ≥130/80 mm Hg with target-organ damage,[b] preclinical CVD,[c] or the presence of CVD[d]	Lifestyle modification + drug therapy	<130/80

Abbreviations: BP, blood pressure; CVD, cardiovascular disease.

[a] Up to 3 months of comprehensive lifestyle modification without drugs if BP is <145/90 mm Hg without target-organ damage or other risk-enhancing comorbidities.

[b] Target-organ damage is defined as albumin:creatinine ratio >200 mg/g, estimated glomerular filtration rate <60 mL/min/1.73 m², or electrocardiographic or echocardiographic evidence of left ventricular hypertrophy.

[c] Indicators of preclinical CVD include metabolic syndrome; Framingham risk score >20%; prediabetes (impaired fasting glucose [100–125 mg/dL] or impaired glucose tolerance [2-h postload glucose ≥140 mg/dL]); or diabetes mellitus.

[d] CVD includes heart failure (systolic or diastolic); coronary heart disease/postmyocardial infarction; peripheral arterial disease; stroke; transient ischemic attack; or abdominal aortic aneurysm.

From Flack JM, Sica DA, Bakris G, et al. International Society on Hypertension in Blacks (ISHIB) consensus statement on the treatment of hypertension in African Americans. Hypertension, in press; with permission.

vessels to dilate in response to dilatory stimuli. A plausible effect of higher central BP leads to exposure of the heart and cerebral vessels to a higher pressure load, predisposing these structures to injury despite relatively normal-appearing brachial pressures.

Pressure-related Target Organ Injury

African Americans with hypertension have markedly more CVD-renal pressure-related target-organ damage (retinopathy, stroke, left ventricular hypertrophy and heart failure, CKD) than whites.[74,89–91] The excessive prevalence of

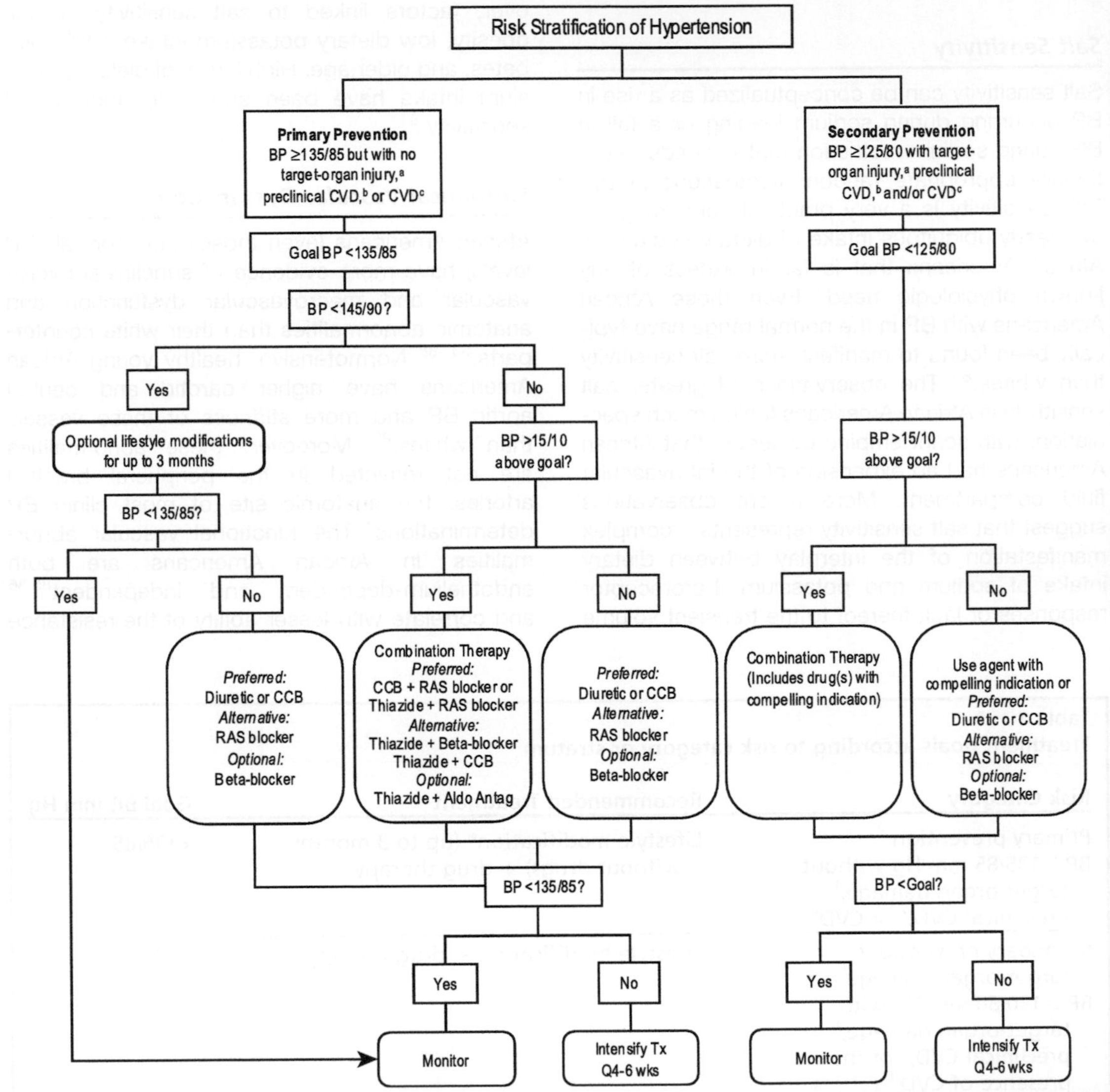

Fig. 1. Risk stratification and treatment algorithm for African Americans with hypertension. Aldo Antag, aldosterone antagonist; BP, blood pressure; CCB, calcium channel blocker; CVD, cardiovascular disease; RAS, renin-angiotensin system; Tx, treatment. [a] Target organ damage is defined as albumin:creatinine ratio >200 mg/g, estimated glomerular filtration rate <60 mL/min/1.73 m^2, or electrocardiographic or echocardiographic evidence of left ventricular hypertrophy. [b] Indicators of preclinical CVD include metabolic syndrome; Framingham risk score >20%; prediabetes (impaired fasting glucose [100–125 mg/dL] or impaired glucose tolerance [2-h postload glucose ≥140 mg/dL]); or diabetes mellitus. [c] CVD includes heart failure (systolic or diastolic); coronary heart disease/postmyocardial infarction; peripheral arterial disease; stroke; transient ischemic attack; or abdominal aortic aneurysm. (*From* Flack JM, Sica DA, Bakris G, et al. International Society on Hypertension in Blacks (ISHIB) consensus statement on the treatment of hypertension in African Americans. Hypertension, in press; with permission.)

target-organ damage in African Americans, in all likelihood, is a consequence of BP elevations of longer duration, a much higher prevalence of severe hypertension greater than or equal to 180/110 mm Hg, lesser long-term BP control, and higher rates of concurrent risk-augmenting comorbidities, such as DM. Not only are manifestations of target-organ injury, such as left ventricular hypertrophy, albuminuria, and depressed estimated GFR, likely caused by long-term BP elevations, but these comorbidities also confer resistance to pharmacologic BP lowering thereby contributing to the long-term BP elevations.[7,8,92,93]

Renin Angiotensin System

There has been pervasive and erroneous interpretations of the tendency toward lower circulating renin levels, along with the lesser average reductions in BP to monotherapy RAS antagonist drugs (eg, ACEIs) compared with diuretics, as indicative of relative inactivity of the RAS system in African Americans. Nevertheless, the low circulating renin levels have been linked to augmented vascular production of angiotensin II[94] and normotensive, healthy African Americans have been shown to have greater not lesser activation of the RAS system.[95]

Pharmacologic blockade of the RAS system (eg, ACEIs, ARBs) in African Americans has consistently lowered BP less on average than monotherapy with diuretics or calcium antagonists. Nevertheless, compared with RAS monotherapy responses in whites, the lesser average group BP lowering in African Americans simply represents a shift in the central tendency of the overall BP response distribution with which it mostly overlaps.[96,97] The spread of BP responses within each racial group is much greater than the between-race mean BP responses. Monotherapy responses to any drug class, however, including RAS antagonists, is not terribly important given that most African American (and white) hypertensives need combination drug therapy; there is no racial difference in BP response when a RAS antagonist is combined with either a diuretic or calcium channel blocker.

Treatment

The treatment of hypertension in African Americans should be a combined approach using comprehensive lifestyle modifications (weight loss, salt and alcohol restriction, increased physical activity as appropriate) along with pharmacologic treatments. **Table 1** displays the risk stratification scheme and target BP levels for African American hypertensives from the new International Society on Hypertension in Blacks Consensus Statement on the Treatment of Hypertension in African Americans.[98] It is also noteworthy that the in the lowest risk stratum, the primary prevention group, that BP consistently greater than or equal to 135/85 mm Hg is considered hypertensive. **Fig. 1** displays the treatment algorithm. Examples of drugs with compelling indications include β-blockers in the patient with systolic heart failure.

REFERENCES

1. Available at: http://www.kidney.org/professionals/KDOQI/guidelines_bp/index.htm. Accessed March 19, 2010.
2. Manjunath G, Tighiouart H, Coresh J, et al. Level of kidney function as a risk factor for atherosclerotic cardiovascular outcomes in the community. J Am Coll Cardiol 2003;41:47–55.
3. Franklin SS, Jacobs MJ, Wong ND, et al. Predominance of isolated systolic hypertension among middle-aged and elderly US hypertensives: analysis based on National Health and Nutrition Examination Survey (NHANES) III. Hypertension 2001;37:869–74.
4. Snyder JJ, Foley RN, Collins AJ. Prevalence of CKD in the United States: a sensitivity analysis using the National Health and Nutrition Examination Survey (NHANES) 1999–2004. Am J Kidney Dis 2009;53(2):218–28.
5. Coresh J, Wei GL, McQuillan G, et al. Prevalence of high blood pressure and elevated serum creatinine level in the United States: findings from the Third National Health and Nutrition Examination Survey (1988–1994). Arch Intern Med 2001;161:1207–16.
6. Hillege HL, Fidler V, Diercks GF, et al. Urinary albumin excretion predicts cardiovascular and noncardiovascular mortality in general population. Circulation 2002;106:1777–82.
7. Flack JM, Duncan K, Ohmit SE, et al. Influence of albuminuria and glomerular filtration rate on blood pressure response to antihypertensive drug therapy. Vasc Health Risk Manag 2007;3(6):1029–37.
8. Nasser SA, Lai Z, O'Connor S, et al. Does earlier attainment of blood pressure goal translate into fewer cardiovascular events? Curr Hypertens Rep 2008;10(5):398–404.
9. Weir MR. Hypertension and the kidney: perspectives on the relationship of kidney disease and cardiovascular disease. Clin J Am Soc Nephrol 2009;4(12):2045–50.
10. Jafar TH, Schmid CH, Landa M, et al. Angiotensin-converting enzyme inhibitors and progression of nondiabetic renal disease. A meta-analysis of patient-level data. Ann Intern Med 2001;135:73–87.
11. Jafar TH, Stark PC, Schmid CH, et al. Progression of chronic kidney disease: the role of blood pressure

control, proteinuria, and agniotensin-converting enzyme inhibition: a patient-level meta-analysis. Ann Intern Med 2003;139:244–52.
12. Brenner BM, Cooper ME, de Zeeuw D, et al. Effects of losartan on renal and cardiovascular outcomes in patients with type 2 diabetes and nephropathy. N Engl J Med 2001;345:861–9.
13. Randomised placebo-controlled trial of effect of ramipril on decline in glomerular filtration rate and risk of terminal renal failure in proteinuric, non-diabetic nephropathy. The GISEN Group (Gruppo Italiano di Studi Epidemiologici in Nefrologia). Lancet 1997;349:1857–63.
14. Hoogwerf BJ. Renin-angiotensin system blockade and cardiovascular and renal protection. Am J Cardiol 2010;105(Suppl 1):30A–5A.
15. Lewis EJ, Hunsicker LG, Bain RP, et al. The effect of angiotensin-converting-enzyme inhibition on diabetic nephropathy. The Collaborative Study Group. N Engl J Med 1993;329:1456–62.
16. Lewis EJ, Hunsicker LG, Clarke WR, et al. Renoprotective effect of the angiotensin-receptor antagonist irbesartan in patients with nephropathy due to type 2 diabetes. N Engl J Med 2001;345:851–60.
17. Wright JT, Bakris G, Greene T Jr, et al. Effect of blood pressure lowering and antihypertensive drug class on progression of hypertensive kidney disease: results from the AASK trial. JAMA 2002; 288:2421–31.
18. Wright JT Jr, Agodoa L, Contreras G, et al. Successful blood pressure control in the African American Study of Kidney Disease and Hypertension. Arch Intern Med 2002;162:1636–43.
19. Chobanian AV, Bakris GL, Black HR, et al. The Seventh Report of the Joint National Committee on prevention, detection, evaluation, and treatment of high blood pressure: the JNC 7 report. JAMA 2003;289:2560–72.
20. Bakris GL, Sarafidis PA, Weir MR, et al. Renal outcomes with different fixed-dose combination therapies in patients with hypertension at high risk for cardiovascular events (ACCOMPLISH): a prespecified secondary analysis of a randomized controlled trial. Lancet 2010;375(9721):1173–81.
21. Mann JF, Schmieder RE, Dyal L, et al, TRANSCEND (Telmisartan Randomised Assessment Study in ACE Intolerant Subjects with Cardiovascular Disease) Investigators. Effect of telmisartan on renal outcomes: a randomized trial. Ann Intern Med 2009;151:1–10.
22. Mann JF, Schmeider RE, McQueen M, et al. Renal outcomes with telmisaran, ramipril, or both, in people at high vascular risk (the ONTARGET study): a multicentre, randomised, double-blind, controlled trial. Lancet 2008;372(9638):547–53.
23. Kolesnyk I, Struijk DG, Dekker FW, et al. Effects of angiotensin-converting enzyme inhibitors and angiotensin II receptor blockers in patients with chronic kidney disease. Neth J Med 2010;68(1): 15–23.
24. Parving HH, Persson F, Lewis JB, et al, AVOID Study Investigators. Aliskiren combined with losartan in type 2 diabetes and nephropathy. N Engl J Med 2008;358:2433–46.
25. Karlsson J, Pivodic A, Aguirre D, et al. Efficacy, safety, and tolerability of the cyclooxygenas-inhibiting nitric oxide donator naproxcinod in treating osteoarthritis of the hip or knee. J Rheumatol 2009;36:1290–7.
26. Available at: http://www.cdc.gov/nchs/pressroom/10newreleases/hus09.htm. or http://www.cdc.gov/nchs/data/hus/hus09.pdf. Accessed March 19, 2010.
27. Malyszko J, Małyszko J, Bachórzewska-Gajewska H, et al. Inadequate blood pressure control in most kidney transplant recipients and patients with coronary artery disease with and without complications. Transplant Proc 2009;41(8): 3069–72.
28. Prasad GV, Huang M, Nash MM, et al. Role of dietary salt intake in posttransplant hypertension with tacrolimus-based immunosuppression. Transplant Proc 2005;37(4):1896–7.
29. Sanchez-Lazaro IJ, Martínez-Dolz L, Almenar-Bonet L, et al. Predictor factors for the development of arterial hypertension following heart transplantation. Clin Transplant 2008;22(6):760–4.
30. Aliabadi AZ, Zuckermann AO, Grimm M. Immunosuppressive therapy in older cardiac transplant patients. Drugs Aging 2007;24(11):913–32.
31. Kobashigawa JA, Patel J, Furukawa H, et al. Five-year results of a randomized, single-center study of tacrolimus vs microemulsion cyclosporine in heart transplant patients. J Heart Lung Transplant 2006;25 (4):434–9.
32. Patel JK, Kobashigawa JA. Tacrolimus in heart transplant recipients: an overview. BioDrugs 2007; 21(3):139–43.
33. Morales JM, Dominguez-Gil B. Impact of tacrolimus and mycophenolate mofetil combination on cardiovascular risk profile after kidney transplantation. J Am Soc Nephrol 2006;17(12 Suppl 3):S296–303.
34. Ye F, Ying-Bin X, Yu-Guo W, et al. Tacrolimus versus cyclosporine microemulsion for heart transplant recipients: a meta-analysis. J Heart Lung Transplant 2009;28(1):58–66.
35. Roche SL, Kaufmann J, Dipchand AI, et al. Hypertension after pediatric heart transplantation is primarily associated with immunosuppressive regimen. J Heart Lung Transplant 2008;27(5):501–7.
36. Report of the National High Blood Pressure Education Program (NHBPEP) Working Group on High Blood Pressure in Pregnancy. Am J Obstet Gynecol 2000;183(1):S1–22.

37. Chang J, Elam-Evans LD, Berg CJ, et al. Pregnancy-related mortality surveillance—United States, 1991–1999. MMWR Surveill Summ 2003;52(2):1–8.
38. Friedman EA, Neff RK. Pregnancy, hypertension: a systemative evaluation of clinical diagnostic criteria. Littleton (MA): PSG Publishing; 1977.
39. Page EW, Christianson RE. The mean impact of mean arterial pressure in the middle trimester on the outcome of pregnancy. Am J Obstet Gynecol 1976;125:740–6.
40. Hedderson MM, Ferrara A. High blood pressure before and during early pregnancy is associated with an increased risk of gestational diabetes mellitus. Diabetes Care 2008;31(12):2362–7.
41. Clapp J, Capeless E. Cardiovascular function before, during and after the first and subsequent pregnancies. Am J Cardiol 1997;80:1469.
42. Chronic Hypertension in Pregnancy. ACOG Practice Bulletin No. 29. American College of Obstetricians and Gynecologists. Obstet Gynecol 2001;98:177–85.
43. Podymow T, August P. Hypertension in pregnancy. Adv Chronic Kidney Dis 2007;14(2):178–90.
44. Lindheimer MD, Taler SJ, Cunningham FG. Hypertension in pregnancy. J Am Soc Hypertens 2010;4 (2):68–78.
45. Mongraw-Chaffin ML, Cirillo PM, Cohn BA. Preeclampsia and cardiovascular disease death. prospective evidence from the child health and development studies cohort. Hypertension 2010;56: 166–71.
46. Hladunewich M, Karumanch SA, Lafayette R. Pathyophysiology of the clinical manifestations of preeclampsia. Clin J Am Soc Nephrol 2007;2:543–9.
47. Lindheimer MD, Conrad KP, Karumanchi SA. Renal physiology and disease in pregnancy. In: Alpern RJ, Herbert SC, editors. Seldin and Giebisch's the kidney: physiology and pathophysiology. 4th edition. San Diego (CA): Academic Press, Elsevier; 2008. p. 2339–98.
48. Khalil A, Jauniaux E, Harrington K. Antihypertensive therapy and central hemodynamics in women with hypertensive disorders in pregnancy. Obstet Gynecol 2009;113(3):646–54.
49. Magee LA, Ornstein MP, von Dadelszen P. Fortnightly review: management of hypertension in pregnancy. BMJ 1999;318(7194):1332–6.
50. Von Dadelszen P, Magee LA. Fall in mean arterial pressure and fetal growth restriction in pregnancy hypertension: an updated metaregression analysis. J Obstet Gynaecol Can 2002;24:941–5.
51. Abalos E, Duley L, Steyn DW, et al. Antihypertensive drug therapy for mild to moderate hypertension during pregnancy. Cochrane Database Syst Rev 2007;1:CD002252.
52. Jones DC, Hayslett JP. Outcome of pregnancy in women with moderate or severe renal insufficiency. N Engl J Med 1996;335(4):226–32.
53. Easterling TR, Carr DB, Brateng D, et al. Treatment of hypertension in pregnancy: effect of atenolol on maternal disease, preterm delivery, and fetal growth. Obstet Gynecol 2001;98(3):427–33.
54. McCowan LM, Buist RG, North RA, et al. Perinatal morbidity in chronic hypertension. Br J Obstet Gynaecol 1996;103(2):123–9.
55. Khedun SM, Maharaj B, Moodley J. Effects of antihypertensive drugs on the unborn child. What is known, and how should this influence prescribing? Paediatr Drugs 2000;2(6):419–36.
56. Sica DA. Centrally acting antihypertensive agents: an update. J Clin Hypertens (Greenwich) 2007;9 (5):399–405.
57. Small MJ, Hayslett JP. Chronic hypertension in pregnancy. In: Evans MI, Funai EF, Lockwood CJ, editors. High risk obstetrics: the requisites in obstetrics and gynecology. Philadelphia: Mosby; 2008. p. 241–56.
58. Sibai BM. Hypertension. In: Gabbe SG, Niebyl JR, Simpson JL, editors. Obstetrics: normal and problem pregnancies. Philadelphia: Elsevier; 2007. p. 863–912.
59. Ferrer RL, Sibai BM, Mulrow CD, et al. Management of mild chronic hypertension during pregnancy: a review. Obstet Gynecol 2009;6(5 Pt 2):849–60.
60. Sibai BA, Mabie WC, Shamsa F, et al. A comparison of no medication versus methyldopa or labetalol in chronic hypertension during pregnancy. Am J Obstet Gynecol 1990;162:960–7.
61. Lip GYH, Beevers M, Churchill D, et al. Effect of atenolol on birth weight. Am J Cardiol 1997;79:1436–8.
62. Lydakis C, Lip GYH, Beevers M, et al. Atenolol and fetal growth in pregnancies complicated by hypertension. Am J Hypertens 1999;12:541–7.
63. Sibai BM, Grossman RA, Grossman HG. Effects of diuretics on plasma volume in pregnancies with long-term hypertension. Am J Obstet Gynecol 1984;150(7):831–5.
64. Cooper WO, Hernandez-Diaz S, Arbogast PG, et al. Major congenital malformations after first-trimester exposure to ACE inhibitors. N Engl J Med 2006; 354(23):2443–51.
65. Robertson D, Beck C, Gary T, et al. Classification of autonomic disorders. Int Angiol 1993;12(2): 93–102.
66. Ketch T, Biaggioni I, Robertson R, et al. Four faces of baroreflex failure: hypertensive crisis, volatile hypertension, orthostatic tachycardia, and malignant vagotonia. Circulation 2002;105(21):2518–23.
67. Floras JS, Aylward PE, Victor RG, et al. Epinephrine facilitates neurogenic vasoconstriction in humans. J Clin Invest 1988;81(4):1265–74.
68. Eisenhofer G, Friberg P, Goldstein DS, et al. Differential actions of desipramine on sympathoadrenal release of noradrenaline and adrenaline. Eur J Clin Pharmacol 1995;40:263–5.

69. Timmers HJ, Wieling W, Karemaker JM, et al. Baroreflex failure: a neglected type of secondary hypertension. Neth J Med 2004;62:151–5.
70. Jordan J, Shannon JR, Black BK, et al. Malignant vagotonia due to selective baroreflex failure. Hypertension 1997;30:1072–7.
71. Zar T, Peixoto AJ. Paroxysmal hypertension due to baroreflex failure. Kidney Int 2008;74(1):126–31.
72. Heusser K, Tank J, Luft FC, et al. Baroreflex failure. Hypertension 2005;45:834–9.
73. Muntner P, He J, Cutler JA, et al. Trends in blood pressure among children and adolescents. JAMA 2004;291(17):2107–13.
74. Lloyd-Jones D, Adams R, Carnethon M, et al. Heart disease and stroke statistics–2009 update: a report from the American Heart Association Statistics Committee and Stroke Statistics Subcommittee. Circulation 2009;119(3):480–6.
75. Cooper RS, Wolf-Maier K, et al. An International comparative study of blood pressure in populations of European vs. African descent. BMC Med 2005;3:2.
76. Cutler JA, Sorlie PD, Wolz M, et al. Trends in hypertension prevalence, awareness, treatment, and control rates in United States adults between 1988-1994 and 1999–2004. Hypertension 2008;52(5):818–27.
77. Giles T, Aranda JM Jr, Suh DC, et al. Ethnic/racial variations in blood pressure awareness, treatment, and control. J Clin Hypertens (Greenwich) 2007;9 (5):345–54.
78. Hughes JW, Kobayashi I, Deichert NT. Ethnic differences in sleep quality accompany ethnic differences in night-time blood pressure dipping. Am J Hypertens 2007;20:1104–10.
79. Flack JM, Staffileno BA. Hypertension in blacks. In: Oparil S, Weber MA, editors. Hypertension: a companion to Brenner and Rector's the kidney. Philadelphia (PA): WB Saunders; 2000. p. 558–63.
80. Flack JM, Ensrud KE, Mascioli S, et al. Racial and ethnic modifiers of the salt-blood pressure response. Hypertension 1991;17(Suppl 1):I115–21.
81. Schmidlin O, Forman A, Tanaka M, et al. NaCl-induced renal vasoconstriction in salt-sensitive African Americans: antipressor and hemodynamic effects of potassium bicarbonate. Hypertension 1999;33(2):633–9.
82. Schmidlin O, Sebastian AF, Morris RC Jr. What initiates the pressor effect of salt in salt-sensitive humans? Observations in normotensive blacks. Hypertension 2007;49(5):1032–9.
83. Heffernan KS, Jae SY, Wilund KR, et al. Racial differences in central blood pressure and vascular function in young men. Am J Physiol Heart Circ Physiol 2008;295(6):H2380–7.
84. Din-Dziethan R, Couper D, Evans G, et al. Arterial stiffness is greater in African Americans than in whites: evidence from the Forsyth County, North Carolina, ARIC cohort. Am J Hypertens 2004;17(4):304–13.
85. Stein CM, Lang CC, Nelson R, et al. Vasodilation in black Americans: attenuated nitric oxide-mediated responses. Clin Pharmacol Ther 1997;62(4):436–43.
86. Stein CM, Lang CC, Singh I, et al. Increased vascular adrenergic vasoconstriction and decreased vasodilation in blacks. Additive mechanisms leading to enhanced vascular reactivity. Hypertension 2000;36(6):945–51.
87. D'Agostino RB Jr, Burke G, O'Leary D, et al. Ethnic differences in carotid wall thickness. The Insulin Resistance Atherosclerosis Study. Stroke 1996;27 (10):1744–9.
88. Zion AS, Bond V, Adams RG, et al. Low arterial compliance in young African-American males. Am J Physiol Heart Circ Physiol 2003;285(2): H457–62.
89. Wong TY, Klein R, Duncan BB, et al. Racial differences in the prevalence of hypertensive retinopathy. Hypertension 2003;41(5):1086–91.
90. Flack JM, Neaton JD, Daniels B, et al. Ethnicity and renal disease: lessons from multiple risk factor intervention trial and the treatment of mild hypertension study. Am J Kidney Dis 1993;21(Suppl 4):31–40.
91. Mensah GA, Mokdad AH, Ford ES, et al. State of disparities in cardiovascular health in the United States. Circulation 2005;111:1233–41.
92. Plantinga LC, Miller ER III, Stevens LA, et al. Blood pressure control among persons without and with chronic kidney disease: US trends and risk factors 1999-2006. Hypertension 2009;54:47–56.
93. Cushman WC, Ford CE, Cutler JA, et al. ALLHAT Collaborative Research Group. Success and predictors of blood pressure control in diverse North American settings: the Antihypertensive and Lipid-Lowering Treatment to Prevent Heart Attack Trial (ALLHAT). J Clin Hypertens (Greenwich) 2002; 4(6):393–404.
94. Boddi M, Poggesi L, Coppo M, et al. Human vascular renin-angiotensin system and its functional changes in relation to different sodium intakes. Hypertension 1998;31(3):836–42.
95. Price DA, Fisher ND, Osei SY, et al. Renal perfusion and function in healthy African Americans. Kidney Int 2001;59(3):1037–43.
96. Mokwe E, Ohmit SE, Nasser SA, et al. Determinants of blood pressure response to quinapril in black and white hypertensive patients: the Quinapril Titration Interval Management Evaluation trial. Hypertension 2004;43(6):1202–7.
97. Sehgal AR. Overlap between whites and blacks in response to antihypertensive drugs. Hypertension 2004;43(3):566–72.
98. Flack JM, Sica DA, Bakris G, et al. International Society on Hypertension in Blacks (ISHIB) consensus statement on the treatment of hypertension in African Americans. Hypertension, in press.

Resistant Hypertension, Secondary Hypertension, and Hypertensive Crises: Diagnostic Evaluation and Treatment

Maria Czarina Acelajado, MD*, David A. Calhoun, MD

KEYWORDS

- Resistant hypertension • Secondary hypertension
- Malignant hypertension • Diagnosis • Treatment

Hypertension (defined as BP >140/90 mm Hg) is a global burden, affecting as many as 1 billion individuals worldwide and causing 7.5 million deaths (12.8% of all deaths) per year.[1] In the United States, hypertension affects 28.9% of the population, or about 85 million individuals.[2] It is an important modifiable risk factor for cardiovascular (CV) morbidity and mortality, particularly for stroke (accounting for 51% of all stroke deaths worldwide), ischemic heart disease (45% of all deaths), chronic kidney disease (CKD), congestive heart failure, aortic aneurysm, and peripheral arterial disease.[1] A mere 5 mm Hg decrease in systolic blood pressure (SBP) in the population is estimated to reduce stroke mortality by 9% and cardiovascular deaths by 12%.[3]

The regulation of BP is a complex interplay of various elements of the cardiovascular, endocrine, renal, and neural systems. Further, compensatory mechanisms to the elevated BP in hypertension result in an array of anatomic and functional derangements (such as left ventricular hypertrophy [LVH]) and complications (such as kidney disease). As a result the hypertensive population, more than having just an elevated BP, is clinically diverse with several subgroups that are not necessarily distinct from one another. Three groups of hypertensive patients merit a closer look and are discussed in this article: patients with secondary hypertension, those with resistant hypertension (RH), and those having a hypertensive crisis. These conditions pose unique challenges to the modern-day clinician, and this review aims to present current diagnostic and therapeutic approaches to these patients.

SECONDARY HYPERTENSION

More than 90% of the adult hypertensive population is considered to have primary (essential) hypertension, for which no identifiable cause is found.[4] In less than 10% of hypertensive individuals, a specific cause wholly or partly explains the elevated BP (secondary hypertension), and consequent antihypertensive therapy; addressing these causes may help reduce the BP further (**Table 1**). Alongside the discovery of potentially reversible causes of elevated BP, the presence

Disclosure: The authors have nothing to disclose.

Vascular Biology and Hypertension Program, Division of Cardiovascular Disease, Department of Medicine, University of Alabama at Birmingham, 1530 3rd Avenue South, Birmingham, AL 35294-2041, USA
* Corresponding author.
E-mail address: czarina.acelajado@ccc.uab.edu

Cardiol Clin 28 (2010) 639–654
doi:10.1016/j.ccl.2010.07.002

of secondary causes warrants a referral to the appropriate specialist.

Chronic Kidney Disease

Renal parenchymal disease is a common secondary cause of hypertension, and may also be a result of long-standing poorly controlled hypertension. Elevated BP (SBP more than diastolic blood pressure [DBP]) is a strong and independent risk factor for the development of kidney disease, while CKD is a common cause of resistant or difficult to treat hypertension.[5] Among adults with a glomerular filtration rate (GFR) greater than 60 mL/min per 1.73 m^2 and no proteinuria or hematuria at baseline, there was increased risk for developing end-stage renal disease with a higher SBP.[6] On the other hand, prevalence of CKD is higher among those with hypertension or diabetes.[7]

Table 1
Secondary causes of hypertension

Secondary Causes	Screening Tests
Common	
Renal parenchymal disease	Kidney function tests (serum creatinine, estimated GFR) Renal ultrasound
Obstructive sleep apnea	Berlin Questionnaire Epworth Sleepiness Scale Polysomnography
Renal artery stenosis	Renal Doppler CT angiography MR angiography
Primary aldosteronism	Aldosterone-to-renin ratio
Uncommon	
Pheochromocytoma	Plasma metanephrines Urinary metanephrines
Cushing disease	Urine cortisol Late-night salivary cortisol Dexamethasone suppression tests
Hyperparathyroidism	Serum calcium level Parathyroid hormone level
Coarctation of the aorta	2-Dimensional echocardiogram
Intracranial tumors	Brain imaging studies (eg, cranial CT, MR imaging)

Abbreviations: CT, computed tomography; GFR, glomerular filtration rate; MR, magnetic resonance.

Data from Acelajado MC, Calhoun DA, Oparil S. Reduction of blood pressure in patients with treatment-resistant hypertension. Exp Opin Pharmacother 2009; 10:2959–71.

The BP in patients with CKD is elevated and difficult to control owing to several factors, most notably an increase in intravascular volume and inappropriate activity of the renin-angiotensin-aldosterone system (RAAS), leading to sodium retention. Other mechanisms also contribute, such as increased activity of the sympathetic nervous system, endothelial dysfunction, and increased vascular stiffness, which are found in patients with CKD.[8] The estimated prevalence of CKD in the United States is 16.8% based on National Health and Nutrition Examination Survey (NHANES) data from 1999 to 2004, an increase from 14.5% in 1990 to 1994.[9] The presence of CKD substantially raises the risk for cardiovascular (CV) morbidity and mortality, with the risk increasing proportionately as the GFR falls below 60 mL/min.

Assessing kidney function in hypertensive individuals is important not only in determining BP goals (<130/80) but also in choosing appropriate antihypertensive medications. Estimated glomerular filtration rate (eGFR) based on the Modified Diet in Renal Disease (MDRD) formula or the Cockcroft-Gault equation provides more information about kidney function than serum creatinine alone, and it is preferably paired with a urine sample to check for albuminuria or proteinuria.[10] Patients are classified between CKD stages 1 and 5, depending on the GFR and the presence and degree of proteinuria.

Antihypertensive therapy in patients with CKD aims to reduce CV risk and prevent further deterioration of kidney function. Angiotensin-converting enzyme (ACE) inhibitors and angiotensin receptor blockers (ARB) are recommended as first-line agents to reduce proteinuria and lower BP in patients without hyperkalemia or other contraindications. Diuretics are usually required for BP control, and nondihydropyridine calcium channel blockers may be added for additional BP lowering and an even greater antiproteinuric effect.[11]

Primary Aldosteronism

Primary aldosteronism (PA) is characterized by excess production of the mineralocorticoid aldosterone by the adrenal gland and suppressed secretion of renin by the kidneys. The elevated aldosterone level is nonsuppressible by sodium loading, and leads to sodium retention, hypertension, and increased potassium excretion. High levels of aldosterone mediate CV injury via nonepithelial mineralocorticoid receptors in the brain, heart, and blood vessels, promote oxidative stress, inflammation and fibrosis, and cause endothelial dysfunction, possibly contributing to resistance to treatment and portending a poorer prognosis.[12–14] Indeed, in hypertensive patients with PA there is a greater incidence of target organ damage (LVH, proteinuria, and retinal hemorrhage) compared with hypertensive patients without biochemical evidence of PA.[15]

The aldosterone-to-renin ratio (ARR) is the best screening test available to check for PA. This test is more sensitive than plasma aldosterone alone and more specific than an isolated plasma renin activity (PRA) level.[16] Mid-morning samples of plasma aldosterone and PRA taken after a patient has been seated for 5 to 15 minutes and while on a diet that is unrestricted in salt before testing is considered to be ideal. Potassium levels, if low, should be corrected before measurement of PRA and plasma aldosterone. An ARR greater than 20 with the plasma aldosterone expressed in ng/dL and PRA in ng/ml/h is considered to be a positive test result. In the authors' studies involving patients with RH and confirmed PA, the ARR had a sensitivity of 78% to 89% and a specificity of 71% to 83%.[17,18] Further, the test is valid for both African American and Caucasian patients on a stable antihypertensive regimen.[17] Once a positive screening test is obtained, any 1 of 4 confirmatory tests may be performed, which include oral sodium loading, saline infusion, fludrosortisone suppression, and captopril challenge.[16] An adrenal computed tomography (CT) scan performed after obtaining a positive confirmatory test can then be the initial step to distinguish between the subtypes of PA (bilateral idiopathic hyperaldosteronism, aldosterone-producing adenoma, unilateral adrenal hyperplasia, and the familial forms of PA).

Hypokalemia appears to be a late manifestation of PA. In 20 patients with RH and a high ARR, serum potassium levels ranged from 3.7 to 4.7 mmol/L.[19] The presence of PA was confirmed in this study using intravenous saline loading. In another study, 71% of hypertensive patients with biochemical PA (based on an elevated ARR) were normokalemic.[15] These results suggest that hypokalemia is often a late manifestation of PA, and should not be used as a criterion for its diagnosis or as a prerequisite for screening.

Renovascular Hypertension

Narrowing of the renal arteries is most commonly the result of atherosclerosis. Obstruction of the renal arteries results in increased renin activity, leading to activation of the RAAS, vasoconstriction, volume overload, and hypertension. In unilateral lesions the opposite kidney responds with a pressure-dependent diuresis, but cannot fully compensate for the volume-overloaded state.[20] The at-risk patient is elderly, with exacerbation of previously well-controlled hypertension, declining kidney function, dyslipidemia, evidence of diffuse atherosclerotic disease, and a history of smoking. Duplex renal artery sonography, CT angiography, or magnetic resonance angiography are all used to detect the lesions of renal artery stenosis, but arteriography remains the gold standard in its diagnosis (**Fig. 1**).[20] In younger patients (particularly women <50 years old), fibromuscular dysplasia has to be considered as well. Treatment options for renovascular lesions are angioplasty with stenting, or medical therapy.

Obstructive Sleep Apnea

Obstructive sleep apnea (OSA) is strongly associated with the possibility of having concomitant hypertension and the risk of developing hypertension.[21] The intermittent episodes of hypoxia are

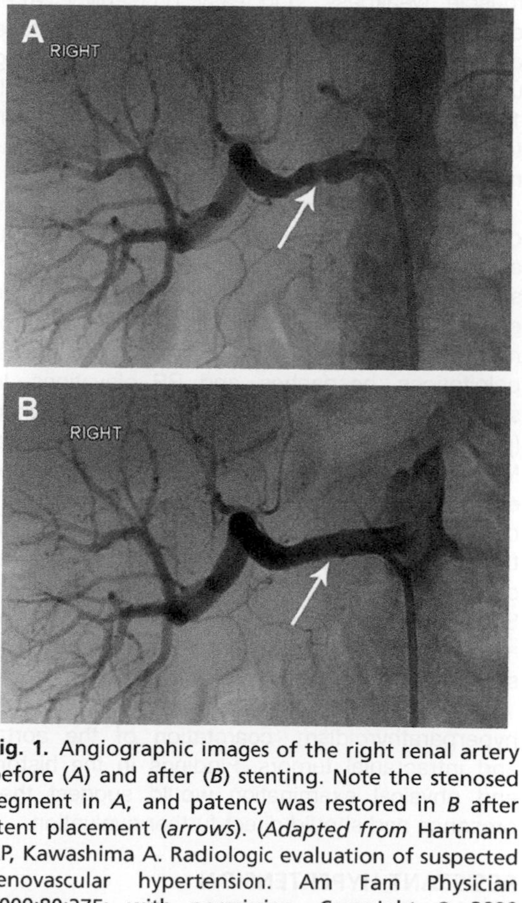

Fig. 1. Angiographic images of the right renal artery before (*A*) and after (*B*) stenting. Note the stenosed segment in *A*, and patency was restored in *B* after stent placement (*arrows*). (*Adapted from* Hartmann RP, Kawashima A. Radiologic evaluation of suspected renovascular hypertension. Am Fam Physician 2009;80:275; with permission. Copyright © 2009 American Academy of Family Physicians. All Rights Reserved.)

thought to activate sympathetic nervous system activity, which contribute to elevation of BP. Overnight polysomnography (PSG) is the diagnostic test of choice for OSA, but expense and lack of facilities limit its use. Screening for OSA is usually done using validated questionnaires such as the Berlin Questionnaire and the Epworth Daytime Sleepiness Scale, or through the use of algorithms found in some sleep centers, all of which attempt to identify patients who may be at risk for having OSA. However, no single questionnaire or clinical prediction model has been found to be an ideal screening test because there is a high false-negative rate, particularly in those with mild disease.[22] OSA is best treated using continuous positive airway pressure, which dramatically improves sleep quality, albeit with overall modest effects on BP.[23]

Other Secondary Causes

Cushing syndrome should be suspected in a hypertensive patient with purplish abdominal striae, buffalo hump, truncal obesity, moon facies, menstrual irregularities, hyperglycemia, proximal muscle weakness, and easy bruisability. After excluding exogenous causes (mainly from intake of glucocorticoids), screening is performed using urine free cortisol, late-night salivary cortisol, 1-mg overnight dexamethasone suppression test, or longer (48 hours) low-dose (2 mg/d) dexamethasone suppression test.[24]

Pheochromocytomas are neuroendocrine tumors derived from adrenal chromaffin cells and extra-adrenal paraganglia, and are characterized by over-secretion of catecholamines, resulting in an elevated BP. The classic presentation of pheochromocytoma consists of paroxysms of diaphoresis, palpitations, headaches, and BP elevations. In some patients, a family history may be obtained (pheochromocytoma, von-Hippel-Lindau disease, Multiple Endocrine Neoplasia type II). Pheochromocytoma is a rare cause of secondary hypertension, but may be more common in patients with uncontrolled BP, as suggested by numerous case reports of difficult to control or severe hypertension. Screening is done using plasma metanephrine and normetanephrine levels, which have a combined sensitivity of 98% and specificity of 92%.[25]

Other rare secondary causes of RH include hyperparathyroidism, coarctation of the aorta, and intracranial tumors. Findings in the history and physical examination would suggest their presence and should direct further evaluation.

RESISTANT HYPERTENSION

RH is an elevated BP despite use of 3 or more antihypertensive medications, ideally one of which is a diuretic, and prescribed at optimal doses.[26] This definition of RH has several implications. First, patients whose BP is controlled with 4 or more medications are still considered to have RH. Second, patients who are on at least 3 antihypertensive medications but not taking a diuretic (due to medication intolerance, for example) are still classified as having RH. Lastly, patients have to be on optimal (as opposed to maximal) doses of antihypertensive medications to be considered to have RH, as higher doses may increase the incidence of adverse effects in some patients. These patients, who will not otherwise be considered as having RH based on previous definitions, still merit the same diagnostic and therapeutic considerations given to patients with RH.

Prevalence

The exact prevalence of RH is unknown. Data from the NHANES reveal that 61.4% of patients with hypertension are receiving antihypertensive medications, and only 35.1% have BP values that are less than 140/90 (controlled).[2] These data imply that a large number of hypertensive individuals still have uncontrolled BP levels even while the majority receive some form of antihypertensive treatment. Uncontrolled BP, however, is not synonymous with RH. Factors such as nonadherence to antihypertensive therapy contribute to the incidence of uncontrolled hypertension. Large randomized trials of antihypertensive drugs minimize this problem because adherence is closely monitored. Data from these large clinical trials on hypertension suggest that RH is a fairly common problem, affecting as many as 20% to 30% of the hypertensive population. In the Antihypertensive and Lipid-Lowering Treatment to Prevent Heart Attack Trial (ALLHAT), which randomized 42,419 ethnically diverse hypertensive patients (mean age 66.9 years, 35% black, 16% Hispanics, and 47% women), approximately 30% of the study patients were taking a minimum of 3 antihypertensive drugs at year 5.[27] In tertiary care hypertension clinics, the prevalence of RH was estimated to be 11% to 18% and was noted to increase over time.[28,29]

Prognosis

Patients with RH have increased CV risk relative to the general hypertensive population. Using 24-hour ambulatory blood pressure monitoring (ABPM) data to exclude a white-coat effect, patients with true RH (defined as elevated office BP and 24-hour ABPM readings while taking a minimum of 3 antihypertensive medications) had a higher serum creatinine at baseline, and were more likely to have LVH, nephropathy, and diabetes as compared with patients without true RH (including those with false RH, or white-coat RH whereby office BP is elevated but 24-hour ABPM readings are within the normal range).[30,31] Further, patients with RH were more likely to experience a CV event such as myocardial infarction, stroke, or heart failure than patients without RH. RH was an independent predictor of CV events, along with age, smoking, LVH, low-density lipoprotein (LDL) cholesterol level, and diabetes (the so-called traditional CV risk factors). Moreover, using 24-hour ABPM data, patients with RH were found to have a higher incidence of the nondipping pattern (nocturnal SBP and DBP reduction <10% compared with daytime BP readings), a larger 24-hour pulse pressure,[31] and a higher 24-hour mean heart rate[32] as compared with their non-RH counterparts. In patients with RH, a nondipping pattern is an independent predictor of CV risk, particularly in younger patients,[33] whereas a higher pulse pressure and heart rate have been found to increase CV risk in the general hypertensive population.[34,35]

Patients' Characteristics

Patients with RH tend to be older, have higher baseline BP (particularly SBP) and body mass index, and have comorbid conditions such as diabetes or CKD. Further, patients with RH are more likely to have evidence of target organ damage such as LVH. African American race and residence in the southeastern United States are also associated with RH.

Based on NHANES data, older age (>70 years) and female gender were associated with poorer control rates for hypertension.[36] In the same cohort, the presence of diabetes or CKD was also correlated with less hypertension control, based on the recommended BP goal of less than 130/80 mm Hg in those with diabetes mellitus or CKD.[37] In the Framingham study, which is a longitudinal observational study evaluating CV risk factors, patients who are older than 75 years were 25% less likely to achieve BP control as those younger than 60 years. Further, obesity and the presence of LVH also independently predicted the presence of uncontrolled BP.[38]

BP that is higher than goal is most often due to an elevated SBP. In the Framingham study, only 49% of patients had controlled SBP (<140 mm Hg), whereas 90% of patients had DBP less than 90 mm Hg. Similar trends were seen in ALLHAT, where persistent elevations in SBP accounted for uncontrolled hypertension for most cases (33% of patients had SBP >140 mm Hg) while the DBP goal was achieved in 92% of patients.[27] Further, a higher baseline SBP was associated with the likelihood of never realizing the BP goal.[39]

Patients with RH are also more likely to have secondary causes of hypertension, particularly OSA, PA, and CKD. OSA is found in 71% to 83% of patients with RH, and is more severe in men than in women.[40–42] The prevalence of PA in patients with RH is estimated to be 17% to 23%, based on different prospective trials, which is higher than reported for the general hypertensive population.[18,43–45] It is interesting that combined PA and OSA are also common in patients with RH. In study patients who were identified to have high risk for OSA based on the Berlin Questionnaire, patients with RH were twice as likely to have PA as those without RH. Further, patients with RH tended to have a lower PRA and a higher 24-hour urinary aldosterone secretion than patients without RH.[46] In patients with CKD, as much as 85% failed to achieve BP goal of less than 130/80 mm Hg even while on an average of 3 antihypertensive medications.[47]

Patients with RH have a higher plasma aldosterone level and lower levels of PRA and serum potassium than patients without RH.[48] Even in the absence of clinical PA, an elevated aldosterone level is associated with development of RH.[49] Low renin levels were also found in a group of patients with RH in Norway, where a suppressed PRA (≤0.4 nmol/L) was found in 67% of patients, 75% of whom had levels below 0.2 nmol/L.[44] Also, patients with RH and a high urinary aldosterone level (≥12 μg/24 h) have a higher daytime, nighttime, and 24-hour BP on ABPM, and this effect was more pronounced with increasing age.[50]

Pseudoresistance

Not all cases of uncontrolled hypertension are RH. Lack of BP control even while prescribed 3 or more antihypertensive drugs is often attributable to medication nonadherence, improper BP measurement technique, or white-coat effect (where office BP is elevated while out-of-office BP readings are at goal). These causes of pseudoresistance need to be sought and corrected before making a diagnosis of RH. Further, suboptimal BP control can result from concomitant intake of drugs or substances that raise the BP or interfere with the effects of antihypertensive medications (**Table 2**) and, if possible, consumption of these interfering substances should be limited or stopped altogether to help bring the BP to goal.

Improper BP measurement technique

Using an improper BP measurement technique is a very common cause of elevated BP, and also

Table 2
Parenteral agents for hypertensive emergencies

Agent	Dose	Onset and Duration of Action	Precautions
Sodium nitroprusside	0.25–10 μg/kg/min as intraventricular (IV) infusion	Immediate/2–3 min after infusion	Nausea, vomiting, muscle twitching; prolonged use cause thiocyanate intoxication, methemoglobinemia acidosis, cyanide poisoning; light-sensitive
Nitroglycerine	5–100 μg as IV infusion	2–5 min/5–10 min	Headache, tachycardia, vomiting, flushing, methemoglobinemia; needs special delivery system due to drug's binding to PVC tubing
Clevidipine butyrate	1–2 mg/h infusion, may double infusion rate every 90 s until goal BP nearly achieved	2–4 min/5–15 min	Avoid in patients with lipid metabolism defects and soy allergy, use no more than 21 mg/h for a 24 h period
Nicardipine	5–15 mg/h IV infusion	1–5 min/15–30 min, may extend for 12 h after prolonged infusion	Tachycardia, nausea, vomiting, headache, increased intracranial pressure, prolonged hypotension after extended infusions
Verapamil	5–10 mg IV; can follow with infusion of 3–25 mg/h	1–5 min/30–60 min	Heart block (first, second, and third degrees), especially with concomitant digitalis or β-blockers, bradycardia
Diazoxide	50–150 mg IV bolus, repeated, or 15–30 mg/min	2–5 min/3–12 h	Hypotension, tachycardia, aggravation of angina pectoris, nausea and vomiting, hyperglycemia with repeated injections
Fenoldopam mesylate	0.1–0.3 mg/kg/min IV infusion	<5 min/30 min	Headache, tachycardia, flushing, local phlebitis
Hydralazine	10–20 mg as IV bolus or 10–40 mg intramuscularly (IM), repeat every 4–6 h	10 min IV/>1–4 h IV 20–30 min IM/4–6 h IM	Tachycardia, headache, vomiting, aggravation of angina pectoris
Enalaprilat	0.625–1.25 mg every 6 h IV	15–60 min/12–24 h	Renal failure in patients with bilateral renal artery stenosis, hypotension
Labetalol	20–80 mg as IV bolus every 10 min; up to 2 mg/min as IV infusion	5–10 min/2–6 h	Bronchoconstriction, heart block, orthostatic hypotension
Esmolol	500 μg/kg IV bolus or 25–100 μg/kg/min by infusion; may repeat bolus after 5 min or increase infusion rate to 300 μg/kg/min	1–5 min/15–30 min	First-degree heart block, congestive heart failure, asthma
Phentolamine	5–15 mg as IV bolus	1–2 min/10–30 min	Tachycardia, orthostatic hypotension

very easy to correct. Falsely high readings may result from using a cuff size that is too small for the patient, and by not allowing the patient to sit quietly for about 5 minutes before taking the BP. The bladder cuff should encircle at least 80% of the bare upper arm (which is the preferred site of measurement), and if so, the large adult cuff is suitable for most persons. Patients should be seated in a chair with both feet on the floor, uncrossed, with the back supported and the arm resting on a table at the level of the heart. Caffeine, exercise, and cigarette smoking may affect the BP; hence, patients are counseled to avoid these when coming into the clinic for a BP check. The Korotkoff sound technique (auscultatory method) using a mercury sphygmomanometer is considered as the gold standard in clinic BP measurements, but concerns regarding the potential toxicity of mercury in these devices has led some clinicians to prefer aneroid or oscillometric devices, which are regarded as less satisfactory in obtaining accurate BP measurements.[51] Patients should also be instructed on proper BP measurement techniques at home.

Nonadherence to antihypertensive medications

Medication nonadherence is a significant contributor to uncontrolled BP. As many as 40% of hypertensive individuals discontinue their prescribed antihypertensive medications within the first year of treatment.[52] Medication adherence is difficult to ascertain, and most clinicians rely on self-report to assess a patient's adherence to treatment. Other methods available to the clinician to monitor adherence are pill counts, pharmacy reports, and monitoring of serum drug levels, but all of these have limitations and may be subject to patient manipulation. Assessment of medication adherence should be made to avoid unnecessary dosage or medication adjustments. Clinicians should inquire about medication intake during every clinic visit, as well as adverse effects, cost of medications, perceptions about drug efficacy, and ease of dosage, all of which may affect adherence. In addition to simplifying the antihypertensive regimen, more frequent follow-ups and asking the patient to keep a home BP log improves adherence rates.[53,54]

Patients with RH who are seen in tertiary care clinics appear to have better adherence rates, despite an increased pill burden and, presumably, cost of treatment. In one study done at a university-based hypertension clinic, only 16% of patients with RH were nonadherent to their antihypertensive regimen.[28] In this group, however, the attainment of goal BP was least satisfactory compared with other causes of uncontrolled BP (suboptimal regimen, interfering substances, secondary causes of hypertension), with only 22% of patients having a BP less than 140/90 (<130/80 if with CKD or diabetes) after 2 follow-ups.

Improving adherence rates is associated with better BP control. In patients with RH whose adherence was monitored electronically (via pillbox openings that are presumed to correspond to medication intake), the BP improved from an average of 156/106 to 145/97 after 2 months, even without modifying the antihypertensive regimen.[55] In another study where adherence was monitored via pill counts, a higher adherence rate after 4 visits (from a baseline of 64% to 96%) in patients with RH (taking a mean of 5.4 antihypertensive drugs) was associated with a significantly lower BP as measured by ABPM (from 142/91 to 132/84 at the end of follow-up).[56] Further, 41% of these patients had controlled BP (office BP <140/90 and 24-hour ABPM values <130/80 mm Hg) at the end of the study period. It is clear that nonadherence is a significant contributor to pseudoresistance, and should be minimized to attain BP goals. Patients should be motivated enough to adhere to a treatment plan. Physicians and other health care providers (pharmacists, nurses, and so forth) should reinforce the importance of adherence to medications to achieve BP control in patients with RH.

White-coat effect

The phenomenon of an elevated BP in the physician's office while out-of-office BPs are lower or normal is termed the white-coat effect, which may result from anxiety, anticipation of BP levels, or a conditioned response. White-coat RH should be suspected in an adherent patient who is taking a minimum of 3 antihypertensive drugs, with an elevated office BP, but manifests signs and symptoms of overtreatment (such as dizziness, syncope, or postural hypotension), or lacks evidence of target organ damage (such as LVH, retinopathy, or CKD). White-coat hypertension is common in patients with RH, as is in the general hypertensive population. Twenty-four-hour ABPM studies in patients with RH have determined that the white-coat effect is responsible for 20% to 30% of elevated office BP in these patients.[31,50] While office BP measurements using the auscultatory method is the traditional way to diagnose and follow up on patients with hypertension, this should be supplemented by out-of-office measurements (from the home or the workplace) to give the physician a more accurate picture of the patient's BP and the effect of antihypertensive treatment.

There has been increasing use of 24-hour ABPM in hypertensive patients, both for diagnostic purposes and to assess BP control. It is currently the best method available to estimate an individual's CV risk in relation to the BP elevation, as CV risk is more tightly correlated to ABPM measurements than to office BP.[57] In patients with RH, 24-hour ABPM measurements were found to predict CV morbidity and mortality, whereas office BP was found to have no prognostic value.[58] The expense of using 24-hour ABPM to rule out a white-coat effect and assess BP control precludes its use in certain populations, or for multi-session use in patients with persistently uncontrolled BP. Properly performed office BP measurements remain the traditional method to assess BP control and guide therapy in hypertensive patients. This practice should be coupled with home BP measurements obtained using validated devices, with patients instructed regarding the correct BP measurement technique. The use of 24-hour ABPM is recommended for patients with RH whose office and home or workplace BP are not sufficient to drive a clinical decision.

Interfering substances

Several substances can interfere with BP control (**Box 1**). Exogenous steroid intake (glucocorticoids and mineralocorticoids, including those that lead to stimulation of the mineralocorticoid receptor, such as licorice) lead to systolic hypertension in a dose-dependent manner, and represent a fairly common cause of elevated BP. Ketoconazole, by altering steroid metabolism, raises BP by enhancing endogenous mineralocorticoid activity.[59] Sex hormones, particularly those in oral contraceptive pills containing at least 50 µg of estrogen and 1 to 4 mg of progestin, have also been found to raise BP,[60] but this effect was not seen in normotensive women receiving hormone replacement therapy.

Probably the most common substances that interfere with BP control are nonsteroidal anti-inflammatory drugs (NSAIDs) and selective cyclooxygenase-2 (COX-2) inhibitors, which provide pain control and anti-inflammatory action. These drugs worsen BP control in hypertensive patients by inhibiting prostaglandin E_2 and prostacyclin production by the kidney, resulting in sodium retention and vasoconstriction,[61] as well as by interfering with the actions of many antihypertensive drug classes, causing SBP elevations as great as 6 mm Hg.[62] Aspirin can produce the same BP elevations as NSAIDs by virtue of its similar inhibitory effects on vasodilator prostaglandins. However, low-dose aspirin, most commonly used in primary and secondary prevention of CV outcomes, has not been shown to have a significant influence on BP control in hypertensive patients.[63]

Box 1
Substances that can interfere with BP control

- Nonsteroidal anti-inflammatory drugs (nonselective and COX-2 selective drugs)
- Sympathomimetic agents (weight loss pills, decongestants, cocaine)
- Amphetamine and amphetamine-like substances, including modafinil
- Exogenous glucocorticoids and mineralocorticoids
- Ketoconazole
- Antidepressants (monoamine oxidase inhibitors, buspirone, tricyclic antidepressants)
- Alcohol
- Caffeine
- Oral contraceptive pills and exogenous estrogen, including danazol
- Immunosuppressants (especially cyclosporine)
- Erythropoietin
- Antiemetics (metoclopramide, alizapride)
- Natural licorice (usually found in oral tobacco products)
- Ephedra or ma huang

Eliciting a complete and current medication history is required for every hypertensive patient. Further, information about intake of certain substances, such as herbal compounds and over-the-counter agents, should be obtained, as this may not be volunteered by the patient. The use of these substances or drugs should be stopped or minimized, if possible, if they are deemed to be contributory to poor BP control.

Treatment

Lifestyle modification

There is abundant evidence linking consumption of excess dietary salt and an elevated BP, and sodium reduction is a proven intervention to reduce BP[64,65] and the attendant increased CV risk in hypertensive individuals.[66] In patients with RH, who tend to be volume expanded, aggressive dietary sodium reduction has been shown to reduce BP. The authors conducted a randomized study in their clinic comparing low (50 mmol/24 h) or high (250 mmol/24 h) sodium diet in 12 patients with RH (females n = 8, African American n = 6) in the setting of a stable multidrug antihypertensive regimen (average of 3.4 antihypertensive medications), which includes a diuretic (hydrochlorothiazide conventionally dosed at 25 mg/d) and a RAAS blocker.[67] One of the 2 dietary interventions was given for 7 days, after which the participants were crossed over to the opposite diet after a 2-week washout period during which they consumed their regular or usual diet. The achieved 24-hour urinary sodium excretion was 46.1 mmol/d in the low-sodium group, and 252.2 mmol/d in the high-sodium group. Patients consuming a low-sodium diet had lower office SBP (−22.7 mm Hg) and DBP (−9.1 mm Hg) than those on a high-sodium diet. This BP-lowering effect of a reduced sodium diet was confirmed by the 24-hour ABPM results, with a reduction in daytime BP by 20.7/9.6 mm Hg and similar reductions in nighttime BP (**Fig. 2**). The importance of dietary sodium reduction (<2 g per day) should be emphasized in all patients with RH.

Other lifestyle interventions have not been evaluated specifically in patients with RH. In a study that enrolled 45 sedentary African American males with BP greater than 180/110, comparisons between antihypertensive medication alone (control) or exercise (stationary biking) plus antihypertensive medication were made. The results showed that after 16 weeks, mean BP had decreased by 7/5 mm Hg in the exercise group compared with the control. The exercise group had a significantly larger regression of LVH than the control group, as measured by echocardiogram, which may have important implications on prognosis. Although the study did not specifically enroll patients with RH, it did demonstrate that moderate-intensity exercise is a safe and effective intervention to help lower BP in patients with severe hypertension (requiring as many as 3 antihypertensive medications). Low- to moderate-intensity aerobic exercise, which is better tolerated and sustained by patients than high-intensity exercise, should be part of the treatment of patients with RH.

In addition to dietary salt restriction and increased physical activity, weight loss in obese individuals, moderation of alcohol intake, and consuming a diet that is rich in fiber, low fat dairy products, potassium, magnesium, and calcium, and low in saturated fat should be part of a comprehensive treatment plan to decrease BP in patients with RH.[26]

Pharmacologic treatment

Once potentially correctible causes of uncontrolled BP have been ruled out or eliminated (pseudoresistance, interfering substances, secondary causes), the patient's antihypertensive medication regimen should be evaluated. Patients with RH, by definition, are on a multidrug regimen prescribed at optimal doses. Optimal dosage of antihypertensive drugs does not always mean maximal dosage, as the dose may be affected by a person's

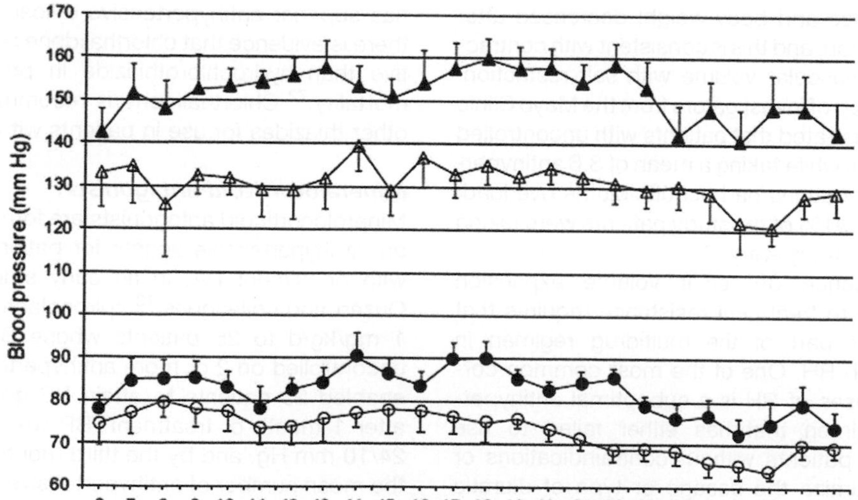

Fig. 2. Comparison of 24-hour ambulatory blood pressure values during low- and high-salt diet. SBP, systolic blood pressure; DBP, diastolic blood pressure. (*From* Pimenta E, Gaddam KK, Oparil S, et al. Effects of dietary sodium reduction on blood pressure in subjects with resistant hypertension. Hypertension 2009;54:478; with permission.)

age, the presence of comorbidities such as CKD or congestive heart failure, and the presence of adverse reactions, particularly those that are dose dependent. Further, the regimen should combine antihypertensive agents with complementary mechanisms of action, to maximize their BP reducing capacity while minimizing side effects, as lower doses may be given than when an antihypertensive agent is used by itself. Combining a RAAS blocker, a calcium channel blocker (CCB), and a thiazide diuretic represents a rational approach and is common in the authors' practice. Whereas initial antihypertensive drug choices are easy to make and are guided by expert recommendations, selecting a fourth, fifth, sixth, or seventh drug may be challenging to the clinician dealing with RH patients. These choices should also take into account a patient's profile (age, race, comorbidities, concomitant drug intake), presence of adverse reactions, and drug cost and availability. Lastly, referral to a hypertension specialist should be considered for patients with RH, and guidelines recommend this option if the BP remains uncontrolled after 6 months of close follow-up.[26]

Diuretics

In patients with RH there is evidence of persistent intravascular volume expansion, as shown by elevated levels of brain natriuretic peptide (BNP) and atrial natriuretic peptide.[48] Further, in the authors' study of patients with RH whose dietary sodium was restricted to 50 mmol/d, both creatinine clearance and body weight decreased after the intervention, and this is consistent with contraction of intravascular volume with salt restriction. Another group of investigators from the Mayo Clinic have demonstrated that patients with uncontrolled BP (>140/90) while taking a mean of 3.6 antihypertensive medications had occult volume overload, even though 91% of the study patients were taking a diuretic on study entry.[68]

The presence of occult volume expansion contributing to treatment resistance requires that diuretics be part of the multidrug regimen in patients with RH. One of the most common correctible causes of RH is a suboptimal antihypertensive regimen that has either failed to use diuretics in patients without contraindications or did not optimize the dosage or type of diuretic prescribed. In a retrospective study done at a university-based hypertension clinic involving patients with BP uncontrolled by 3 or more antihypertensive drugs, a suboptimal medication regimen, most notably the inappropriate use of diuretics, explained the apparent treatment resistance in 58% of cases.[48] Modifying the diuretic regimen by adding a diuretic, optimizing diuretic dose, or changing the diuretic class to a more appropriate agent based on a patient's renal function allowed 65% of patients to achieve goal BP (<140/90 or <130/80 if with kidney disease or diabetes).

Among the diuretic classes, thiazide diuretics, particularly chlorthalidone, are preferred. This preference is based on extensive evidence from randomized controlled trials demonstrating that thiazides reduce the risk of CV mortality and morbidity in hypertensive patients. Moreover, thiazides have favorable effects on calcium and bone mineral metabolism by promoting calcium reabsorption and reducing tubular calcium excretion, thereby preventing formation of calcium-containing renal stones, osteoporosis, and hip fractures.[69,70] In patients with RH and stage 4 CKD (estimated GFR <30 mL/min) where thiazides cannot be used, loop diuretics may be needed to treat volume overload.

In ALLHAT, the thiazide diuretic chlorthalidone was comparable to lisinopril and amlodipine, and superior to doxazosin in preventing CV outcomes (fatal coronary heart disease, nonfatal myocardial infarction, and other CV disease, including angina, peripheral arterial disease, and stroke), and was superior to the other agents in reducing the risk of heart failure.[27] Compared with hydrochlorothiazide, which is more widely available in fixed-dose drug combinations in the United States and is prescribed more frequently, chlorthalidone is more potent, has a longer duration of action, and has superior antihypertensive efficacy.[71] Further, there is evidence that chlorthalidone is more effective than hydrochlorothiazide in preventing CV mortality.[72] Chlorthalidone is recommended over other thiazides for use in patients with RH.[26]

Mineralocorticoid antagonists

Mineralocorticoid antagonists are formidable add-on antihypertensive agents for patients with RH, with or without PA. In an early study done by Ouzan and colleagues,[73] spironolactone given at 1 mg/kg/d to 25 patients whose BP remained uncontrolled on 2 or more antihypertensive drugs enabled 23 patients to attain BP goal (<140/90) after 1 month of treatment. BP was reduced by 24/10 mm Hg, and by the third month of therapy, the mean number of antihypertensive medications needed for BP control was decreased from 3.2 to 2.1 per day. In the Anglo-Scandinavian Cardiac Outcomes Trial—Blood Pressure Lowering Arm (ASCOT-BPLA), spironolactone was used as a fourth-line antihypertensive agent, with a mean starting dose of 35 mg/d, increasing to a mean of 41 mg/d at the end of the trial period.[74] A subgroup analysis in 1411 patients who received spironolactone showed that it effectively lowered BP by 21.9/9.5 mm Hg among patients with uncontrolled hypertension who were already receiving a mean of 2.9 antihypertensive agents.[75]

In patients with PA, even low doses of spironolactone produced dramatic reductions in BP. In 76 subjects referred to the authors' tertiary care hypertension clinic, nearly half of whom had biochemical evidence of aldosterone excess, spironolactone at 12.5 to 50 mg/d decreased BP by an additional 21/10 mm Hg at 6 weeks of follow-up and by 25/12 mm Hg after 6 months.[76] The BP response was similar in subjects with or without PA, but there was a greater tendency for subjects with PA to be titrated to 50 mg/d to achieve BP control. Lastly, the study enrolled 45 African American patients, and did not see a difference in the effect of spironolactone on BP between African American and Caucasian patients.

Adverse effects of spironolactone include hyperkalemia, which may be pronounced in patients with CKD or diabetes, and in those receiving RAAS blockers. Spironolactone use was also associated with elevations in serum creatinine (13.2–19.3 μmol/L) in the setting of a significant reduction in BP, but not with the development of overt kidney failure.[74,76] The affinity of spironolactone for androgen and progesterone receptors produce the more common but less severe adverse effects including menstrual irregularities, gynecomastia, breast tenderness, erectile dysfunction, and decreased libido, which may pose problems in the treatment of a young male hypertensive patient. Eplerenone, another mineralocorticoid receptor blocker, does not have these effects, and has been used as an alternative to spironolactone in this setting.

Lastly, mineralocorticoid antagonists have also been found to decrease proteinuria by blocking the aldosterone-mediated expansion in intravascular volume, which leads to hyperfiltration in the kidneys and increased protein excretion.[77,78] Hence, spironolactone may have an important role in patients with both RH and diabetes or CKD, with benefits that extend beyond BP lowering.

Other agents

In a group of patients with RH (n = 38, 17 of whom had PA based on urinary aldosterone excretion) and low PRA levels (≤0.4 nmol/L), the potassium-sparing diuretic amiloride plus hydrochlorothiazide as a replacement diuretic to an otherwise stable antihypertensive drug regimen reduced the office BP by 31/15 mm Hg and 24-hour BP by 17/11 mm Hg during treatment compared with placebo, without an increased incidence of hyperkalemia.[44] Seven patients manifested an escape phenomenon, whereby BP levels rose to pretreatment levels within 6 to 12 months of follow-up, and this was effectively treated by doubling the dose of amiloride plus hydrochlorothiazide. Plasma aldosterone and PRA increased significantly during treatment.

Selective α-receptor blockers such as doxazosin and terazosin reduce BP by blocking the post-synaptic α1 receptor in vascular smooth muscle and inducing vasodilation. Doxazosin is not recommended as a first-line agent in the treatment of hypertension based on findings from ALLHAT, where it was associated with an increased risk of heart failure.[27] On the other hand, in ASCOT-BPLA, where doxazosin was used as a third-line antihypertensive agent, it reduced mean BP by 11.7/6.9 mm Hg during a median of 12 months of treatment, thereby enabling 29.7% of the participants to achieve target BP.[79] Further, this was achieved without an excess in incidence of heart failure. In a retrospective study done in a Hypertension Clinic in the Czech Republic, doxazosin (dose range 2–16 mg/d, mean dose of 6.9 mg/d) given as part of a combination of 4 to 8 antihypertensive drugs effectively reduced the BP from 159 ± 20/92 ± 14 to 126 ± 16/73 ± 10.[80] Doxazosin was well tolerated by the study participants, even at higher doses (12–16 mg/d). Randomized controlled trials are needed to determine whether the BP-lowering effect of α-receptor blockers translates to reduced overall CV risk, and to establish its role and indications for treating patients with RH.

An uncontrolled and unblinded case series of 17 male patients with RH referred to a tertiary clinic in Ireland who were given the vasodilator minoxidil as an add-on agent to an antihypertensive regimen that included a diuretic, β-blocker, and either an ACE inhibitor or an ARB showed that the addition of minoxidil at a mean dose of 20 mg/d reduced the BP by 20/13 mm Hg after 6 months of treatment.[81] Minoxidil is rarely used due to its adverse effects, which include reflex tachycardia, fluid retention, hair growth, and development of diabetes, but may still be useful in patients whose options are limited due to medication intolerances. Minoxidil should always be paired with a β-blocker and a diuretic to prevent some adverse effects that are associated with its use.

The newer vasodilating β-blockers (labetalol, carvedilol, and nevibolol) are preferred in the authors' clinics, because some data suggest that they may be better antihypertensive agents than β1-selective antagonists.[82] Other antihypertensive classes (eg, centrally acting agents, vasodilators) have not been evaluated specifically for use in patients with RH. Further, there is a higher incidence of adverse events associated with their use. These agents may be considered if conventional antihypertensive combinations fail to control the BP, or in patients who have adverse reactions to usual treatment.

Surgical treatment

Surgical methods have also been explored to control BP in patients with RH. Stimulation of the carotid baroreflex by means of an implantable device (the Rheos system) lowers BP by activating the carotid baroreflex and the intrinsic neurohormonal pathways, leading to increased parasympathetic flow and decrease in peripheral vascular resistance, heart rate, and stroke volume, resulting in a reduction in BP.[83] Phase 2 trial data in the United States involving 10 patients with RH taking a mean of 6 antihypertensive medications showed that the device reduced SBP by 41 mm Hg without causing significant bradycardia.[84] Phase 3 trials have been recently completed.

Surgical sympathectomy of the renal sympathetic nerves via percutaneous radiofrequency catheter ablation has also been evaluated as a possible treatment option for patients with RH. In 45 patients with RH, whose baseline BP was 177/101 while on a mean of 4.7 antihypertensive medications, renal sympathetic denervation was effective in reducing BP, again without profoundly affecting heart rate.[85] Office BP decreased significantly by the first month (−14/−10 mm Hg), was further reduced by the third month (−21/−10 mm Hg), and the reduction persisted for 12 months (−27/−17 mm Hg). Advantages of this approach include catheter-based intervention, and minimal effects on the innervation of other abdominal organs and the lower extremities. Phase 2 trials are underway.

HYPERTENSIVE CRISES

An episode of DBP elevation above 120 mm Hg is considered a hypertensive crisis. It is further classified into hypertensive emergency or hypertensive urgency, depending on the presence or absence of acute target organ damage. If there is associated target organ damage, including unstable angina, myocardial infarction, stroke, encephalopathy, subarachnoid hemorrhage, acute renal failure, microangiopathic hemolytic anemia, acute aortic dissection, or eclampsia, it is considered a hypertensive emergency. If there is no ongoing end-organ deterioration,, it is considered an hypertensive urgency. Hypertensive emergencies historically have been further classified based on retinal findings from accelerated hypertension, where cotton wool exudates or flame-shaped hemorrhages are present, and malignant hypertension, where bilateral papilledema is the predominant finding. These terms, however, are being used less often.

The distinction between hypertensive emergencies and urgencies is important in determining treatment. Hypertensive emergencies require intravenous antihypertensive drugs to lower the BP within the first few hours of presentation, with a primary objective of reversing or reducing target organ damage. A general rule is that BP should be reduced by 10% in the first hour, then by another 15% in the next 2 to 3 hours (except in aortic dissection, where an SBP of <120 mm Hg should be attained within 20 minutes). Once stable, transition to oral antihypertensive therapy can be made after 6 to 12 hours. On the other hand, hypertensive urgencies are managed in a monitored outpatient setting using oral antihypertensive agents to lower BP in the next 24 hours to 2 to 3 days.

A hypertensive crisis is generally viewed to result from inadequate treatment of hypertension, or poor adherence to antihypertensive medications. Although its incidence is low (<1%), the sheer number of hypertensive individuals makes this a formidable problem for clinicians worldwide.

Various intravenous antihypertensive agents are accepted in the initial treatment of a patient presenting with a hypertensive emergency (see **Table 2**). At present, there is insufficient evidence to show that one drug is superior to another in reducing morbidity or mortality in patients presenting with a hypertensive emergency.[86] There are minor differences in the degree of BP lowering between the drug classes, but the clinical significance of this is difficult to ascertain.[87] Often, the choice of parenteral antihypertensive agents is dictated by the clinical picture and the presence of contraindications.

SUMMARY

Hypertension is a global problem affecting as many as 1 billion individuals worldwide. It is an important modifiable risk factor for CV morbidity and mortality. The hypertensive population, apart from having BP greater than 140/90 mm Hg, is a heterogeneous group. Within this group are patients with secondary forms of hypertension, RH, and hypertensive emergencies. Patients with secondary forms of hypertension have an identifiable cause that contributes to or explains the elevated BP. Common causes include CKD, PA, and OSA. Patients with RH are taking 3 or more antihypertensive medications to control BP. These patients have higher CV risk than the general hypertensive population and have a higher incidence of secondary causes of hypertension. Elements of pseudoresistance (white-coat effect, improper BP measurement technique, and medication nonadherence) need to be ruled out and corrected. Intake of interfering substances has to be eliminated or regulated. Thiazide diuretics, especially chlorthalidone, are recommended for patients without contraindications. Mineralocorticoid antagonists are formidable add-on agents to lower BP in patients with RH. Patients with a hypertensive emergency have an episode of severe BP elevation that is associated with target organ damage. These episodes are best treated by intravenous antihypertensive agents, and no evidence exists to recommend one agent over another.

REFERENCES

1. Global health risks: mortality and burden of disease attributable to selected major risks. Geneva (Switzerland): World Health Organization; 2004. Available at: http://www.who.int/healthinfo/global_burden_disease/global_health_risks/en/index.html. Accessed December 23, 2009.
2. Cutler JA, Sorlie PD, Wolz M, et al. Trends in hypertension prevalence, awareness, treatment, and control rates in United States adults between 1988-1994 and 1999-2004. Hypertension 2008;52:818–27.
3. Whelton PK, He J, Appel LJ, et al. Primary prevention of hypertension: clinical and public health advisory from the National High Blood Pressure Education Program. JAMA 2002;288:1882–8.
4. Oparil S, Zaman MA, Calhoun DA. Pathogenesis of hypertension. Ann Intern Med 2003;139:761–76.
5. Young JH, Klag MJ, Muntner P, et al. Blood pressure and decline in kidney function: findings from the Systolic Hypertension in the Elderly Program (SHEP). J Am Soc Nephrol 2002;13:2776–82.
6. Hsu CY, McCulloch CE, Darbinian J, et al. Elevated blood pressure and risk of end-stage renal disease in subjects without baseline kidney disease. Arch Intern Med 2005;165:923–8.
7. Lloyd-Jones D, Adams R, Carnethon M, et al. American Heart Association Statistics Committee and Stroke Statistics Subcommittee. Heart Disease and Stroke Statistics 2009 Update: a report from the American Heart Association Statistics Committee and Stroke Statistics Subcommittee. Circulation 2009;119:e21–181.
8. Campese VM, Mitra N, Sandee D. Hypertension in renal parenchymal disease: why is it so resistant to treatment? Kidney Int 2006;69:967–73.
9. Centers for Disease Control and Prevention (CDC). Prevalence of chronic kidney disease and associated risk factors: United States, 1999–2004. MMWR Morb Mortal Wkly Rep 2007;56:161–5.
10. National Kidney Foundation. K/DOQI clinical practice guidelines for chronic kidney disease: evaluation, classification and stratification. Am J Kidney Dis 2002;39:S1–266.
11. National Kidney Foundation. K/DOQI clinical practice guidelines on hypertension and antihypertensive agents in chronic kidney disease. Am J Kidney Dis 2004;43:S1–268.
12. Nishizaka MK, Zaman MA, Green SA, et al. Impaired endothelium-dependent flow-mediated vasodilation in hypertensive subjects with hyperaldosteronism. Circulation 2004;109:2857–61.
13. Lombes M, Farman N, Bonvalet JP, et al. Identification and role of aldosterone receptors in the cardiovascular system. Ann Endocrinol (Paris) 2000;61:41–6.
14. Marney AN, Brown NJ. Aldosterone and end-organ damage. Clin Sci 2007;113:267–78.
15. Rayner BL, Opie LH, Davidson JS. The aldosterone/renin ratio as a screening test for primary aldosteronism. S Afr Med J 2000;90:394–400.
16. Funder JW, Carey RM, Fardella C, et al. Case detection, diagnosis, and treatment of patients with primary aldosteronism: an Endocrine Society clinical practice guideline. J Clin Endocrinol Metab 2008;93:3266–81.
17. Nishizaka MK, Pratt-Ubunama M, Zaman MA, et al. Validity of plasma aldosterone to renin activity ratio in African American and white subjects with resistant hypertension. Am J Hypertens 2005;18:805–12.
18. Calhoun DA, Nishizaka MK, Zaman MA, et al. High prevalence of primary aldosteronism among black and white subjects with resistant hypertension. Hypertension 2002;40:892–6.
19. Benchetrit S, Bernheim J, Podjarny E. Normokalemic hyperaldosteronism in patients with resistant hypertension. Isr Med Assoc J 2002;4:17–20.
20. Garovic VD, Kane GC, Schwartz GL. Renovascular hypertension: balancing the controversies in diagnosis and treatment. Cleve Clin J Med 2005;72:1135–47.
21. Nieto FJ, Young TB, Lind BK, et al. Sleep Heart Health Study. Association of sleep-disordered breathing, sleep apnea, and hypertension in a large community-based study. JAMA 2000;283:1829–36.
22. Ramachandran SK, Josephs LA. A meta-analysis of clinical screening tests for obstructive sleep apnea. Anesthesiology 2009;110:928–39.
23. Haentjens P, Meerhaeghe AV, Moscariello AV, et al. The impact of continuous positive airway pressure on blood pressure in patients with obstructive sleep apnea syndrome. Arch Intern Med 2007;167:757–65.
24. Nieman LK, Biller BM, Findling JW, et al. The diagnosis of Cushing's syndrome: an Endocrine Society

clinical practice guideline. J Clin Endocrinol 2008; 93:1526–40.
25. Eisenhofer G, Siegert G, Kotzerke J, et al. Current progress and future challenges in the biochemical diagnosis and treatment of pheochromocytomas and paragangliomas. Horm Metab Res 2008;40: 329–37.
26. Calhoun DA, Jones D, Textor S, et al. Resistant hypertension: diagnosis, evaluation, and treatment: a scientific statement from the American Heart Association Professional Education Committee of the Council for High Blood Pressure Research. Hypertension 2008;51:1403–19.
27. Furberg CD, Wright JT, Davis BR, et al. ALLHAT Collaborative Research Group. Major outcomes in high-risk hypertensive patients randomized to angiotension converting enzyme inhibitor or calcium channel blocker vs. diuretic. JAMA 2002;288:2981, 2977.
28. Garg JP, Elliott WJ, Folker A, et al. Resistant hypertension revisited: a comparison of two university-based cohorts. Am J Hypertens 2005;18:619–26.
29. Leotta G, Rabbia F, Canade A, et al. Characteristics of the patients referred to a Hypertension Unit between 1989 and 2003. J Hum Hypertens 2008; 22:119–21.
30. Pierdomenico SD, Lapenna D, Bucci A, et al. Cardiovascular outcome in treated hypertensive patients with responder, masked, false resistant and true resistant hypertension. Am J Hypertens 2005;18:1422–8.
31. Muxfeldt ES, Bloch KV, Nogueira AR, et al. Twenty four hour ambulatory blood pressure monitoring pattern of resistant hypertension. Blood Press Monit 2003;8:181–5.
32. Veglio F, Rabbia F, Riva P, et al. Ambulatory blood pressure monitoring and clinical characteristics of the true and white-coat resistant hypertension. Clin Exp Hypertens 2001;23:203–11.
33. Muxfeldt ES, Cardoso CR, Salles GF. Prognostic value of nocturnal blood pressure reduction in resistant hypertension. Arch Intern Med 2009;169: 874–80.
34. Verdecchia P, Schillaci G, Borgioni C, et al. Ambulatory pulse pressure. A potent predictor of total cardiovascular risk in hypertension. Hypertension 1998;32:983–8.
35. Gillman MW, Kannel WB, Belanger A, et al. Influence of heart rate on mortality among patients with hypertension: the Framingham Heart Study. Am Heart J 1993;125:1148–54.
36. Ostchega Y, Dillon CF, Hughes JP, et al. Trends in hypertension prevalence, awareness, treatment and control in older US adults: data from the National Health and Nutrition Examination Survey 1998-2004. J Am Geriatr Soc 2007;55:1056–65.
37. Chobanian AV, Bakris GL, Black HR, et al. The seventh report of the joint national committee on prevention, detection, evaluation, and treatment of high blood pressure: The JNC 7 report. JAMA 2003;289:2560–72.
38. Lloyd-Jones DM, Evans JC, Larson MG, et al. Differential control of systolic and diastolic blood pressure: factors associated with lack of blood pressure control in the community. Hypertension 2000;36:594–9.
39. Lloyd-Jones DM, Evans JC, Larson MG, et al. Treatment and control of hypertension in the community: a prospective analysis. Hypertension 2002;40:640–6.
40. Pratt-Ubunama MN, Nishizaka MK, Boedefeld RL, et al. Plasma aldosterone is related to severity of obstructive sleep apnea in subjects with resistant hypertension. Chest 2007;131:453–9.
41. Logan AG, Perlikowski SM, Mente A, et al. High prevalence of unrecognized sleep apnoea in drug-resistant hypertension. J Hypertens 2001;19: 2271–7.
42. Goncalves SC, Martinez D, Gus M, et al. Obstructive sleep apnea and resistant hypertension. A case control study. Chest 2007;132:1858–62.
43. Gallay BJ, Ahmad S, Xu L, et al. Screening for primary aldosteronism without discontinuing hypertensive medications: plasma aldosterone-renin ratio. Am J Kidney Dis 2001;37:699–705.
44. Eide IK, Torjesen PA, Drolsum A, et al. Low-renin status in therapy-resistant hypertension: a clue to efficient treatment. J Hypertens 2004;22:2217–26.
45. Štrauch B, Zelinka T, Hampf M, et al. Prevalence of primary hyperaldosteronism in moderate to severe hypertension in the Central Europe region. J Hum Hypertens 2003;17:349–52.
46. Calhoun DA, Nishizaka MK, Zaman MA, et al. Aldosterone excretion among subjects with resistant hypertension and symptoms of sleep apnea. Chest 2004;125:112–27.
47. Saelen MG, Prøsch LK, Gudmundsdottir H, et al. Controlling systolic blood pressure is difficult in patients with diabetic kidney disease exhibiting moderate-to-severe reductions in renal function. Blood Press 2005;14:170–6.
48. Gaddam KK, Nishizaka MK, Pratt-Ubunama MN, et al. Characterization of resistant hypertension. Association between resistant hypertension, aldosterone, and persistent intravascular volume expansion. Arch Intern Med 2008;168:1159–64.
49. Sartori M, Calo LA, Mascagna V, et al. Aldosterone and refractory hypertension: a prospective cohort study. Am J Hypertens 2006;19:373–9.
50. Pimenta E, Gaddam KK, Pratt-Ubunama MN, et al. Aldosterone excess and resistance to 24 hour blood pressure control. J Hypertens 2007;25:2131–7.
51. Pickering TG. Principles and techniques of blood pressure measurement. Cardiol Clin 2002;20:207–23.
52. Caro JJ, Speckman JL, Salas M, et al. Effect of initial drug choice on persistence with antihypertensive

therapy: the importance of actual practice data. CMAJ 1999;160:41–6.
53. Ogedegbe G, Schoenthaler A. A systematic review of the effects of home blood pressure monitoring on medication adherence. J Clin Hypertens 2006; 8:174–80.
54. Stason WB, Shepard DS, Perry HM Jr, et al. Effectiveness and costs of veterans affairs hyper-tension clinics. Med Care 1994;32:1197–215.
55. Burnier M, Santschi V, Favrat B, et al. Monitoring compliance in resistant hypertension: an important step in patient management. J Hypertens 2003;31: S37–42.
56. De Souza WA, Yugar-Toledo JC, Bergsten-Mendes G, et al. Effect of pharmaceutical care on blood pressure and health related quality of life in patients with resistant hypertension. Am J Health Syst Pharm 2007;64:1955–61.
57. Pickering TG, White WB. When and how to use self (home) and ambulatory blood pressure monitoring. J Am Soc Hypertens 2008;2:119–24.
58. Rodrigues CS, Bloch KV, Noguiera AR. Office blood pressure and 24-h ambulatory blood pressure measurements: high proportion of disagreement in resistant hypertension. J Clin Epidemiol 2009;62: 745–51.
59. Grossman E, Messerli FH. Secondary hypertension: interfering substances. J Clin Hypertens (Greenwich) 2008;10:556–66.
60. Chasan-Taber L, Willett WC, Manson JE, et al. Prospective study of oral contraceptives and hypertension among women in the United States. Circulation 1996;94(3):483–9.
61. Frishman WH. Effects of nonsteroidal anti-inflammatory drug therapy on blood pressure and peripheral edema. Am J Cardiol 2002;89:18D–25D.
62. Ishiguro C, Fukita T, Omori T, et al. Assessing the effects of non-steroidal anti-inflammatory drugs on anti-hypertensive drug therapy using post-marketing surveillance database. J Epidemiol 2008;18(3):119–24.
63. Avancini F, Palumbo G, Alli C, et al. Effects of low-dose aspirin on clinic and ambulatory blood pressure in treated hypertensive patients. Am J Hypertens 2000;13:611–6.
64. Vollmer WM, Sacks FM, Ard J, et al. DASH-Sodium Trial Collaborative Research Group. Effects of diet and sodium intake on blood pressure: subgroup analysis of the DASH-sodium trial. Ann Intern Med 2001;135:1019–28.
65. He FJ, MacGregor GA. Effect of modest salt reduction on blood pressure: a meta-analysis of randomized trials. Implications for public health. J Hum Hypertens 2002;16:761–70.
66. Cook NR, Cutler JA, Obarzanek E, et al. Long term effects of dietary sodium reduction on cardiovascular disease outcomes: observational follow-up of the trials of hypertension prevention (TOHP). BMJ 2007;334:885–8.
67. Pimenta E, Gaddam KK, Oparil S, et al. Effects of dietary sodium reduction on blood pressure in subjects with resistant hypertension: results from a randomized trial. Hypertension 2009;54:475–81.
68. Taler SJ, Textor SC, Augustine JE. Resistant hypertension. Comparing hemodynamic management to specialist care. Hypertension 2002;39:982–8.
69. Ray WA, Griffin MR, Downey W, et al. Long-term use of thiazide diuretics and risk of hip fracture. Lancet 1989;1:687–90.
70. Wanich R, Davis J, Ross P, et al. Effects of thiazides on rates of bone mineral loss: a longitudinal study. Br Med J 1990;310:1303–5.
71. Ernst ME, Carter BL, Goerdt CJ, et al. Comparative antihypertensive effects of hydrochlorothiazide and chlorthalidone on ambulatory and office blood pressure. Hypertension 2006;47:352–8.
72. Multiple Risk Factor Intervention Trial Research Group. Mortality after 10 ½ years for hypertensive participants in the Multiple Risk Factor Intervention Trial. Circulation 1990;82:1616–28.
73. Ouzan J, Perault C, Lincoff AM, et al. The role of spironolactone in the treatment of patients with refractory hypertension. Am J Hypertens 2002;15:333–9.
74. Dahlof B, Sever PS, Poulter NR, et al. Prevention of cardiovascular events with an antihypertensive regimen of amlodipine adding perindopril as required versus atenolol adding benzoflumethiazide as required, in the Anglo-Scandinavian Cardiac Outcomes Trial—Blood Pressure Lowering Arm (ASCOT-BPLA): a multicentre randomised controlled trial. Lancet 2005;366:895–906.
75. Chapman N, Dobson J, Wilson S, et al. Effect of spironolactone on blood pressure in subjects with resistant hypertension. Hypertension 2007;49: 839–45.
76. Nishizaka MK, Zaman MA, Calhoun DA. Efficacy of low-dose spironolactone in subjects with resistant hypertension. Am J Hypertens 2003;16:925–30.
77. Schjoedt KJ, Rossing K, Juhl TR, et al. Beneficial impact of spironolactone in diabetic nephropathy. Kidney Int 2005;68:2829–36.
78. Bianchi S, Bigazzi R, Campese VM. Antagonists of aldosterone and proteinuria in patients with CKD: an uncontrolled study. Am J Kidney Dis 2005;46: 45–51.
79. Chapman N, Chang CL, Dahlof B, et al, on behalf of the ASCOT investigators. Effect of doxazosin gastrointestinal therapeutic system as third-line antihypertensive therapy on blood pressure and lipids in the Anglo-Scandinavian Cardiac Outcomes Trial. Circulation 2008;118:42–8.
80. Ceral J, Solar M. Doxazosin: safety and efficacy in the treatment of resistant arterial hypertension. Blood Press 2009;18:74–7.

81. Black RN, Hunter SJ, Atkinson AB. Usefulness of the vasodilator minoxidil in resistant hypertension [research letter]. J Hypertens 2007;25:1102–3.
82. Townsend RR, DiPette DJ, Goodman R, et al. Combined alpha/beta blockade versus beta 1-selective blockade in essential hypertension in black and white patients. Clin Pharmacol Ther 1990;48:665–75.
83. Filippone JD, Bisognano JD. Baroreflex stimulation in the treatment of hypertension. Curr Opin Nephrol Hypertens 2007;16:403–8.
84. Illig KA, Levy M, Sanchez L, et al. An implantable carotid sinus stimulator for drug-resistant hypertension: surgical technique and short-term outcome from the multicenter Phase II Rheos feasibility trial. J Vasc Surg 2006;44:1213–8.
85. Krum H, Schlaich M, Whitbourn R, et al. Catheter-based renal sympathetic denervation for resistant hypertension: a multicentre safety and proof-of-principle cohort study. Lancet 2009;373:1275–81.
86. Perez MI, Musini VM, Wright JM. Pharmacological interventions for hypertensive emergencies. Cochrane Database Syst Rev 2008;1:CD003653.
87. Perez MI, Musini VM. Pharmacological interventions for hypertensive emergencies: a Cochrane systematic review. J Hum Hypertens 2008;22:596–607.

Patient Self-Management Support: Novel Strategies in Hypertension and Heart Disease

Hayden B. Bosworth, PhD[a,b,*]
Benjamin J. Powers, MD, MHSc[a,b]
Eugene Z. Oddone, MD, MHSc[a,b]

KEYWORDS

• Cardiovascular disease • Hypertension
• Self-management • Lifestyle

Chronic diseases, specifically cardiovascular diseases (CVDs), have become the leading cause of death and disability in most countries in the world.[1,2] In the United States, an estimated 81.1 million persons have CVD, and coronary heart disease (CHD) and stroke remain the first and third leading causes of death, respectively. CVD also carries an enormous personal and financial burden (the total direct and indirect cost of heart disease and stroke in the United States for 2010 is estimated at $503.2 billion).[3] These epidemiologic data integrated within the context of unsustainable health care expenses define a burning platform for the prevention and incorporation of strategies that allow patients to take more control over their illnesses. In this article, the authors discuss patient self-management of hypertension and CVD as a crucial component of effective high-quality health care for chronic diseases.

WHAT IS SELF-MANAGEMENT OF HYPERTENSION AND CVD?

Managing a chronic illness is a time-consuming and complex process. Patients and their informal caregivers are required to make day-to-day decisions about actions, such as how to respond to new symptoms, what and how much to eat, whether to take their medication, or whether to exercise, which can all have substantial effects on their clinical outcomes, particularly when the decisions are aggregated over months and years. These day-to-day decisions and tasks are referred to as self-management, which was formally defined by Barlow and colleagues[4] as "the individual's ability to manage the symptoms, treatment, physical and psychosocial consequences and lifestyle changes inherent in living with a chronic condition." All patients with hypertension

This research is supported by an Established Investigator Award from the American Heart Association and Career Scientist Award from Health Services Research and Development, Veterans Affairs Medical Center to the first author (HBB). The second author (BJP) is supported by a KL2 career development award RR024127-02, Duke University. No authors have conflicts of interest. The views expressed in this article are those of the authors and do not necessarily represent the views of the Department of Veterans Affairs.
[a] Center for Health Services Research in Primary Care, Durham Veterans Affairs Medical Center, HSR&D (152), Suite 600, 411 West Chapel Hill Street, Durham, NC 27701, USA
[b] Division of General Internal Medicine, Department of Medicine, Duke University, 2424 Erwin Road, Hock Plaza, Durham, NC 27703, USA
* Corresponding author. Division of General Internal Medicine, Department of Medicine, Duke University, 2424 Erwin Road, Hock Plaza, Durham, NC 27703.
E-mail address: hboswort@acpub.duke.edu

Cardiol Clin 28 (2010) 655–663
doi:10.1016/j.ccl.2010.07.003
0733-8651/10/$ – see front matter. Published by Elsevier Inc.

self-manage; the question is how well they self-manage, and the influence of self-management on the patient's experience of chronic disease and health outcomes. An important goal for the health system is to discover effective interventions that improve patients' ability to self-manage and implement those interventions into practice.

The potential benefit of interventions to improve patients' self-management and subsequent health behaviors exceeds that of interventions aimed at health care providers, in part, because unhealthy behaviors may contribute to poor health and premature death more than inadequate health care. Unhealthy behaviors, such as smoking, poor diet, and sedentary lifestyles, account for as much as 40% of premature deaths in the United States, whereas deficiencies in health care delivery account for only 10%.[5] Thus, with recent discussions of health care reform, the focus on self-management in chronic diseases, particularly hypertension, is likely to increase.

Self-management is more than simple adherence to provider recommendations because it also incorporates the psychological and social management of living with a chronic condition. Self-management consists of the following components: engaging in activities that promote physical and psychological health, interacting with health care providers and adhering to treatment recommendations, monitoring health status and making associated care decisions, and managing the effect of the illness on physical, psychological, and social functioning.[6] To a great extent, patients' outcomes are dictated by the degree to which these choices lead to improved risk reduction.

Studies conducted among individuals with chronic conditions demonstrate that many patients struggle with self-management[7–11] and therefore suffer from inadequate disease control, reduced quality of life, and poor psychological well-being.[12–14] Patients' ability to self-manage may be influenced by the demands of their illnesses and their social and economic circumstances.[6] For patients with multiple or complex conditions (multimorbidity), the time, effort, and cost of effective self-management can be challenging from the patient's perspective.[15] From the provider's perspective, improving patients' adherence to medication and timely initiation or intensification of medications as well as counseling on self-management behaviors are complex and time consuming. Time limitations, competing demands,[16,17] the burden of comorbid illness,[18] and inadequate mechanisms for follow-up constitute the barriers to effective self-management of CVD.

Research and practice of self-management has been improved by a larger understanding of the context or framework in which these health care decisions are made. One framework that contextualizes patient self-management the larger health systems and the larger community is the Chronic Care Model.[19] This model emphasizes the role of patients with chronic conditions as being their own principal caregiver and the importance of support from the provider, family, and community in self-management.[7,20] In effect, patients are at the center of this model with the providers, family, and community interacting in different ways to influence and support health care decisions. This model of care recognizes a collaborative partnership between patients and providers, each with their own expertise in managing that person's health, to share in the decision-making process. This collaborative partnership between patients and providers is important in supporting the patient's management of chronic diseases over multiple encounters and adjustments in the treatment plan to achieve optimal care.

WHAT ARE THE GOALS OF EFFECTIVE SELF-MANAGEMENT?

One important goal of self-management support is to provide the patient with problem-solving skills to recognize challenges in chronic disease management and to generate a plan to forge a solution.[21] Although traditional patient education offers information and technical skills, self-management programs include education as well as problem-solving skills. Self-management programs focus on helping patients develop self-efficacy and the confidence to carry out behavior change necessary to reach a desired goal. Self-management education programs are distinct from simple patient education or skills training in that they are designed to allow people with chronic conditions to take an active part in the management of their own condition.

Effective self-management of hypertension and CVD consists of (1) self-monitoring disease control and symptoms; (2) knowing when blood pressure (BP) levels or symptoms indicate a problem; (3) responding with appropriate actions (adjust medications, initiate call to a health care provider); (4) making major lifestyle changes (eg, stop smoking, reduce alcohol consumption, modify diet, lose weight, and increase exercise); (5) adhering to medication regimens (even in the absence of symptoms), some of which are inconvenient or produce side effects; (6) identifying and responding to the psychosocial contributors of chronic disease management; and (7) maintaining regular contact with a health care provider for monitoring progress. Thus, self-management programs designed to reduce the effect of CVD might include components to address each of the problems listed earlier by (1) promoting patient-centered care and improving physician-patient communication,[22,23] (2) increasing patients' adherence to recommended medications and self-care regimens, (3) facilitating greater communication between physicians and patients, (4) making medical care more evidence-based through proven health behaviors,[24,25] and (5) increasing focus on self-monitoring (eg, balancing weight, BP, glucose levels, and so on).

HOW DOES SELF-MANAGEMENT FIT INTO THE LARGER CONTEXT OF THE HEALTH SYSTEM?

Driven largely by the methods of reimbursement, traditional health care, both primary and specialty, has been office or clinic based, requiring a direct encounter between a provider and the patient. Although providers have always done what they could to teach patients how to manage their conditions in this setting, it is increasingly recognized that the model of care is not sufficient, particularly for chronic illnesses. There has been an increased focus on self-management with the incorporation of the patient-centered medical home into medical practice. The Veterans Health Administration, Medicare, and other large health care insurers are exploring the medical home as a way to improve quality, satisfaction, and outcomes for patients with chronic medical illnesses. According to the Joint Principles of the Patient-Centered Medical Home, individuals have a personal physician who provides first-contact care, which is continuous, comprehensive, and accessible, while being coordinated with the care offered by other providers.[26] Thus, the core features of the medical home include a physician-directed medical practice, a personal doctor for every patient, the capacity to coordinate high-quality accessible care, and payments that recognize a medical home's added value for patients.[27] Such strategies require an evidence base to understand which components should be included to maximize benefit yet limit cost.

Although self-management is an important component of the medical home, a goal of self-management support programs is to reduce health care costs and workplace costs related to the reduced productivity of chronically ill workers. Offering better support to patients may help them stay healthier, prevent expensive exacerbations and complications, and decrease the use of health care services, thereby reducing costs for providers, insurers, employers, and other large purchasers of health care services as well as for the patients themselves. However, data thus far suggest that self-management programs that are not well integrated with patients' providers are not all that efficacious.[28]

WHAT ARE THE EFFECTIVE COMPONENTS OF SELF-MANAGEMENT SUPPORT?

A key requirement of self-management for chronic conditions such as hypertension is that patients must be empowered and motivated to take an active role in their care and ownership of patient-centered management plans. Self-management programs typically emphasize patients being their own principal caregiver and the importance of support of the provider, family, and community in the self-management process. Despite this common goal, the methods by which self-management programs have worked to empower the patient have varied significantly.

One important tool in supporting self-management of hypertension has been the use of home BP self-monitoring. Home monitoring is inexpensive, is accurate, and has gained wider acceptance as an important component in managing hypertension.[29] Patients' home BP measurement is more prognostically important than measurement at office in predicting clinical events and represents an important target in reducing risks attributable to hypertension.[30] Furthermore, home BP monitoring allows patients to gauge BP responses to their health behaviors and also overcomes the fact that hypertension is an asymptomatic disease. Home BP monitoring alone has also been shown to have a modest effect in lowering BP.[31]

A second effective method of promoting patient self-management is collaborative goal setting,[32] which is the process by which providers and patients agree on a health goal related to the target disease. The goal can be general (eg, getting more exercise) or may involve a specific action plan (eg, walking 1 mile 3 times a week). Establishing specific action plans allows the patient and provider to agree on discrete actionable goals as well as in establishing accountability for the proposed goal. Goals identified through this process then become the basis for future conversations that address methods to help patients achieve their goals.

An additional tool used by members of the health care team for enhancing the effectiveness of patient self-management is motivational interviewing (MI). There has been considerable interest in adapting MI, which may be used by various providers (eg, nurses, health care coaches) to address health behaviors such as treatment adherence.[33] A key goal of MI is to assist individuals to work through their ambivalence about behavior change. In MI, the goal is not simply to exchange information with the patient but to promote behavior change by helping the patient to explore and resolve ambivalence.[34] Effective MI results in the patients' ability to make the right choice and follow through.

More recently, self-management has been studied in the context of more direct reward mechanisms through introducing financial, or other, incentives to help patients achieve a meaningful change. Many patients have strong health incentives to engage in healthy behaviors, but they fail to do so, in part, because the benefits tend to be delayed and intangible. Rewards can provide immediate and tangible benefits for reducing such costs by improving health behavior, leading patients to internalize the future costs they impose on themselves.[35] One study found a significant effect when patients were provided with financial incentives to improve smoking cessation rates[36] as well as to promote weight loss.[37] Policy decisions concerning who would provide such financial incentives to patients are complex. These incentives may make the most sense in an insurance model or for payers of health care. However, further research into the use of financial incentives and their operationalization are needed.

The timing and sequencing of interventions to support patient self-management may also be important. Hypertension control, for example, is known to involve long-term sustained changes in multiple behaviors, including increased medication adherence, dietary modification, increased exercise, weight loss, reduced sodium intake, alcohol moderation, and smoking cessation.[38] Ongoing work suggests that self-management interventions may differ depending on whether there is a focus on initiating one or multiple behaviors as compared with maintaining single or multiple behaviors. A recent hypertension intervention study (PREMIER) demonstrated that after 6 months, change in multiple risk factors improved systolic BP. The improvement was linked specifically to weight loss, greater physical activity, greater adherence to dietary-approaches-to-stop-hypertension dietary changes, and reduced sodium intake.[39] Because changes in the various lifestyle factors were generally not associated with each other (eg, few dietary changes were linked to increased exercise), it seems that some patients successfully controlled hypertension through exercise, others through diet, and still others through sodium reduction. These results suggest that counseling that simultaneously addresses multiple paths to improved behavior and is tailored to individuals' level of change (initiating or successfully maintaining behaviors) may be a promising approach when multiple risk behaviors are present, as is often the case with patients with complex chronic conditions.

An important component of self-management is also the consideration of individuals' culture and environment; patients' health beliefs and health-related behaviors are grounded, at least in part, in their cultures' values and norms. Cultural competence is a dynamic, continuous process by which an individual provider, health care system, or health care agency finds meaningful and useful care-delivery strategies based on the knowledge of the cultural heritage, beliefs, attitudes, and behaviors of those receiving care.[20] Self-management interventions to improve CVD outcomes are more likely to be accepted if the intervention can be adapted to (1) the norms of the specific culture and community of which the patient is a part and (2) the health decision making in that culture. Competency can involve asking questions to determine cultural beliefs or practices that may influence health behavior, listening closely, and using information about the patient to tailor an intervention to local context.[20]

WHERE DOES SELF-MANAGEMENT SUPPORT OCCUR?

Most patients with hypertension receive most of the information about their disease and all of the treatment in the ambulatory clinic settings. Paradigms of self-management support have been developed in the recognition that treating chronic illness requires more than simple face-to-face clinic visits. Thus, relying on the outpatient provider to deliver the needed self-management support is often limited by the competing issues that arise during routine office visits or due to the lack of accessibility to primary care. Although critically important, improving patients' hypertension management behaviors and medication adherence can be complex and time consuming. In a typical office setting, time limitations, competing demands,[16,17] and inadequate mechanisms for follow-up constitute barriers to effective hypertension risk factor management. Moreover, the primary care office visit is often filled with multiple tasks, including cancer screening, medication refill, and payment issues, making it even more difficult to concentrate on any given disease. Perhaps for these reasons, prior interventions that sought to influence physician medication prescribing (through education, reminders, and academic detailing) in a clinic setting have been mostly ineffective.[22,40] Current reimbursement models also inhibit alternative mechanisms to improve self-management, such as telephone or e-visits. In addition, focusing solely on patients receiving treatment in health care settings may lead to underrepresenting patients with chronic diseases who are disenfranchised from the health care system or who have limited access to health care because of transportation issues. Novel approaches to test treatment interventions outside the office setting and their effects on quality indicators as well as costs need to be considered.

An initial step in choosing or building a self-management program is to decide where it can be positioned. Should it be managed and administered within the patient's primary care setting or external to it? The distinction often has important ramifications for the degree to which self-management support is integrated with other aspects of the patient's chronic care and thus on who the players are, the quantity and kind of data available to support it, and the nature of the administrative oversight and support. However, most aspects of hypertension risk reduction do not require a physical examination or laboratory evaluation and could therefore be accomplished through encounters that happen outside the traditional office visit. Recent data suggest that incorporating self-management into clinical care as opposed to an added layer of care may be preferred.[28]

Modes of administering hypertension interventions and programs include the use of landline or cellular telephones. As of 2003, most homes in the United States have phones (>97%),[41] making it a useful tool to deliver self-management programs. Telephone care has an established track record as an acceptable[42] and often-preferred method of receiving care by patients.[43]

Telemedicine or remote monitoring in patients' homes has also been offered as a plausible solution to improving ambulatory medical care. In the case of hypertension, advances in home BP telemonitoring are likely to have a significant effect in the way health care is provided for those with CVD. In home BP telemonitoring, hypertensive persons self-monitor their BP at home and then transmit their BP readings over telephone lines to a central server.[44,45] Adults, particularly those who are the most vulnerable (eg, greater comorbidities, lower social economic status, lower literacy), may have barriers to receiving care in the traditional clinic-based model, given the relatively longer distances they live from their usual source of care. One way to improve BP control is to facilitate access to care by incorporating BP telemonitoring in patients' homes; this monitoring may be more acceptable and effective than clinic-based monitoring and management. The use of telecommunications has been increasing but is still comparatively rare, and few trials have assessed the efficacy of such technology for improving BP control in patients.[46]

Several Internet and Web-based information management tools have emerged in the health care marketplace enabling communication between patients and providers and among providers.[47] Web-based monitoring may be more acceptable and effective than clinic-based monitoring and management as well as more scalable and cost-effective than traditional disease management programs. The American Heart Association has developed a Web-based interactive communication tool, Heart360 (http://www.heart360.org), based on Microsoft's HealthVault (http://www.healthvault.com) electronic health record platform. Heart360 is designed to facilitate better information exchange between patients and their providers as well as to promote patient engagement in their own disease management. The authors conducted a novel study, Secondary Prevention Risk Interventions via Telemedicine and Tailored Patient Education (SPRITE), to simultaneously evaluate 2 risk-reduction interventions of CHD via a randomized controlled trial. One group received ambulatory BP monitors and was enrolled into Heart360 for Web-based data transmission, tracking, and communication of BP measurements with a nurse-based tailored education and disease management via telephone. A second group also received home BP monitors to use with Heart 360, but tailored education and disease management were given in a Web-based format. This study design provides information on whether Web-based communication coupled with a Web-based tailored disease management and education program improves risk factor control beyond telemedicine disease management provided by health care personnel as well as considers the costs of implementing this program.

WHO DELIVERS SELF-MANAGEMENT SUPPORT?

Many different individuals can take part in self-management support. In the health system, the patients' primary care or specialty care provider play central roles in defining the care plan. Office nursing staff typically provides much of the educational components and strategies for success. The patients' social network, particularly those living with them at home, are also central components.

More recently, health care coaches and even lay personnel (eg, community health workers) may engage patients in effective self-management. Despite that a traditional office visit may not be the best place to conduct all self-management practices, an effective patient-provider relationship is a central component of effective self-management. There must be a commitment to self-management on the part of the individual and the provider, trust that decisions are being made with requisite information, and willingness to make adjustments in the treatment plan to achieve optimal care and appropriate hypertension management. Thus, the patient-provider relationship is based on shared decision making between patients and other members of the health care team.

Alternative members of the health care team may be more effective in improving patients' self-management practices than physicians.[48] The use of nonphysicians to implement interventions may enhance the ability to achieve high-quality care. For example, nurses as interventionists in clinical trials have been found to be more effective than physicians at bringing hypertensive individuals in concordance with national guideline goals[49–54] and can improve both patient adherence to BP medications and BP control.[55–58] Nurses have also been shown to significantly improve self-management practices and BP control, even when their only interaction with patients is over the telephone.[31,59]

Self-management education programs led by lay leaders (rather than health professionals, such as doctors or nurses) are becoming common as a way of trying to promote self-care for people with chronic conditions. In a Cochrane review of lay-led self-management programs for people with chronic conditions, 7 studies showed a small, statistically significant increase in self-reported aerobic exercise (standardized mean difference −0.20; 95% confidence interval [CI], −0.27 to −0.12). There were no statistically significant differences between groups for hospital visits (6 studies). Patients' confidence to manage their condition showed a small statistically significant improvement (10 studies; standardized mean difference −0.30; 95% CI, −0.41 to −0.19). Lay-led self-management education programs may lead to small short-term improvements in the participants' self-efficacy, self-rated health, cognitive symptom management, and frequency of aerobic exercise.[60]

Self-management programs that do not include members of the patients' social network typically exhibit changes that are short lived, with less-healthy behaviors returning after brief periods,[61–63] which is particularly true when behaviors such as diet, exercise, and smoking are the focus of self-management. What is needed, then, are interventions that can enhance the social support provided by spouses/significant others to help patients adhere better to the treatment recommendations.

WHAT IS THE EVIDENCE SUPPORTING SELF-MANAGEMENT INTERVENTIONS?

In general, self-management interventions have achieved modest success in clinical trials. In the most recent updated Cochrane review of hypertension self-management interventions, 56 randomized controlled trials met inclusion criteria and assessed mean systolic and diastolic BP, control of BP, and the proportion of patients followed up at clinic. The range of interventions used included (1) self-monitoring, (2) educational interventions directed to the patient, (3) health professional–led care (by the nurse or pharmacist), (5) organizational interventions that aimed to improve the delivery of care, and (6) appointment reminder systems. Self-monitoring was associated with moderate net reductions in diastolic BP but not with significant relationships with systolic BP or BP control. Trials of educational interventions directed at patients or health professionals seemed unlikely to be associated with large net reductions in BP by themselves. Health professional–led care (by the nurse or pharmacist) seems to be a promising way of delivering care but requires further evaluation. The investigators conclude that an organized system of registration, recall, and regular review allied to a vigorous stepped care approach to antihypertensive drug treatment seems the most likely way to improve the control of high BP.[64]

SUMMARY

The daily decisions patients make regarding what to eat, whether to exercise, or whether to take medications substantially affect CVD outcomes and, ultimately, quality and quantity of life. Supporting patient self-management is therefore one of the most important aspects of high-quality hypertension care. The patient must be a collaborator in this process, and methods of improving patients' ability and confidence for self-management are needed. Successful self-management programs have often supplemented the traditional patient-physician encounter by using nonphysician providers, remote patient encounters (telephone or Internet), group settings, and peer support for promoting self-management.

Implementing effective self-management support within the current health care system remains an important challenge for improving hypertension and CVD care.

Most work to date has focused on how people initiate change in health behaviors. Only rarely has research considered the factors that promote long-term maintenance of these behavioral changes. New approaches are needed to address maintenance of behavior change. Innovative methods are needed to identify the mechanisms that lead to long-term maintenance of the change produced by health interventions.

Factors to consider in self-management include staffing, content of the program, patient population served, supporting material, protocols for how staff members are to provide support, staff training, communication with patients, and communication between health care providers and self-management support. For a program that seeks to change patient behavior, a key underlying consideration is the need to include both supportive coaching interventions and educational interventions along with incorporating the patient's social network as a part of the program content. Rather than being prescriptive or hierarchical, self-management programs should be patient centered and tailored to the needs and concerns defined by the patient and their situation.

Given our health care systems' inability to achieve several quality indicators using traditional office-based physician visits, interventions that use novel methods for the delivery of quality health care could increase the quality of care, potentially at a lower cost than the current methods of care. Research is needed to determine the degree to which these interventions can be integrated into primary care, their effectiveness in different groups, and their sustainability for improving chronic disease care.

REFERENCES

1. World Health Organization. The global burden of disease: 2004 update. Geneva (Switzerland): World Health Organization; 2008.
2. Kearney PM, Whelton M, Reynolds K, et al. Global burden of hypertension: analysis of worldwide data. Lancet 2005;365(9455):217–23.
3. Lloyd-Jones D, Adams RJ, Brown TM, et al. Heart disease and stroke statistics—2010 update: a report from the American Heart Association. Circulation 2010;121(7):e46–215.
4. Barlow J, Wright C, Sheasby J, et al. Self-management approaches for people with chronic conditions: a review. Patient Educ Couns 2002;48(2):177–87.
5. Schroeder SA. Shattuck lecture. We can do better—improving the health of the American people. N Engl J Med 2007;357(12):1221–8.
6. Clark NM, Becker MH, Janz NK, et al. Self-management of chronic disease by older adults. J Aging Health 1991;3:3–27.
7. Bodenheimer T, Lorig K, Holman H, et al. Patient self-management of chronic disease in primary care. JAMA 2002;288(19):2469–75.
8. Kinmonth AL, Woodcock A, Griffin S, et al. Randomised controlled trial of patient centered care of diabetes in general practice: impact on current wellbeing and future disease risk. The Diabetes Care From Diagnosis Research Team. BMJ 1998;317(7167):1202–8.
9. Steven K, Morrison J, Drummond N. Lay versus professional motivation for asthma treatment: a cross-sectional, qualitative study in a single Glasgow general practice. Fam Pract 2002;19(2):172–7.
10. World Health Organization. Adherence to long-term therapies: evidence for action. Geneva (Switzerland): World Health Organization; 2003.
11. DiMatteo MR. Variations in patients' adherence to medical recommendations: a quantitative review of 50 years of research. Med Care 2004;42(3):200–9.
12. Rubin RR, Peyrot M. Quality of life and diabetes. Diabetes Metab Res Rev 1999;15(3):205–18.
13. Pincus T, Griffith J, Pearce S, et al. Prevalence of self-reported depression in patients with rheumatoid arthritis. Br J Rheumatol 1996;35(9):879–83.
14. Juenger J, Schellberg D, Kraemer S, et al. Health related quality of life in patients with congestive heart failure: comparison with other chronic diseases and relation to functional variables. Heart 2002;87(3):235–41.
15. Bayliss EA, Bosworth HB, Noel PH, et al. Supporting self-management for patients with complex medical needs: recommendations of a working group. Chronic Illn 2007;3(2):167–75.
16. Rost K, Nutting P, Smith J, et al. The role of competing demands in the treatment provided primary care patients with major depression. Arch Fam Med 2000;9(2):150–4.
17. Bernard AM, Anderson L, Cook CB, et al. What do internal medicine residents need to enhance their diabetes care? Diabetes Care 1999;22(5):661–6.
18. Redelmeier DA, Tan SH, Booth GL. The treatment of unrelated disorders in patients with chronic medical diseases. N Engl J Med 1998;338(21):1516–20.
19. Bodenheimer T, Wagner EH, Grumbach K. Improving primary care for patients with chronic illness: the chronic care model, part 2. JAMA 2002;288(15):1909–14.
20. Scisney-Matlock M, Bosworth HB, Giger JN, et al. Strategies for implementing and sustaining therapeutic lifestyle changes as part of hypertension

management in African Americans. Postgrad Med 2009;121(3):147–59.
21. Coleman K, Austin BT, Brach C, et al. Evidence on the Chronic Care Model in the new millennium. Health Aff (Millwood) 2009;28(1):75–85.
22. Stanford-UCSF Evidence-based Practice Center. Closing the quality gap: a critical analysis of quality improvement strategies. Available at: http://www.ahrq.gov/downloads/pub/evidence/pdf/qualgap2/qualgap2.pdf. Accessed August 6, 2010.
23. Institute of Medicine. Crossing the quality chasm: a new health system for the 21st century. Washington, DC: National Academy Press; 2001.
24. Bodenheimer T. Coordinating care—a perilous journey through the health care system. N Engl J Med 2008;358(10):1064–71.
25. Clark AM, Hartling L, Vandermeer B, et al. Meta-analysis: secondary prevention programs for patients with coronary artery disease. Ann Intern Med 2005;143(9):659–72.
26. American College of Physicians. American College of Physicians. Joint principles of the patient-centered medical home. Available at: http://www.acponline.org/advocacy/where_we_stand/medical_home/approve_jp.pdf. Accessed January 19, 2010.
27. Iglehart JK. No place like home—testing a new model of care delivery. N Engl J Med 2008;359(12):1200–2.
28. Peikes D, Chen A, Schore J, et al. Effects of care coordination on hospitalization, quality of care, and health care expenditures among Medicare beneficiaries: 15 randomized trials. JAMA 2009;301(6):603–18.
29. Pickering TG, Miller NH, Ogedegbe G, et al. Call to action on use and reimbursement for home blood pressure monitoring: executive summary: a joint scientific statement from the American Heart Association, American Society Of Hypertension, and Preventive Cardiovascular Nurses Association. Hypertension 2008;52(1):1–9.
30. Bobrie G, Chatellier G, Genes N, et al. Cardiovascular prognosis of "masked hypertension" detected by blood pressure self-measurement in elderly treated hypertensive patients. JAMA 2004;291(11):1342–9.
31. Bosworth HB, Olsen MK, Grubber JM, et al. Two self-management interventions to improve hypertension control: a randomized trial. Ann Intern Med 2009;151(10):687–95.
32. Bodenheimer T, Handley MA. Goal-setting for behavior change in primary care: an exploration and status report. Patient Educ Couns 2009;76(2):174–80.
33. Bosworth HB, Voils CI. Theoretical models to understand treatment adherence. In: Bosworth HB, Oddone EZ, Weinberger M, editors. Patient treatment adherence: concepts, interventions, and measurement. Mahwah (NJ): Lawrence Erlbaum Associates; 2006. p. 13–48.
34. Rollnick S, Miller W. What is motivational interviewing? Behav Cogn Psychother 1995;23:325–34.
35. Volpp KG, Pauly MV, Loewenstein G, et al. P4P4P: an agenda for research on pay-for-performance for patients. Health Aff (Millwood) 2009;28(1):206–14.
36. Volpp KG, Troxel AB, Pauly MV, et al. A randomized, controlled trial of financial incentives for smoking cessation. N Engl J Med 2009;360(7):699–709.
37. Volpp KG, John LK, Troxel AB, et al. Financial incentive-based approaches for weight loss: a randomized trial. JAMA 2008;300(22):2631–7.
38. Chobanian AV, Bakris GL, Black HR, et al. Seventh report of the joint national committee on prevention, detection, evaluation, and treatment of high blood pressure. Hypertension 2003;42(6):1206–52.
39. Obarzanek E, Vollmer WM, Lin PH, et al. Effects of individual components of multiple behavior changes: the PREMIER trial. Am J Health Behav 2007;31(5):545–60.
40. Goldstein MK, Lavori P, Coleman R, et al. Improving adherence to guidelines for hypertension drug prescribing: cluster-randomized controlled trial of general versus patient-specific recommendations. Am J Manag Care 2005;11(11):677–85.
41. United States Census Bureau. American community survey, 2003 selected housing characteristics. Available at: http://factfinder.census.gov. Accessed March 28, 2009.
42. Wasson J, Gaudette C, Whaley F, et al. Telephone care as a substitute for routine clinic follow-up. JAMA 1992;267(13):1788–93.
43. Beaver K, Tysver-Robinson D, Campbell M, et al. Comparing hospital and telephone follow-up after treatment for breast cancer: randomised equivalence trial. BMJ 2009;338:a3147.
44. Bosworth HB, Olsen MK, McCant F, et al. Hypertension Intervention Nurse Telemedicine Study (HINTS): testing a multifactorial tailored behavioral/educational and a medication management intervention for blood pressure control. Am Heart J 2007;153(6):918–24.
45. Friedman RH, Kazis LE, Jette A, et al. A telecommunications system for monitoring and counseling patients with hypertension. Impact on medication adherence and blood pressure control. Am J Hypertens 1996;9(4 Pt 1):285–92.
46. Bosworth HB, Oddone EZ. Telemedicine and hypertension. J Clin Outcomes Manag 2004;11(8):517–22.
47. Green BB, Cook AJ, Ralston JD, et al. Effectiveness of home blood pressure monitoring, web communication, and pharmacist care on hypertension control: a randomized controlled trial. JAMA 2008;299(24):2857–67.

48. Ostbye T, Yarnall KS, Krause KM, et al. Is there time for management of patients with chronic diseases in primary care? Ann Fam Med 2005;3(3):209–14.
49. Borenstein JE, Graber G, Saltiel E, et al. Physician-pharmacist comanagement of hypertension: a randomized, comparative trial. Pharmacotherapy 2003;23(2):209–16.
50. Denver EA, Barnard M, Woolfson RG, et al. Management of uncontrolled hypertension in a nurse-led clinic compared with conventional care for patients with type 2 diabetes. Diabetes Care 2003;26(8): 2256–60.
51. New JP, Mason JM, Freemantle N, et al. Specialist nurse-led intervention to treat and control hypertension and hyperlipidemia in diabetes (SPLINT): a randomized controlled trial. Diabetes Care 2003; 26(8):2250–5.
52. Vivian EM. Improving blood pressure control in a pharmacist-managed hypertension clinic. Pharmacotherapy 2002;22(12):1533–40.
53. Mehos BM, Saseen JJ, MacLaughlin EJ. Effect of pharmacist intervention and initiation of home blood pressure monitoring in patients with uncontrolled hypertension. Pharmacotherapy 2000;20(11): 1384–9.
54. Boulware LE, Daumit GL, Frick KD, et al. An evidence-based review of patient-centered behavioral interventions for hypertension. Am J Prev Med 2001;21(3):221–32.
55. Bosworth HB, Olsen MK, Gentry P, et al. Nurse administered telephone intervention for blood pressure control: a patient-tailored multifactorial intervention. Patient Educ Couns 2005;57(1):5–14.
56. Bosworth HB, Olsen MK, Oddone EZ. Improving blood pressure control by tailored feedback to patients and clinicians. Am Heart J 2005;149(5):795–803.
57. Bosworth HB, Olsen MK, Goldstein MK, et al. The veterans' study to improve the control of hypertension (V-STITCH): design and methodology. Contemp Clin Trials 2005;26(2):155–68.
58. Krass I, Taylor SJ, Smith C, et al. Impact on medication use and adherence of Australian pharmacists' diabetes care services. J Am Pharm Assoc (2003) 2005;45(1):33–40.
59. Bosworth HB, Olsen MK, Dudley T, et al. Patient education and provider decision support to control blood pressure in primary care: a cluster randomized trial. Am Heart J 2009;157(3):450–6.
60. Foster G, Taylor SJ, Eldridge SE, et al. Self-management education programmes by lay leaders for people with chronic conditions. Cochrane Database Syst Rev 2007;4:CD005108.
61. Sherman AM, Bowen DJ, Vitolins M, et al. Dietary adherence: characteristics and interventions. Control Clin Trials 2000;21(Suppl 5):206S–11S.
62. Gallant MP. The influence of social support on chronic illness self-management: a review and directions for research. Health Educ Behav 2003; 30(2):170–95.
63. Carmody TP, Fey SG, Pierce DK, et al. Behavioral treatment of hyperlipidemia: techniques, results, and future directions. J Behav Med 1982;5(1):91–116.
64. Fahey T, Schroeder K, Ebrahim S. Interventions used to improve control of blood pressure in patients with hypertension. Cochrane Database Syst Rev 2006;4:CD005182.

The Role of Diets, Food, and Nutrients in the Prevention and Control of Hypertension and Prehypertension

Michelle L. Slimko, MPH, RD[a,b,*],
George A. Mensah, MD, FACC, FACP, FACN[c]

KEYWORDS

• Diet • Food • Nutrients • Hypertension • Prehypertension

Hypertension is the leading risk factor for death worldwide, even surpassing tobacco use, high blood glucose, high blood cholesterol, and obesity.[1] Globally, the estimated prevalence of hypertension is nearly 1 billion persons with an annual mortality of almost 7.5 million deaths.[1] In the United States, hypertension affects an estimated 65 million Americans,[2] and it is the leading risk-factor cause of death in women and only second to tobacco use as a contributory cause of death in men.[3] Multiple sources of data from prospective observational, cohort, and randomized controlled clinical trials show that hypertension and its complications are highly preventable when the raised blood pressure (BP) is prevented, or treated and controlled.[4,5] In fact, average reductions of just 5 to 6 mm Hg of diastolic BP in large, randomized, placebo-controlled trials resulted in an approximate reduction of 38% in stroke, 16% in incident coronary heart disease events, 21% in composite cardiovascular events, and 12% in death from all causes.[6]

A fundamental component of effective prevention, treatment, and control of hypertension is the adoption of recommended behavioral and lifestyle changes among which dietary intake of foods and nutrients play crucial roles. In this article, the authors focus on the role that diet, foods, and nutrients play in the prevention and control of hypertension and prehypertension. The report of the 2010 Dietary Guidelines Advisory Committee (DGAC) is reviewed, and its recommendations relevant to the promotion of nutrition education and the prevention and control of hypertension are summarized. The role of the dietitian, as a critical member of the care team for the management of hypertension, is also discussed. Finally, the role of the food system, including food manufacturers and restaurants, in addressing dietary sodium intake, calorie density, and other strategies in support of energy balance to support the prevention and control of hypertension and prehypertension is discussed.

DEFINITIONS AND CLASSIFICATIONS

The Seventh Report of the Joint National Committee on Prevention, Detection, Evaluation, and Treatment of High Blood Pressure (JNC 7 Report) provides present criteria for the definitions of normal BP, prehypertension, and hypertension.[7] Among these terms, the newest is

[a] Global Research & Development, PepsiCo, Inc, 617 West Main Street, Barrington, IL 60010, USA
[b] School of Public Health, University of Illinois-Chicago, 1603 West Taylor, Chicago, IL 60612, USA
[c] Heart Health and Global Health Policy, Global Research and Development, 700 Anderson Hill Road, PepsiCo, Inc, Building 6-2, Purchase, NY 10755, USA
* Corresponding author.
E-mail address: michelle.slimko@pepsico.com

Cardiol Clin 28 (2010) 665–674
doi:10.1016/j.ccl.2010.08.001

prehypertension, defined as BP that ranges from 120 to 139 mm Hg systolic BP and/or 80 to 89 mm Hg diastolic BP.[7] Prehypertension is not a disease. The purpose of this designation is to identify those individuals for whom early intervention by adoption of recommended behavioral and lifestyle changes could lower BP, decrease the rate of progression of BP to hypertensive levels with age, or prevent hypertension entirely.[7] Persons with BP levels in this range have a greater risk of developing clinical hypertension than persons with lower BP levels.[8]

For persons aged 18 years and older, normal BP is defined as systolic BP less than 120 mm Hg and diastolic BP less than 80 mm Hg, although the JNC 7 Report makes it clear that the risk of cardiovascular disease (CVD) begins at systolic BP of 115 and diastolic BP of 75 mm Hg, and doubles with each increment of 20 mm Hg (systolic) and 10 mm Hg (diastolic).[7] Hypertension is defined as systolic BP of greater than or equal to 140 mm Hg or diastolic BP greater than or equal to 90 mm Hg. Hypertension is further classified as Stage 1 or 2 depending on the level of BP (Stage 1 is systolic BP of 140–159 mm Hg and diastolic BP of 90–99 mm Hg; Stage 2 is systolic BP of 160 mm Hg or higher or diastolic BP of 100 mm Hg or higher). The treatment goal for persons with hypertension and no other compelling conditions is less than 140/90 mm Hg. The goal BP for individuals with prehypertension and no compelling indications is to lower BP to the normal range using lifestyle changes.[7] The lifestyle changes of most interest in the prevention and control of hypertension are interventions in dietary sodium, potassium, and energy intake, alcohol use, physical activity, and weight management.

DIET, FOODS, AND NUTRIENTS

Diet plays a major role in overall health and wellness. A diet appropriate for healthy living provides adequate, but not excessive, levels of energy and nutrients.[9] Foods and beverages make up the total diet and provide both macronutrients and micronutrients. The 6 major classes of nutrients include carbohydrates, lipids, proteins, water, vitamins, and minerals. Together, these macronutrients and micronutrients in the diet provide energy as well as provide for growth, maintenance, and repair of cells. Consumed in excess or in insufficient amounts, they can contribute to poor health or nutrition-related morbidity and mortality.

Diet-Related Lifestyle Modifications

Several lifestyle modifications and changes are important in the prevention and control of hypertension and prehypertension. These changes include adopting a lifelong commitment to healthy eating, engaging in regular physical activity, limiting alcohol consumption, and learning about any comorbidities and its specific treatment. This personal commitment poses as paramount importance to improved health overall. It is essential to work closely with a comprehensive health care team to ensure a proper diet is prescribed with appropriate medical and/or pharmacotherapy along with any relevant counseling such as options for smoking cessation. Of the nondrug approaches, a greater emphasis on dietary interventions is important because of the critical role diet therapy plays in the prevention and control of hypertension and prehypertension.[10]

Research has shown that reducing sodium consumption, losing weight, engaging in regular physical activity, and taking antihypertensive medications can lower high BP. The prehypertensive category highlights an even greater need for early intervention to lower BP through lifestyle changes. Persons with prehypertension had a higher prevalence of other risk factors for stroke and heart disease, including hypercholesterolemia, overweight, obesity and diabetes, than persons with normal BP. These risk factors did not include smoking.[8]

The 2010 DGAC Report

The Dietary Guidelines for Americans (DGA) were first published in 1980, with revisions every 5 years. The dietary guidelines are jointly issued by the US Departments of Agriculture, Health, and Human Services. The reports provide authoritative advice targeted toward the healthy, general public, aged 2 years and older, with an emphasis on how good dietary habits can promote health and reduce risk for major chronic diseases. The 2005 *Dietary Guidelines* remain the present guidance until the final *Dietary Guidelines* are published later in 2010.[11]

The report of the DGAC has placed appropriate emphasis on the concept of the total diet approach to healthy living. The total diet approach is defined as the combination of foods and beverages that provide energy and nutrients and comprises an individual's complete dietary intake, on average, over time.[12] This does not translate into recommending compliance of a strict diet prescription; rather it translates into considerations of various diet patterns allowing for flexibility and individual tastes and preferences.

The 2010 DGAC report's recommendations can serve as an important tool for practitioners and all health care providers in helping individuals prevent and control hypertension and prehypertension. The recommended dietary patterns within the 2010 DGAC report are anchored by the dietary approaches to stop hypertension (DASH) diet and Mediterranean-style diets. It is important to understand how to use the DGA as a practitioner and recognize the role of diets in preventing the progression of elevated BP in various populations. Patterns of eating that have been shown to be healthful include the DASH diet and certain Mediterranean-style dietary patterns. The DGAC report concludes that achieving good health and vitality across the life span is achievable for Americans but requires a lifestyle approach that includes a total diet that is:

- Energy-balanced, limited in calories, and portion controlled
- Nutrient-dense including: vegetables, fruit, high-fiber whole grains, fat-free or low-fat fluid milk and milk products, seafood, lean meat and poultry, eggs, soy products, nuts, seeds, and oils, very low in solid fats and added sugars and reduced in sodium.

ROLE OF VARIOUS DIETARY PATTERNS

A significant body of evidence supports the important association between many aspects of the diet and the pathogenesis of hypertension. The 2010 DGAC report provides a review of the scientific evidence supporting the DASH-style dietary patterns and Mediterranean-style dietary patterns. The committee also examined traditional Asian dietary patterns and vegetarian diets. Traditional Asian dietary patterns (eg, Japanese and Okinawan dietary patterns) have been associated with a reduced risk of coronary heart disease. A comparison of the characteristics of dietary patterns using present United States intake and the DASH-sodium diet, and United States Department of Agriculture food patterns is shown in **Table 1**.[12] The table has been adjusted to reflect a daily intake of 2000 calories.

DASH and DASH-style Dietary Patterns

The DASH Collaborative Group provided compelling data to show that a diet rich in fruits, vegetables, and low-fat dairy foods and with reduced saturated and total fat can substantially lower BP.[5] This DASH diet and other DASH-style dietary patterns emphasize vegetables, fruits, and low-fat dairy products; include whole grains, poultry, seafood, and nuts; and are reduced in fats, red meat, sweets, sodium, and sugar-containing beverages.[10,12] These diets are also rich in potassium, magnesium, calcium, and fiber and reduced in total fat, saturated fat, and cholesterol.[10] The DASH diet is primarily composed of a reduction in total fat (27% of kcal) with total protein intake of 18% of calories and carbohydrate intake of 55% of calories. The original DASH dietary patterns are considered safe and broadly applicable to the general population. However, they are higher in potassium, phosphorus, and protein content, and thus are not recommended for persons with chronic kidney disease.[10]

The DGA report emphasizes the DASH-style eating pattern. It is likely that many aspects of the DASH diet, rather than any one nutrient or food, collectively reduce BP. Within all participants of the DASH diet, it significantly lowered mean systolic/diastolic BP by 5.5/3.0 mm Hg. Another diet lowered BP as well, but to a lesser extent, showing about half of the effect of the DASH diet.[10] Other variations of the DASH diet have been applied, in which carbohydrate is partially replaced with protein (about half from plant sources) or unsaturated fat (predominantly monounsaturated fat [MUFA]). This replacement of carbohydrates is important because nutrient adequacy and a reduced saturated fat intake (6% of kcal) were both achieved in the setting of high MUFA (21% of kcal) and total fat (37% of kcal) intake.

In a free-living setting, care is needed to meet but not exceed energy needs to avoid weight gain.[12] The DASH dietary pattern has shown to reduce systolic BP by 8 to 14 mm Hg.[13] A 1600 mg sodium DASH dietary pattern had BP effects similar to single drug therapy in some individuals, and combinations of more than 2 lifestyle modifications could potentially achieve greater results.[5,13] Each of these DASH-style diets was found to lower BP, improve blood lipids, and reduce CVD risk. Successful BP reduction corresponds best when the DASH diet is consumed and the patient can adhere to a reduced sodium intake. However, not many adults, with or without hypertension, eat a diet that is consistent with the DASH dietary pattern.[12]

Obesity and weight loss effects are important considerations for patients using the DASH diet. In overweight or obese persons with more than normal BP, the addition of exercise and weight loss to the DASH diet resulted in even larger BP reductions, greater improvements in vascular and autonomic function, and reduced left ventricular mass.[14–17] It has also been reported that the potential use of a low-sodium vegetable juice consumed with a calorie-restricted diet may help with weight loss in overweight individuals with metabolic syndrome.

A high adherence to the DASH diet is most likely to lead to most benefits.[18–22] It seems to work

Table 1
Characteristics of selected dietary patterns with documented cardiovascular health benefits (adjusted to 2000 calories)

Dietary Pattern	DASH with Reduced Sodium	Mediterranean Diet (Greece)	Mediterranean Diet (Spain)	Mediterranean Diet (USA)	Japanese	Okinawan
Citation	Karanja et al, 1999 and Lin et al, 2003	Trichopoulou et al, NEJM 2003	Nunez-Cordoba 2008 (SUN Study; MAI high score)	Fung et al, 2009	Wilcox et al, 2007 (Circa 1950)	Wilcox et al, 2007 (Circa 1949)
Qualitative Description						
Emphasizes	Potassium-rich vegetables, fruits, and low-fat dairy products	Plant foods, vegetables, fruits, grains, beans, nuts and seeds, olive oil, and fish	Plant foods, vegetables, fruits, breads, other cereals potatoes, bears, nuts and seeds, olive oil, and fish	Plant foods, vegetables, fruits, whole grains, legumes, fish	Rice, legumes, soy foods, vegetables, seaweed, and fish	Plant foods, primarily Okinawan sweet potatoes, rice, legumes, soy foods, other vegetables, and nutrient rich foods of low energy density
Includes	Whole grains, poultry, fish, and nuts	Lean meat, red wine	Cheese, yogurt, red wine	Lean meat	Fruit, meat, and eggs	
Limits (small amount)	Red meats, sweets, and sugar-containing beverages		Red meat, sweets	Potatoes	Milk products	Fruit, meat, eggs, milk products
Nutrients						
Calories (kcal)	2000	2000	2000	2000	2000	2000
Carbohydrates (% total kcal)	58%	nd	47%	39.1%	79%	85%
Protein (% total kcal)	18%	nd	18%	15.1%	13%	9%
Total fat (% total kcal)	27%	~42.7 (summed)	33%	nd	8%	6%
Saturated fat (% total kcal)	7%	13.1%	10%	10% (Incl trans)	2.0%	1.9%
Monounsaturated (% total kcal)	10%	22.7%	15%	9.5%	2.3%	1.8%
Polyunsaturated (% total kcal)	8%	6.9%	5.1%	nd	3.5%	2.4%
Cholesterol (mg)	143	nd	nd	nd	nd	nd
Fiber (g)	29	nd	29	20	22	26
Potassium (mg)	4371	nd	4589	nd	2623	5826
Sodium (mg)	1095	nd	2532	nd	2370	1269

Food Groups						
Vegetables: total (c)	2.1	4.1	1.2	2.2	nd	nd
Dark green (c)	nd	nd	nd	nd	<0.1 (seaweed)	<0.1 (sea weed)
Legumes (c)	nd	<0.1	0.4	0.3	0.3	0.5
Red orange (c)	nd	nd	nd	nd	0.5 (Asian sweet potatoes)	6.6 (Asian sweet potatoes)
Other veg (c)	nd	nd	nd	nd	1.3; + 0.3 (pickled veg)	0.9
Starchy veg (c)	nd	0.6	nd	No potatoes	0.3 (other potatoes)	<0.1 (other potatoes)
Fruit & juices (c)	2.5	1.0 (fruit & nuts) 1.5 (juice & other beverages)	1.3 (fruit & juice) 0.1 (dried fruit & nuts)	1.6	0.2 (papaya & tomato = veg)	<0.1 (papaya & tomato = veg)
Grains: total (oz)	7.3	5.4	2.0	nd	2.4; 1.7 (rice)	1.1; 0.9 (rice)
Whole grains (oz)	3.9	nd	nd	1.6	nd	nd
Milk & milk products, whole	0.7	1.0	0.8	nd	<0.1	<0.1
Low-fat (c)	1.9	nd	1.3	nd	nd	nd
Animal proteins:						
Meat (oz)	14	3.5	3.6	2.4	0.4	0.1
Poultry (oz)	1.7	nd	nd	nd	nd	nd
Eggs (oz)	nd	nd	1.9	nd	0.3	<0.1
Fish (total) (oz)	1.4	0.8	2.4	1.5	2.1	0.6
High N3 (oz)	nd	nd	nd	nd	nd	nd
Low N3 (oz)	nd	nd	nd	nd	nd	nd
Plant proteins:						
Legumes (oz)	0.4	nd	0.4	nd	0.4 (Incl soy)	0.3 (Incl soy)
Nuts & seeds (oz)	0.9	See fruit earlier	See fruit earlier	0.5	<1 g	<0.1
Soy products (oz)	nd	nd		nd	See legumes	See legumes
Oils (g)	24.8	40.3 (olive oil)	19.0 (olive oil)	nd	nd	nd
Solid fats (g)	nd	nd	nd	nd	nd	nd
Added sugar (g)	12	24.3	nd	nd	7.7	3.4
Alcohol (g)	nd	7.9^2	7.1 (red wine)	7.3	30.0 (flavors and alcohol)	7.8 (flavors and alcohol)

Abbreviation: nd, not determined.

Data from Report of the Dietary Guidelines Advisory Committee on the Dietary Guidelines for Americans, 2010. USDA Press; 2010.

independently of peripheral mechanisms as well as lower homocysteine,[14] reduces oxidative stress, and improve vascular function in salt-sensitive subjects.[23–25]

Mediterranean-Style Dietary Patterns

The Mediterranean-style dietary pattern is another pattern that has shown positive health outcomes. Because there are several Mediterranean cultures and agricultural patterns that border the Mediterranean Sea, the Mediterranean diet is centered on only one dietary pattern.[12] Thus, there is no well-accepted set of criteria that exist. A traditional Mediterranean diet can be described as one that emphasizes breads and other cereal foods usually made from wheat, vegetables, fruits, nuts, unrefined cereals, and olive oil; includes fish and wine with meals (in non-Islamic countries); and is reduced in saturated fat, meat, and full-fat dairy products.[12] Results from observational studies and clinical trials suggest that consumption of a traditional Mediterranean diet, similar to that of Crete in the 1960s, is associated with one of the lowest risks of coronary heart disease in the world.[12] The scientific review of these studies on dietary patterns is also included in **Table 1**.

Vegetarian Dietary Patterns

Vegetarian diets are associated with reduced BP.[10] In some observational studies, vegetarian diets and lifestyle have been associated with improved health outcomes such as experiencing a lower age-related increase in BP. Different variations of the vegetarian diets exist in the United States. Individuals who do not consume any animal products are termed vegans. Lacto-ovo vegetarians consume milk and egg products. Some individuals may not be strict vegetarians, but consume small or minimal amounts of animal products.

On average, vegetarians consume fewer calories from fat than nonvegetarians, particularly saturated fat, and have a higher consumption of carbohydrates than nonvegetarians. In addition, vegetarians tend to consume fewer overall calories and have a lower body mass index (BMI; calculated as the [weight in kg] divided by [height in $m]^2$) than nonvegetarians.[12]

Several characteristics of a vegetarian lifestyle may contribute to lower BP. These characteristics may include nondietary factors (eg, physical activity), established dietary risk factors (eg, reduced weight, increased potassium, and low-to-moderate alcohol intake), and other aspects of the vegetarian diet (eg, high-fiber, meatless diet).[10,26] In 2 trials, one in individuals without hypertension and another in individuals with hypertension, lacto-ovo vegetarian diets reduced systolic BP by approximately 5 mm Hg but had equivocal effects on diastolic BP.[26]

Other Dietary Patterns

Other considerations for other various dietary patterns have recently been reviewed because of the increasing diversity of the United States population. Special interest in the potential health effects of non–Unites States diets remains an opportunity for further exploration. One group of diets with potential health benefits are those diets traditionally consumed in Asia, which has experienced some of the lowest rates of coronary heart disease in the world. Both traditional Japanese and Okinawan dietary patterns have been associated with a low risk of coronary heart disease.[12] Compared with the evidence supporting the DASH and Mediterranean diets, data related to diet composition as well as epidemiologic and clinical trial evidence on health benefits, similar to that available for the other types of diets, is sparse. Also, over time, dietary intakes in these countries have changed and may no longer reflect the healthiest options.

ROLE OF MACRONUTRIENTS

Carbohydrates, fat, protein, and alcohol provide the energy supplied by all foods and are generally referred to as macronutrients. Some evidence suggests that the amount and type of carbohydrate intake affect BP.[26] Increasing emphasis on the type of fats rather than on total fat consumption has been raised. The type of protein, increased intakes of protein, or result from substitution for reduced carbohydrates has also been studied. Lastly, observational and clinical trials suggest that moderation of alcohol intake may be an effective approach to lower BP.

Carbohydrates

Carbohydrates provide 4 calories per gram. Bodies of evidence suggest that both the amount and type of carbohydrate affect BP.[10] Americans who are mostly sedentary should aim to decrease energy-dense carbohydrates, especially refined, sugar-dense foods, to help balance energy and maintain an ideal weight.[12] The results of observational studies that specifically examined the effect of carbohydrate intake on BP have been inconsistent.[26] The results have been mixed, showing a direct relationship in one study, no association in another, and an inverse relationship in another. In the OmniHeart feeding trial, partial substitution of carbohydrate either with protein or MUFA lowered BP.[26] More research is needed before making recommendations about the amount and type of carbohydrate required to lower BP.[10]

Fiber

The establishment of a definition for dietary fiber has historically depended on a balance between nutritional knowledge and analytical method capabilities.[27] There are 2 types of fiber. Some sources of insoluble fiber include oats, apples, and beans. Sources of insoluble fiber include wheat and rye bran, broccoli, and celery. Some observational studies and clinical trials suggest that increased fiber may reduce BP.[10] More than 40 randomized trials of dietary fiber supplementation have been done. However, most did not have BP as the primary outcome and included a multicomponent intervention.[26] A meta-analysis of these trials, restricted to the 20 trials that only increased fiber intake, showed that supplemental fiber (an average increase of 14 g/d) was associated with net systolic BP and diastolic BP reductions of 1.6 and 2.0, respectively.[26] The effect to reduce BP is unclear and further research is needed. Overall, fiber is still recommended to be included as part of an overall healthy diet.

Protein

Protein provides 4 calories per gram. Animal sources of protein include meat, poultry, seafood, milk, and eggs. Plant proteins can be eaten in combination to form complete proteins in the forms of legumes and grains.[12] Some studies have shown that protein from plants was associated with lower BP, whereas protein from animal sources had no significant effect.[10] Some trials have also looked at increased protein intake using soy interventions, which reduced BP. However, on aggregate, data from clinical trials, with evidence from observational studies, support the hypothesis that consuming increased intakes of vegetable proteins instead of carbohydrates lowers BP. It is still unclear whether the effects are derived from reduced carbohydrate or increased protein. Data in the United States also show that protein intake is adequate.[12]

Fat

Fat provides 9 calories per gram. Total fat includes saturated fat, omega-3 polyunsaturated fatty acids (PUFAs), omega-6 PUFAs, and MUFA. Strong evidence indicates that the type of fat consumed is more important than the total fat consumed for reducing metabolic and cardiovascular risk.[26] This is a major change of recommendation from past DGA.

Saturated fat

Several observational studies and a few clinical trials looked at the impact of saturated fat on BP. In many cases, including 2 prospective observational studies (the Nurses Health Study and Health Professional Follow-up Study), saturated fat intake was not associated with incident hypertension.[26] In the few trials that exist, dietary interventions that focused only on reducing saturated fat had no significant effect on BP.

Omega-3 PUFA

Several small clinical trials and meta-analysis of these trials documented that high-dose omega-3 PUFA supplements can lower BP in individuals with hypertension. In individuals without hypertension, BP reductions were small or not significant. The effect of omega-3 fish oil supplementation seems to be dose dependent, with BP reductions occurring at relatively high doses, particularly more than 3 g/d. In individuals with hypertension the average systolic BP and diastolic BP reductions were 4.0 and 2.5 mm Hg, respectively.[26] Typical side effects occurred with the fish oil supplementation such as belching and fish aftertaste. Due to the high dose required to lower BP and their noted side effects, fish oil supplements cannot be routinely recommended as a means to prevent or lower hypertension.[26]

Omega-6 PUFA

Dietary intake of omega-6 PUFA has little effect on BP.[26] In an overview of cross-sectional studies that correlated BP with tissue or blood levels of omega-6 PUFA, no apparent relationship was found. Additional prospective observational studies and clinical trials have also been unsupportive of a relationship.[26]

MUFA

Not many studies have assessed the relationship between MUFA intake and BP. Other cross-sectional and prospective studies did not detect a relationship on the effect of MUFA on subsequent hypertension. Some trials have shown that diets rich in MUFA lower BP.[26]As mentioned, the OmniHeart Study used a partial substitution of carbohydrate with MUFA to lower BP. Despite a lowering of BP from MUFA intake, this reduction may be confounded by the reduction in carbohydrate. Thus, the effect of MUFA intake on BP warrants further research.

Alcohol

Alcohol provides 7 calories per gram. For those who can safely consume alcohol, consumption should be limited to no more than 2 drinks (24 oz beer, 10 oz wine, or 3 oz of 80-proof liquor) per day in most men and no more than 1 drink per day in women. A reduction in alcohol consumption may reduce systolic BP by approximately 2 to 4 mm Hg.[7,13]

ROLE OF MICRONUTRIENTS

Micronutrients include vitamins and minerals and are not needed as much as macronutrients. The following micronutrients have been studied in relation to the prevention and control of hypertension and prehypertension.

Sodium

Excessive dietary sodium consumption increases BP, which increases the risk for stroke, coronary heart disease, heart failure, and renal disease.[28] The main source of sodium in food is salt (NaCl). Uniodized salt is 40% sodium by weight. In the United States, an estimated 77% of dietary sodium intake comes from processed and restaurant foods. About 10% of dietary sodium comes from table salt and cooking.[28] Major sources of foods include breads, mixed dishes, pizza, deli meats, cheese, and grain-based desserts. Special populations (blacks, the middle-aged, and the elderly) now comprise 70% of the population of the United States. The general recommendation for sodium intake has been lowered to 2300 mg/d (equal to about 1 teaspoon of salt) to 1500 mg/d.[28] However, this recommendation is to be taken over time, which has not been specified. Consumers and health care providers should be aware of the lower sodium recommendation, and health care providers should inform their patients of the evidence linking greater sodium intake to increased BP. Sodium reduction is recommended for persons with hypertension and as first-line interventions for persons with prehypertension.

Potassium

A high intake of potassium can be achieved through the diet because potassium-rich foods are usually made with other nutrients, such as bicarbonate precursors. Patients benefit from potassium intake through diet rather than supplementation via pills. The level of BP reduction from consumption of potassium depends on concurrent levels of salt intake, mostly a high-salt intake compared with a low-salt intake.[10] Present desirable levels of potassium intake as a means to lower BP do not exist because of the lack of dose response trials. A level of 4.7 g/d (120 mmol/d) was found to be reasonable as the level corresponded to the average total potassium intake in clinical trials of potassium supplements, the highest dose in the one available dose response trial, potassium content of the DASH intake diet, and the adequate intake level set by the Institute of Medicine Committee.[10] Not many Americans achieve this level of intake.

Calcium and Magnesium

The effect of calcium as a single nutrient used as a therapy to reduce BP is unclear.[13] The body of evidence showing magnesium as a major determinant of BP is inconsistent. In a meta-analysis of 20 trials, there was no clear effect of magnesium intake on BP.[10] The effect of magnesium as a single nutrient on BP in adults who are healthy or who have hypertension is unknown.[13]

ROLE OF CALORIES

Energy Balance and Maintenance of Ideal Weight

Energy balance is an important principle in the maintenance of ideal body weight and in the prevention and control of hypertension and prehypertension. All persons with hypertension and prehypertension should be encouraged to lower their overall energy intakes to match their individual energy needs. Nutrient-dense foods such as vegetables, fruits, whole grains, low-fat milk, and milk products should replace energy-dense foods, which tend to be higher in sodium, fat, and calories. Consumption of nutrient-dense foods improves the intake of shortfall nutrients, and other nutrients of concern such as vitamin D, calcium, potassium, and dietary fiber.

In addition, sedentary persons should engage in regular aerobic physical activity for at least 30 min/d on most days of the week.[7]

Calorie Restriction and Weight Loss

Weight gain is associated with increased BP level. Almost 65% of United States adults are classified as overweight or obese.[10] Weight loss of as little as 10 pounds (4.5 kg) reduces BP and/or prevents hypertension in a large proportion of overweight persons, although the ideal is to maintain a normal body weight.[7] For overweight or obese persons, the goal is to attain a BMI of less than 25 kg/m^2. For nonoverweight persons, maintenance of a desirable BMI of less than 25 kg/m^2 is also recommended. Some trials have documented that modest weight loss, with or without sodium reduction, can prevent hypertension by almost 20% among individuals with prehypertension and facilitate gradual reduction of medications and drug withdrawal.[10]

ROLE OF DIETITIANS ON THE TREATMENT AND CARE TEAM

The registered dietitian plays an integral role in the interdisciplinary health care team by creating the ideal nutrition prescription to support a plan including physical activity, behavioral changes, and drug therapy when appropriate. Based on the patient's treatment plan and comorbid conditions, other nutritional practice guidelines such as those recommended for the management of type 2 diabetes, lipid disorders, and obesity may be warranted to provide optimal treatment.[13]

ROLE OF THE FOOD SYSTEM, INCLUDING FOOD MANUFACTURERS AND RESTAURANTS, IN ADDRESSING DIETARY SODIUM INTAKE

The American Public Health Association, along with the National High Blood Pressure Education Program Coordinating Committee, recommends that the food industry (including manufacturers and restaurants), reduce sodium in the food supply by 50% over the next decade.[7] It is well established that Americans consume an excess of sodium and not enough potassium in the diet. For example, a recent report from the US Centers for Disease Control and Prevention shows that 9 out of 10 Americans exceed the limit recommended for daily sodium intake.[28] In fact, for the group of Americans for whom a lower dietary intake of sodium is important, the amount of sodium consumed was more than double the recommended limit. Only 9.6% of adults in the United States met the recommended dietary limit of 2300 mg per day for sodium, and only 5.5% among the group recommended to limit sodium intake to less than 1500 mg per day achieved that target. Overall, the average sodium consumption for United States adults was 3466 mg per day, far in excess of the 2300 mg per day recommended. In the group of adults recommended to limit sodium intake to less than 1500 mg per day, the actual intake averaged 3366 mg per day.

It is also well established that in most of the developed world and many developing countries, most of the sodium consumed comes from processed and restaurant food.[29] In the United States, about 77% of dietary sodium intake comes from processed foods while another 11% comes from salt added at the table or during cooking.[30] Thus, efforts at reducing dietary intake of sodium must go beyond the recommended lifestyle changes for individual patients. These efforts must also engage all members of the food system including ingredient manufacturers, retailers, restaurants, and especially the food industry.

Several companies within the food industry have made commitments to reduce the sodium content of their products.[31] For example, PepsiCo has set a global goal and has made a commitment to reduce the average amount of sodium per serving in key global food brands, in key countries, by 25% by 2015, with a 2006 baseline.[32] For PepsiCo to achieve sodium reductions of 50% and greater, significant scientific and technological breakthroughs are required and engagement of the broader scientific community is crucially needed. The DGAC also recognizes that time is "required to adjust taste perception of the general population." Thus, the reduction from 2300 mg to 1500 mg per day should occur gradually over time.

SUMMARY

Hypertension and prehypertension remain important public health challenges. A substantial body of evidence strongly supports the concept that various dietary factors play a role in lowering BP. Dietary modifications that can effectively lower BP are reduced calorie intake to match energy requirements, reduced salt intake, increased potassium intake, moderation of alcohol consumption (among those who drink), and consumption of an overall diet rich in fruits and vegetables and low in sodium. The DASH diet; the Mediterranean- and vegetarian-style diets; and potentially the Japanese and Okinawan dietary patterns have been associated with lowering BP. Further research is needed to determine the role that the amount and types of carbohydrate, protein, and fats play in lowering BP from dietary intake. Champions of the health care team who emphasize prevention remain vital in nutritional education and patient assessment for dietary intervention and goals. Dietitians play an integral role as members of the patient and care team in working closely with individuals with hypertension or prehypertension. To promote positive behavior change and create a broader impact on public health, it has become necessary to leverage multilevel stakeholders such as all health care providers, researchers, policy makers, schools, the food industry, and the general public to drive policy changes and future innovation from research and development endeavors, and to emphasize the importance of diet-related lifestyle modifications to effectively prevent and control hypertension and prehypertension.

REFERENCES

1. World Health Organization. Global health risks: mortality and burden of disease attributable to selected major risks. Geneva: World Health Organization; 2009.
2. Egan BM, Zhao Y, Axon RN. US trends in prevalence, awareness, treatment, and control of hypertension, 1988-2008. JAMA 2010;303(20):2043–50.
3. Danaei G, Ding EL, Mozaffarian D, et al. The preventable causes of death in the United States: comparative risk assessment of dietary, lifestyle,

and metabolic risk factors. PLoS Med 2009;6(4). [e1000058].
4. Chobanian AV, Bakris GL, Black HR, et al. The seventh report of the joint national committee on prevention, detection, evaluation, and treatment of high blood pressure: the JNC 7 report. JAMA 2003;289(19):2560–72.
5. Appel LJ, Moore TJ, Obarzanek E, et al. A clinical trial of the effects of dietary patterns on blood pressure. DASH Collaborative Research Group [see comments]. N Engl J Med 1997;336(16):1117–24.
6. Mensah GA. The global burden of hypertension: good news and bad news. Cardiology Clinics 2002;20:181–5.
7. National High Blood Pressure Education Program. Seventh report of the Joint National Committee on Prevention, Detection, Evaluation, and Treatment of High Blood Pressure. Rockville, (MD): National, Heart, Lung, Blood Institute; NIH publication; 2003. p. 1206–52.
8. Greenlund KJ, Croft JB, Mensah GA. Prevalence of heart disease and stroke risk factors in persons with prehypertension in the United States, 1999-2000. Arch Intern Med 2004;164:2113–8.
9. Otten JJ, Hellwig JP, Meyers LD. Dietary reference intakes. The essential guide to nutrient requirements. Inst Med 2006.
10. Appel LJ. ASH position paper: dietary approaches to lower blood pressure. J Clin Hypertens (Greenwich) 2009;11(7):358–68.
11. Dietary guidelines for Americans. http://www.cnpp.usda.gov/DGAs2010-DGACReport.htm. Accessed July 15, 2010.
12. Report of the Dietary Guidelines Advisory Committee on the dietary guidelines for Americans. USDA Press; 2010. Available at: http://www.cnpp.usda.gov/Publications/DietaryGuidelines/2010/DGAC/Report/B-2-TotalDiet.pdf. http://www.cnpp.usda.gov/DGAs2010-DGACReport.htm. Accessed July 15, 2010.
13. Hypertension (HTN) evidence based nutrition practice guideline. http://www.adaevidencelibrary.com/topic.cfm?cat=3248. Accessed July 22, 2010.
14. Al-Solaiman Y, Jesri A, Mountford WK, et al. DASH lowers blood pressure in obese hypertensives beyond potassium, magnesium and fibre. J Hum Hypertens 2010;24(4):237–46.
15. Blumenthal JA, Babyak MA, Hinderliter A, et al. Effects of the DASH diet alone and in combination with exercise and weight loss on blood pressure and cardiovascular biomarkers in men and women with high blood pressure: the ENCORE study. Arch Intern Med 2010;170(2):126–35.
16. Moore TJ, Alsabeeh N, Apovian CM, et al. Weight, blood pressure, and dietary benefits after 12 months of a Web-based Nutrition Education Program (DASH for health): longitudinal observational study. J Med Internet Res 2008;10(4):e52.
17. Shenoy SF, Poston WS, Reeves RS, et al. Weight loss in individuals with metabolic syndrome given DASH diet counseling when provided a low sodium vegetable juice: a randomized controlled trial. Nutr J 2010;9:8, 8.
18. Kotchen TA. Does the DASH diet improve clinical outcomes in hypertensive patients? Am J Hypertens 2009;22(4):350.
19. Levitan EB, Wolk A, Mittleman MA. Consistency with the DASH diet and incidence of heart failure. Arch Intern Med 2009;169(9):851–7.
20. Folsom AR, Parker ED, Harnack LJ. Degree of concordance with DASH diet guidelines and incidence of hypertension and fatal cardiovascular disease. Am J Hypertens 2007;20(3):225–32.
21. Doyle L, Cashman KD. The DASH diet may have beneficial effects on bone health. Nutr Rev 2004; 62(5):215–20.
22. Liese AD, Nichols M, Sun X, et al. Adherence to the DASH Diet is inversely associated with incidence of type 2 diabetes: the insulin resistance atherosclerosis study. Diabetes Care 2009;32(8):1434–6.
23. Hodson L, Harnden KE, Roberts R, et al. Does the DASH diet lower blood pressure by altering peripheral vascular function? J Hum Hypertens 2010;24(5): 312–9.
24. Al-Solaiman Y, Jesri A, Zhao Y, et al. Low-Sodium DASH reduces oxidative stress and improves vascular function in salt-sensitive humans. J Hum Hypertens 2009;23(12):826–35.
25. DASH diet lowers homocysteine levels. Harv Heart Lett 2000;11(3):6–7.
26. Appel LJ, Brands MW, Daniels SR, et al. Dietary approaches to prevent and treat hypertension: a scientific statement from the American Heart Association. Hypertension 2006;47:295–308.
27. American Association of Cereal Chemists. The definition of fiber. Available at: http://www.aaccnet.org/definitions/. Accessed July 22, 2010.
28. CDC. Sodium intake among adults—United States, 2005-2006. MMWR Morb Mortal Wkly Rep 2010; 59(24):746–9.
29. Sodium intakes around the world. Background document prepared for the forum and technical meeting on reducing salt intake in populations. Paris: World Health Organization; 2006. Available at: http://www.who.int/dietphysicalactivity/Elliot-brown-2007.pdf. Accessed July 23, 2010.
30. Mattes RD, Donnelly D. Relative contributions of dietary sodium sources. J Am Coll Nutr 1991;10(4): 383–93.
31. Innova Market Insights. Low sodium analysis—Innova market insights for foodingredientsfirst.com. 2010. Available at: http://www.foodingredientsfirst.com/Content/pdf/InnovaMarketInsights_LowSodium_Feb2010.ppt. Accessed July 30, 2010.
32. PepsiCo. 2009 annual report. Performance with purpose —the promise of PepsiCo. 2010. Available at: http://www.pepsico.com/annual09/human_sustainability.html. Accessed July 30, 2010.

Prevention, Diagnosis, and Treatment of Hypertensive Heart Disease

Vasiliki V. Georgiopoulou, MD,
Andreas P. Kalogeropoulos, MD, Paolo Raggi, MD,
Javed Butler, MD, MPH*

KEYWORDS

• Hypertensive heart disease • Prevention • Treatment

Prolonged increase of blood pressure (BP) causes a variety of changes in the myocardial structure, coronary vasculature, and conduction system of the heart, collectively known as hypertensive heart disease (HHD). The resulting left ventricular dysfunction, ischemia, and arrhythmias all contribute to the high morbidity and mortality burden, and health care cost related to HHD. Controlling BP effectively reduces HHD complications, but BP control at the population levels has largely been met with only modest success. Moreover, recent epidemiologic studies continue to shift acceptable BP levels from what is usual in the population to what is optimal for preventing HHD-related complications.[1,2]

DEFINITION

Long-standing hypertension leads to complex changes in cardiac chamber geometry and myocardial composition, which in turn result in the development of left ventricular hypertrophy (LVH), ischemic heart disease, various conduction abnormalities, and heart failure (HF) (with reduced or preserved systolic function) (**Box 1**). These changes are collectively referred to as HHD. In the latest version of International Classification of Diseases (ICD-10), hypertensive diseases have been assigned multiple codes (I10–I15) to classify the various forms of HHD including essential hypertension, HHD with and without HF, combined HHD and renal disease, and secondary hypertension.[3] Pathophysiologically, HHD encompasses both the direct and indirect effects of prolonged uncontrolled hypertension; however, the term HHD is clinically usually reserved for disease states in which patients' symptoms cannot be attributed to an alternate cause. Thus, although hypertension is clearly associated with coronary disease, angina in the presence of obstructive coronary stenosis may not be equated with HHD because coronary disease can be attributable to other simultaneous causes. However, angina related to LVH and microvascular disease in a patient with hypertension in the absence of obstructive epicardial coronary stenosis can be regarded as HHD.

PATHOPHYSIOLOGY

The pathophysiology of HHD is a complex interplay of hemodynamic, structural, cellular, neurohormonal, and molecular factors. Increased BP leads to adverse changes in cardiac structure and function through increased afterload and neurohormonal and vascular changes. According to the nature of the trigger stimulus, signal transduction can occur in 2 directions. Cardiomyocytes either undergo hypertrophy,[4] an adaptive response in an attempt to normalize systolic wall stress of the ventricle, or apoptosis,[5] a maladaptive process resulting in dilatation and failure of the ventricle. Pressure overload of the left ventricle (LV) and loss of reciprocal regulation between profibrotic and antifibrotic molecules is associated with increased

Disclosures: None.
Division of Cardiology, Emory University, 1365 Clifton Road NE, Suite AT-430, Atlanta, GA 30322, USA
* Corresponding author.
E-mail address: javed.butler@emory.edu

Cardiol Clin 28 (2010) 675–691
doi:10.1016/j.ccl.2010.07.005
0733-8651/10/$ – see front matter

Box 1
Components of myocardial structural remodeling

Cellular components

Cardiomyocytes

- Hypertrophy
- Increased apoptosis

Fibroblasts

- Hyperplasia
- Increased apoptosis
- Conversion to myofibroblasts

Other cells

- Vascular smooth-muscle cell hypertrophy and/or hyperplasia
- Monocytes/macrophages infiltration

Noncellular components

Extracellular matrix

- Increased interstitial deposition of collagen types I/III fibers
- Increased perivascular deposition of collagen types I/III fibers
- Increased interstitial accumulation of fibronectin

Intramyocardial vasculature

- Wall thickening of small arteries/arterioles
- Decreased capillary number

collagen synthesis and reduced collagenase activity,[6] contributing to ventricular fibrosis.

Initially, the changes are compensatory and asymptomatic, causing a compromise in relaxation rate, diastolic suction, and passive stiffness of the LV. Later, they become symptomatic as a result of change in the spatial orientation of collagen fibers, which further impairs diastolic filling and transduction of cardiomyocyte contraction into myocardial force development.[7] Cardiomyocyte apoptosis, which is enhanced in the hypertrophied LV and is associated with collagen production, accelerates LV dilatation and dysfunction. Adrenergic and renin-angiotensin-aldosterone system activation that results from ventricular dilatation leads to downregulation of myocardial β receptors and inhibition of sarcolemmal calcium-release channels.[7] These structural changes are also responsible for impaired coronary flow reserve and arrhythmias. When collagen accumulation increases, these changes cause ischemia and ventricular and/or atrial arrhythmias (**Fig. 1**).[7]

EPIDEMIOLOGY

In the World Health Organization (WHO) Monitoring of Trends and Determinants in Cardiovascular Disease (MONICA) project, hypertension prevalence was high in all countries, with a range from 20% to almost 50%, whereas most industrialized countries have a higher prevalence than the United States.[8] The prevalence of LVH is closely associated with age and severity of hypertension. Prevalence of LVH ranges from 6% in people less than 30 years old to 43% in those more than 69 years old, and from 20% to 50% in individuals who have mild to severe hypertension, and reaches 60% in those with more severe hypertension.[9] Coronary artery disease (CAD) is also a common complication of hypertension in individuals of all ages. Unrecognized infarctions are more common among persons who are hypertensive than persons who are normotensive, with as many as 35% of infarctions in men who are hypertensive and 50% in women who are hypertensive being unrecognized.[10] The population attributable risk (PAR) of hypertension for HF ranges from 39% in men and 59% in women in the Framingham Study,[11] whereas uncontrolled BP accounts for 21.3% of cases in white people to 30.1% in black people in the Health, Aging, and Body Composition (Health ABC) Study.[12] This risk increases in a graded continuous fashion with increase in BP.[11,13] The lifetime risk for HF doubles in subjects with BP more than 160/100 mm Hg versus those with less than 140/90 mm Hg, and this gradient of risk is apparent in both men and women in every decade of age from 40 to 70 years.[14] A total of 7.1 million deaths (13% of deaths) may be attributable to hypertension annualy.[15] WHO reports that suboptimal BP is responsible for 62% of cerebrovascular disease and 49% of CAD, with little gender variation.[15]

DIAGNOSTIC EVALUATION

The main purpose of diagnostic evaluation in patients with hypertension is early detection of target organ damage; evaluation for LVH is crucial in this respect.

Electrocardiography

Although LVH can be predicted by surface electrocardiography (ECG), the sensitivity and specificity are suboptimal (25%–60%).[16,17] In a comparative study with cardiac magnetic resonance (CMR) imaging for assessment of LVH, the ECG showed a sensitivity of ~25%. Moreover, there are racial differences in ECG diagnoses of LVH, with ECG having a lower specificity in black people.[18,19]

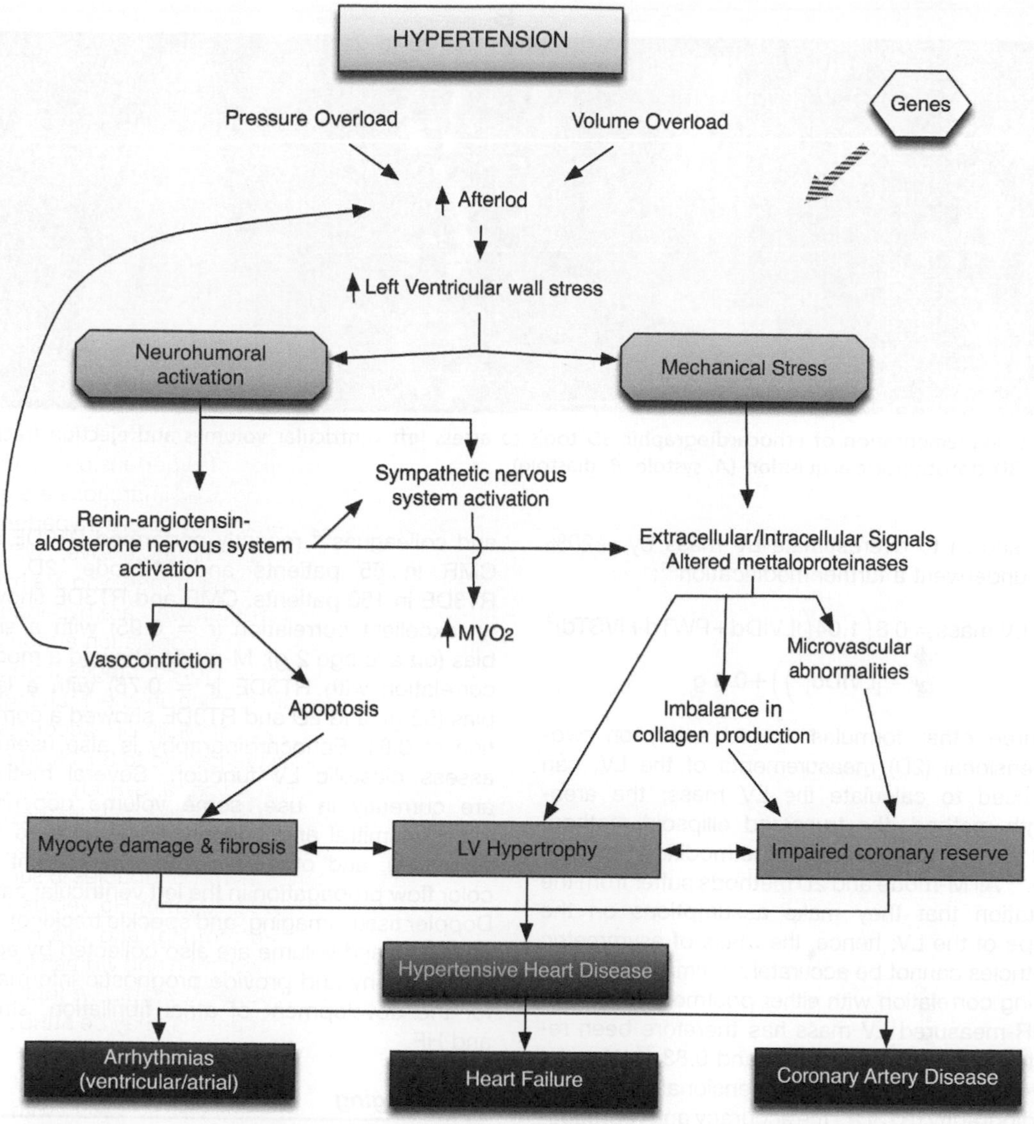

Fig. 1. Pathophysiology of HHD. Hypertension increases cardiac afterload and left ventricular wall stress, leading to mechanical and neurohumoral activation and, in turn, triggering endocellular pathways. This process produces hormones that cause vasoconstriction, enhance apoptosis and myocyte damage and fibrosis, and increase myocardial oxygen demand, leading to loss of reciprocal regulation between profibrotic and antifibrotic mechanisms and an imbalance in collagen production and microvascular abnormalities. These structural alterations of myocardium (fibrosis, hypertrophy, and decreased coronary reserve) lead to HHD and its clinical manifestations.

Although ECG remains an accessible and low-cost tool that may suggest the presence of LVH, its sensitivity and specificity characteristics preclude it from being the definitive test for screening and diagnosis of LVH, necessitating assessment and the use of alternate imaging modalities.

Echocardiography

In most echocardiographic formulas, LV mass is calculated by subtracting the volume of the LV cavity (endocardial volume) from the volume encompassed by the epicardium, multiplied by the estimated specific density of the myocardium. The original formula proposed was[20]:

$$\text{LV mass} = 1.04\left([\text{LVIDd}+\text{PWTd}+\text{IVSTd}]^3 - [\text{LVIDd}]^3\right) - 13.6\ \text{g}$$

where LVIDd is the LV internal diameter at end diastole, PWTd is the posterior wall thickness at end diastole, and IVSTd is the interventricular septal thickness at end diastole. This formula

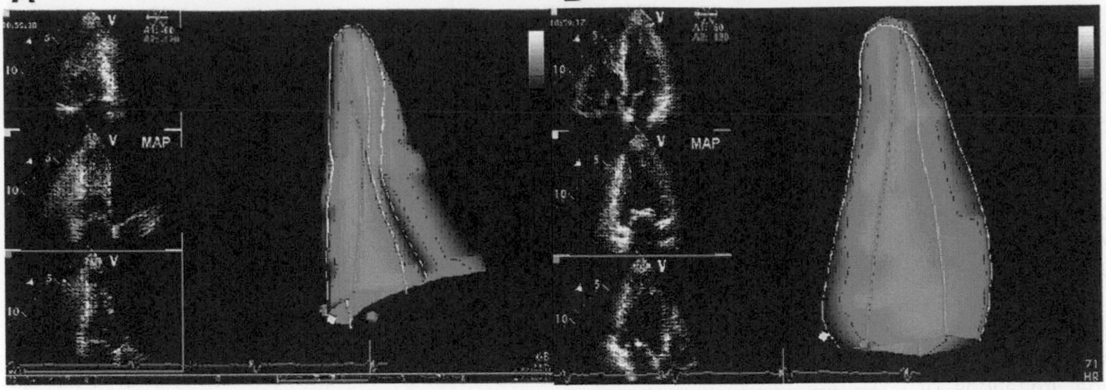

Fig. 2. Implementation of echocardiographic 3D tools to assess left ventricular volumes and ejection fraction from 3D transthoracic acquisition (*A*, systole; *B*, diastole).

was shown to overestimate LV mass by ~20% and underwent a further modification[21]:

$$\text{LV mass} = 0.8\left(1.04\left(\left[\text{LVIDd}+\text{PWTd}+\text{IVSTd}\right]^3 - \left[\text{LVIDd}\right]^3\right)\right) + 0.6\ \text{g}$$

Three other formulas, based solely on two-dimensional (2D) measurements of the LV, can be used to calculate the LV mass: the area-length method, the truncated ellipsoid method, and the disc methods using the modified Simpson rule.[22] All M-mode and 2D methods suffer from the limitation that they make assumptions on the shape of the LV; hence, the mass of asymmetric ventricles cannot be accurately estimated. The resulting correlation with either postmortem data or CMR-measured LV mass has therefore been reported to vary between 0.40 and 0.83.[23] With the advent of real-time three-dimensional (3D) echocardiography (RT3DE) the accuracy and reproducibility of LV volume and mass by echocardiography improved (**Fig. 2**). Takeuchi and colleagues[24] recently performed RT3DE and CMR in 55 patients and M-mode, 2D, and RT3DE in 150 patients. CMR and RT3DE showed an excellent correlation ($r = 0.95$) with a small bias (on average 2 g); M-mode showed a modest correlation with RT3DE ($r = 0.76$) with a large bias (52 g), and 2D and RT3DE showed a correlation of 0.91. Echocardiography is also useful to assess diastolic LV function. Several methods are currently in use, some volume dependent (eg, transmitral and pulmonary veins blood flow velocities), and others volume independent (eg, color flow propagation in the left ventricular cavity, Doppler tissue imaging, and speckle tracking). Left atrial size and volume are also collected by echocardiography and provide prognostic information for the development of atrial fibrillation, stroke, and HF.

CMR Imaging

CMR imaging is considered the gold standard for measurement of LV mass and volumes (**Fig. 3**). It

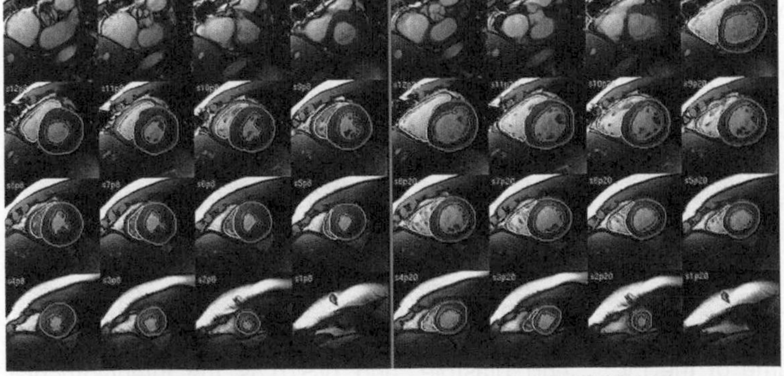

Fig. 3. Multilevel short axis slices of the LV in systole and diastole obtained with CMR imaging. Dedicated software can calculate left ventricular volume, ejection fraction, and mass.

provides a high spatial and acceptable temporal resolution (~20 frames/s); furthermore, it allows acquisition of images in any plane, overcoming the anatomic limitations inherent in other modalities. In addition, there is no radiation or iodine contrast exposure. CMR imaging has the highest reproducibility of all noninvasive modalities; in a study of repeat measurements by 2D echocardiography and CMR, the reproducibility of LV volumes and function was 65% and 98%, and 94% and 99%, respectively.[25] For patients with LVH, the coefficient of variation with CMR and 2D echocardiography were 3.6% and 13.5%, showing the superior reproducibility of CMR.[25] The limitations of CMR include claustrophobia, artifacts caused by arrhythmias and patient's movement, and limitations resulting from patients' size. CMR can be used to assess LV diastolic function by analysis of deformation of tagged myocardium.[26]

Cardiac Computed Tomography

Cardiac computed tomography (CT) imaging began with the introduction of electron beam CT (EBCT), which provided adequate temporal resolution to overcome the issue of cardiac motion. Temporal resolution is an even greater issue with multidetector CT (MDCT), although the latter provides better spatial resolution compared with EBCT. The obvious limitations of cardiac CT include radiation and iodine contrast exposure. Data acquired with CT are generally accurate for LV volume, function, and mass calculations (**Fig. 4**). Raman and colleagues[27] showed a high correlation between 16-row MDCT and CMR for LV volume ($r = 0.97$), and mass ($r = 0.95$) with a mean difference of 6.5 ($\pm$7.5) g. However, Schlosser and colleagues[28] showed a larger average error of ~12 g between 64-row MDCT and CMR, and calculated a significantly lower LV ejection fraction with 64-slice cardiac MDCT than CMR. This systematic error between the techniques may be secondary to the different assumptions between the techniques, as well as the effect of β-blockade before imaging and the effect of contrast. Despite the small measurement error, the additional coronary angiography data provided by CT are important.

Nuclear Cardiology Imaging

The frequent use of exercise nuclear stress testing to diagnose and risk stratify CAD in patients who are hypertensive makes this technique a desirable method to assess LV volumes, function, and mass. Gated tomographic images are typically acquired during the performance of single-photon emission computed tomography (SPECT) and positron emission tomography; volumes as well as mass estimates are provided as part of the final report (**Fig. 5**). Unlike planar blood pool approaches that use decay counts to assess volume and function, tomographic methods use a volume-based approach that requires an accurate identification of the endocardial border. The accuracy of nuclear tomographic techniques has been validated against other gold standards such as CMR and

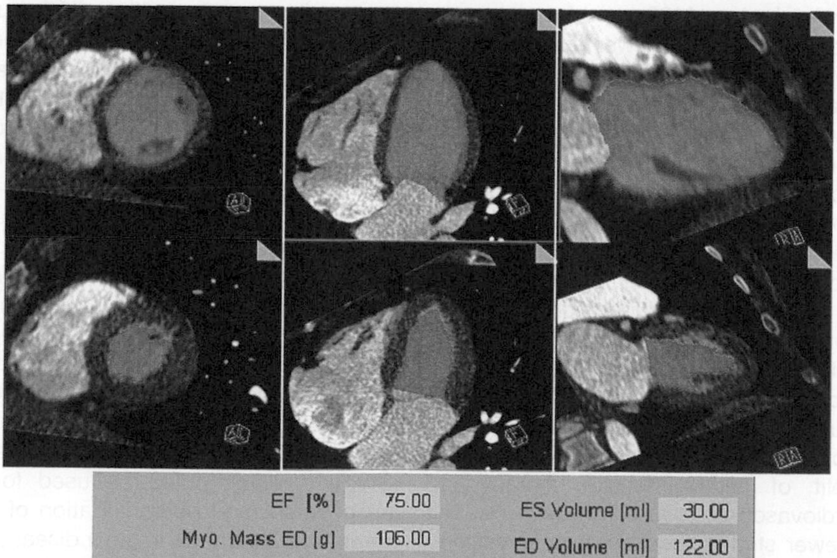

Fig. 4. Left ventricular volume, ejection fraction, and mass obtained with MDCT.

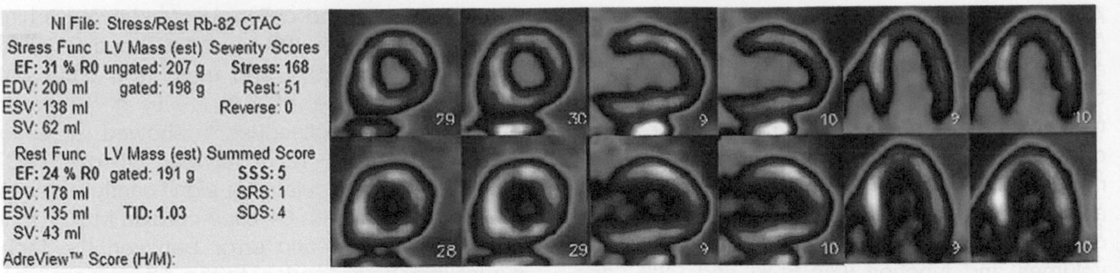

Fig. 5. Positron emission tomography study in a patient with hypertensive cardiomyopathy. Note the low ejection fraction (24% at rest) and the increased mass (191 g at rest).

CT. The reported correlation coefficient varied between 0.7 and 0.97 depending on the comparator used. Recently, Schepis and colleagues[29] compared 64-slice MDCT with gated SPECT and found a correlation of 0.82 for the LV function. The low spatial resolution of SPECT compared with other techniques may cause underestimation of the cavity size in small ventricles and in patients with LVH, with a subsequent overestimation of LV ejection fraction. The limited spatial resolution may also affect LV mass measurement, although fair accuracy is reported. Time-volume curves can be used to assess LV diastolic function.

PREVENTION AND TREATMENT

The prevention and management of hypertension and HHD are major public health challenges. If the increase in BP with age could be prevented or diminished, a substantial proportion of complications might be prevented. Overall, 122 million Americans are overweight or obese,[30] and the mean sodium intake is ~4400 mg/d for men and ~2900 mg/d for women.[31] Fewer than 20% of Americans engage in regular physical activity,[32] and fewer than 25% consume 5 or more servings of fruits and vegetables daily.[33] Primary prevention measures should be introduced to reduce or minimize these causal factors, particularly in individuals with prehypertension. A population-wide approach decreasing the BP level in the general population by even modest amounts has the potential to substantially reduce morbidity and mortality from hypertension; a 5–mm Hg reduction of systolic BP would result in a 14% reduction in mortality caused by stroke, a 9% reduction in mortality caused by CAD, and a 7% decrease in all-cause mortality.[34]

The benefit of antihypertensive therapy in reducing cardiovascular disease has been clearly showed.[35] Fewer studies focused on progression to severe hypertension, prevention of LVH, and development of HF. The Systolic Hypertension in the Elderly Program (SHEP) demonstrated that antihypertensive treatment exerted a strong protective effect on HF,[36] whereas a meta-analysis of 12 trials that included incident HF and 4 that included incident LVH as an outcome showed significant treatment benefits.[37] Incidence of LVH was decreased by 35% and an even greater benefit was observed for incident HF, with a reduction of 52%. Significant reductions were also reported for stroke and CAD.[37]

Global Risk Assessment

At any BP level, cardiovascular risk varies depending on the other accompanying risk factors.[38] Therefore, it may be advantageous to link BP therapy to level of cardiovascular risk. However, no clinical trial data have shown the efficacy of a risk-based approach to date. In an analysis from the SHEP study,[39] cardiovascular event rates in the placebo group were progressively higher in relation to higher quartiles of predicted cardiovascular risk. The protection afforded by treatment was similar across quartiles of risk, but the number needed to treat to prevent 1 event increased progressively at lower predicted cardiovascular disease risk quartiles.[39] Similar findings were observed in other studies.[40] Therefore, in 2005, a writing group of the American Society of Hypertension proposed an alternate classification system that incorporated total cardiovascular risk, considering that only a minority of patients who are hypertensive are devoid of other risk factors.[41] Recently, the European Society of Hypertension and European Society of Cardiology[42] have also embraced the concept of global cardiovascular risk. There are tools for cardiovascular risk prediction derived from the Framingham cohort[43] and for HF derived from the Health ABC Study,[13] which could be used for global risk assessment and personalization of hypertension treatment. Examples in other diseases states exist for such a paradigm (eg, low-density lipoprotein cholesterol treatment is based on the overall risk profile).[40]

Controlling Predisposing Risk Factors

Healthy lifestyle is critical for high BP prevention and is a crucial part of the management of hypertension.[34] Lifestyle interventions are more likely to be cost-effective, and the absolute reductions in risk of hypertension are likely to be greater, when targeted persons are older and at higher risk for hypertension. However, prevention strategies applied early in life provide the greatest long-term potential for avoiding the precursors that lead to hypertension and for reducing the overall burden of BP-related complications in the community.[44] Data from a meta-analysis indicate the important role of lifestyle on hypertension in Western societies.[45] Overweight has the largest contribution to hypertension, with PAR between 11% in Italy and 25% in the United States; for physical inactivity PAR ranges from 5% to 13%, for high sodium intake 9% to 17%, and for low potassium intake 4% to 17%.

Weight loss

Interventions targeting overweight and obesity have shown favorable effects on prevention and control of hypertension. Aggregate results of 25 trials show that mean systolic and diastolic BP reductions from an average weight loss of 5.1 kg were 4.4 and 3.6 mm Hg, respectively; BP reductions are similar for nonhypertensive and hypertensive subjects and greater in those who lose more weight.[46] In other studies, weight loss parallels BP reduction,[47] with a 21% to 35% reduction in incident hypertension.[47] Individuals with sustained weight loss of 4.5 kg (10 lb) for more than 3 years achieved a lower BP.[47]

Physical activity

Persons who are less active and less fit have a 30% to 50% greater risk for developing hypertension.[48] Studies evaluating various forms of physical activity have identified an inverse relation between physical activity and BP. This relation has been noted at all ages, in both sexes, in racial subgroups, and was independent of body weight.[34]

Sodium intake and diet

The Dietary Approaches to Stop Hypertension (DASH) diet is effective in reducing BP in individuals who are hypertensive and those who are nonhypertensive,[49] and it reduces incident hypertension. Reduction in sodium lowered systolic and diastolic BP by 2.0 and 1.0 mm Hg in individuals who were nonhypertensive and by 5.0 and 2.7 mm Hg in individuals who were hypertensive. The combination of DASH diet and low sodium intake lowers BP levels substantially more than each alone.[50] Moreover, a reduced sodium intake lowers risk for hypertension by ~20%,[51] and facilitates hypertension control.[52] The effects of sodium reduction tend to be greater in black people; middle-aged and older persons; and individuals with hypertension, diabetes, or chronic kidney disease. Currently, the recommended amount of sodium is less than 2300 mg/d for healthy adults, but less than 1500 mg/d for specific groups.[53] Because 69.2% of adults in the United States meet the criteria for lower sodium consumption,[54] it is argued that this recommended quantity should be applied for all.[55] Sodium intake has been shown to be a potent determinant of LV growth in hypertensive as well as in normotensive experimental animal models, through complex mechanisms that involve circulating volume expansion and possible activation of the tissue renin-angiotensin system.[56–58]

Treatment Principles and Guidelines for Controlling BP

The care of patients with HHD falls into 2 categories: (1) treatment of increased BP, and (2) prevention and treatment of HHD. Treatment of hypertension is discussed in detail elsewhere in this issue. Briefly, according to the Seventh Report of the Joint National Committee on Prevention, Detection, Evaluation, and Treatment of High Blood Pressure (JNC-7), the BP goal is less than 140/90 mm Hg except for those with diabetes or renal disease for whom the goal is less than 130/85 mm Hg.[59] Treatment includes (1) dietary modifications, (2) regular aerobic exercise, (3) weight loss, and (4) pharmacotherapy. The achievement of the treatment goals depends on timing of treatment initiation, selection of appropriate medications, and adherence to treatment.

Current guidelines recommend antihypertensive medications in all patients with systolic BP greater than or equal to 140 mm Hg or diastolic BP greater than or equal to 90 mm Hg, who have 1 or no risk factors and cannot reach this goal by lifestyle changes alone. However, recent trial data suggest that tight control of systolic BP (<130 mm Hg) in patients who are not diabetic has additional benefit on the composite of all-cause mortality, cardiovascular events, and HF; LVH was also less frequent in the tight control group.[60] A meta-analysis on BP and cardiovascular death also showed similar results,[2] raising the question of whether treatment should be started earlier.

Treatment should follow contemporary guidelines and evidence suggesting the most appropriate agents that reduce the risk for HHD complications. Evidence suggests that antihypertensive medications have important non–BP mediated mechanisms of action that may enhance or diminish the benefit of BP control on HHD. For example, in the Antihypertensive and Lipid-Lowering Treatment to Prevent Heart Attack (ALLHAT) trial, doxazosin-based treatment was associated with a twofold higher risk for HF compared with diuretic-based treatment, despite comparable BP reduction. This risk seems to be associated with increased plasma volume[61] as a result of renin-angiotensin system stimulation and increased plasma norepinephrine levels through sympathetic nerve activation.[62] In a recent study that evaluated the effect of doxazosin on LV structure and function when administered with other antihypertensive medications in patients with morning hypertension, compared with no additional medication, the doxazosin group demonstrated increased LV diastolic diameter and B-type natriuretic peptide levels despite reductions in LV wall thickness.[63] Moreover, LV diastolic function deteriorated without any change in systolic function in the doxazosin group and, although HF developed in a small number of patients, all patients with incident HF had preserved ejection fraction and were from the doxazosin group.[63]

Compelling evidence derived from a meta-analysis of double-blind trials suggests beneficial effects of angiotensin-converting enzyme inhibitors (ACEI) and angiotensin receptor blockers (ARB) on LV mass.[64,65] Moreover, 33% reduction of incident atrial fibrillation was observed in the losartan versus the atenonol-treated group.[66] Also, losartan has favorable effects on recurrent atrial fibrillation[67] and reduces cardiomyocyte apoptosis and myocardial fibrosis in patients with HHD compared with amlodipine.[68] Thiazide-type diuretics are suggested by JNC-7 as initial therapy for most patients with uncomplicated hypertension. Diuretics have been effective in preventing complications of hypertension.[69] β-Blockers are effective in lowering BP, but less effective in the reduction of LV mass[65] and prevention of complications including CAD and cardiovascular and all-cause mortality in patients with hypertension.[70] However, a recent meta-analysis suggested that β-blockers are efficacious for primary prevention of HF in patients with hypertension independent of age when compared with other agents. However, there was an increased risk for stroke (19%) in participants 60 years of age or older associated with β-blocker use.[71] Calcium channel blockers (CCB) are effective for treatment of systolic hypertension in elderly patients. Although a recent meta-analysis suggested that CCBs are less effective in HF risk reduction for the same reduction of BP,[72] the effect of CCBs on LV mass is similar to that of renin-angiotensin system inhibitors.[64] In a recent study, an ACEI/CCB combination proved to be superior to the ACEI/thiazide combination for prevention of cardiovascular events in patients at high-risk with hypertension.[73]

Because most antihypertensive agents with antihypertrophic effects target outside-in signaling cardiac cells, new interventions of targeting intracellular events are investigated. These events include (1) intervention on genetic mechanisms that regulate the hypertrophic or the profibrotic response of myocardium, (2) blockage of detrimental intracellular mechanisms and prevention of inhibition of negative signaling modulators triggered by biomechanical stress, (3) preservation of cardiomyocytes or regeneration of lost cardiomyocytes, (4) restoration of normal turnover of the collagen network, and (5) stimulation of the angiogenic activity of endothelial cells.

Adherence to lifestyle changes (**Table 1**) is crucial before and after medication initiation. Adherence to medications is also important.[74] Barriers to adherence are multifactorial and could be patient specific (eg, forgetfulness, beliefs), medication specific (eg, complexity, dosing frequency), logistic (eg, frequency of clinic visits and pharmacy fills), or disease specific (eg, absence of symptoms for hypertension).[75] Understanding these barriers could provide a framework to facilitate communication with patients about medication adherence in clinical settings and assist in developing multicomponent behavioral interventions. Maneuvers likely to help include (1) providing instruction and instructional materials, (2) simplifying and counseling about the regimen (eg, less-frequent dosing, controlled release dosage forms), (3) support group sessions, (4) reminders (manual and computer) for medications and appointments, (5) cuing medications to daily events, (6) reinforcement and awards, (7) self-monitoring with regular physician review and reinforcement, and (8) involving family members.

Treatment Principles and Guidelines for Cardiac Structural and Functional Abnormalities

LVH

Early detection and aggressive treatment of LVH is crucial, including (1) early identification of patients who are hypertensive and prone to LVH, (2) accurate assessment of LV anatomy and function, and (3) repair of the molecular and cellular alterations of the myocardium. Prevention of LVH attenuates risk for new-onset HF in patients at high risk[76] and regression of LVH with antihypertensive

Table 1
Lifestyle modifications to prevent and manage hypertension

Lifestyle Modification	Recommendation
Weight loss	For overweight/obese: • lose weight (ideal BMI<25 kg/m^2) For nonoverweight: • maintain desirable BMI<25 kg/m^2
Physical activity	Engage in regular aerobic physical activity (at least 30 min/d, most days of the week)
Reduced salt intake	Lower salt intake as much as possible (ideal 1.5 g/d of sodium or 3.8 g/d salt)
DASH-type dietary patterns	Consume a diet rich in fruits and vegetables (8–10 servings/d), low-fat dairy products (2–3 servings/d), and reduced saturated fat/cholesterol
Increased potassium intake	Increase potassium intake 4.7 g/d
Moderation of alcohol intake	For those who drink alcohol: • consume ≤2 alcoholic drinks/d (men) • consume ≤1 alcoholic drink/d (women)

therapy is associated with a lower risk for HF, independent of BP lowering and other risk factors.[77] Regression of LVH leads to reduction in cardiovascular mortality and morbidity.[78] All classes of antihypertensive medications have been shown to reduce LVH. Recent analyses indicated that ARB, ACEI, and CCB were more effective than β-blockers in reversing LVH, but efficacy of diuretics was intermediate (more effective than β-blockers but <ACEI).[42,64,79] Recently, the combination of ARB and hydrochlorothiazide has been shown to be more effective than ARB alone in LVH reduction.[80]

The degree of LVH regression and the time needed for LVH to regress are important issues. To date, few studies have investigated the effects of antihypertensive treatment on LVH for longer than 1 year. Among these, the Losartan Intervention For Endpoint (LIFE) study compared the LVH effects of medications repeatedly for a period of 4 years[79] and the European Lacidipine Study on Atherosclerosis (ELSA) study[81] evaluated the echocardiographic effect of medications for up to 4 years. In both studies, LV mass markedly decreased during the first and second year of treatment and further (but marginally) decreased through the remaining follow-up. These findings suggest that LVH regression occurs mostly during the first 2 years of treatment, despite persistent satisfactory BP control.

Gender-related differences in cardiac structure and function (higher LV mass and worse systolic and diastolic performance in men) and differential LVH regression for similar BP reductions (larger LVH regression in women) have been described.[82] However, the underlying mechanisms are unclear.

Diastolic dysfunction

Limited information is available about the comparative effects of antihypertensive treatments on diastolic function and HF with preserved ejection fraction, both of which are frequently associated with LVH. Although prospective studies on LVH regression did not enroll patients based on diastolic function, differences between treatments on LV diastolic function have been found.[83,84] Moreover, studies with sophisticated methodologies for diastolic function showed a significant improvement in patients treated with ACEI in contrast to diuretics despite similar reductions in LV mass[85] and ARB.[86] In the Regression with the Angiotensin Antagonist Losartan (REGAAL) study,[87] although the early-to-late mitral flow velocity ratio was not differentially affected by ARBs or β-blockers, ARB reduced the more sensitive indicators of myocardial stretch. These findings indicate that changes in myocardial texture may play a major role in reversing diastolic dysfunction. ARBs are the best-studied drug class in HF with preserved ejection fraction. In a crossover study comparing ARB with placebo in patients with dyspnea and exercise-induced hypertension (systolic BP>200 mm Hg),[88] ARB treatment significantly reduced exercise systolic BP, and the patients were able to exercise for a longer period with improved quality of life. Various investigators have recommended the use of drugs that reduce heart rate and prolong diastolic filling time, including β-blockers and verapamil. There are limited human data evaluating the efficacy of this approach. In a small study, verapamil was compared with placebo and was associated with prolongation of exercise duration after a 5-week treatment period.[89] Diuretics are generally required to reduce ventricular preload and relieve symptoms of HF. However, delicate titration is necessary, because they may cause severe hypotension by inappropriately decreasing the preload that is required for adequate LV filling pressures.

Despite these mechanistic data, the clinical trial evidence for the treatment of patients with HF and preserved ejection fraction is modest at best. In the Candesartan in Heart Failure: Assessment of Reduction in Mortality and Morbidity (CHARM)–Preserved trial[90] there was a nonsignificant reduction (11%) in the primary endpoint of cardiovascular death or HF hospitalization. Data from other trials including the Digoxin Investigators Group (DIG) Trial with digoxin,[91] the Perindopril in Elderly People with Chronic Heart Failure (PEP-CHF) trial with the ACEI peridopril in the elderly,[92] and 2 trials with ARBs including the Irbesartan in Heart Failure with Preserved Systolic Function (I-PRESERVE) trial with irbesartan[93]; all failed to show a clinical benefit with the use of these agent in patients with HF and preserved ejection fraction. Another ongoing trial, Aldosterone Antagonist Therapy for Adults with Heart Failure (TOPCAT)[94] is randomizing these patients to aldosterone antagonists and the results are awaited.

There continues to be a debate regarding the modest to no benefit seen in clinical outcomes in trials for patients with HF and preserved ejection fraction, a major manifestation of HHD. Diastolic dysfunction seen on echocardiography, which may be related to hypertension, is not synonymous with HF with preserved ejection fraction, which represents a distinct clinical syndrome. There continues to be uncertainty and difficulty regarding the diagnosis of HF with preserved ejection fraction, leading to detailed but onerous echocardiography and biomarker-based guidelines for the diagnosis of this condition.[95] It is possible that a segment of patients enrolled in these trials who had nonspecific symptoms such as dyspnea in the presence of preserved ejection fraction may not have had the syndrome of HF with preserved ejection fraction in the first place. In addition, patients with HF with preserved ejection fraction tend to have many other comorbidities.[96] Unlike patients with systolic dysfunction, these patients have a significant proportion of their hospitalizations and mortality related to their comorbidity burden as opposed to primary cardiac causes.[96]

Therefore, until further trials data are available, the management of these patients is primarily directed toward underlying manifestations of HHD, including treatment of BP and arrythmias (especially atrial fibrillation), diuretics for volume control, and optimal detection and treatment of ischemia. Primary valvular disease should be treated based on guideline recommendations. Particular emphasis should be placed on adequate management of all comorbidities, especially those associated with worsening HF, including chronic lung disease, diabetes, and chronic kidney disease.

Systolic dysfunction

ACEI are indicated in all patients with asymptomatic or symptomatic LV dilatation and dysfunction unless there is a contraindication or intolerance. ACEI have been shown to decrease morbidity and mortality in patients with HF caused by systolic dysfunction.[97] The aim should be to use the target dose or the maximum tolerable doses. β-Blockers (cardioselective or mixed α and β selective) have been shown to improve LV function and decrease mortality and morbidity from HF, even for patients with New York Heart Association (NYHA) class IV. Clinical improvement may be delayed and may take 2 to 3 months to become apparent. However, long-term treatment with β-blockers can lessen the symptoms of HF and improve clinical status. β-Blockers should be initiated at low doses and titrated to target doses.[97,98] ARB can be considered an alternative to ACEI in cases of intolerance. Although experience with ARB in trials is less than with ACEI, survival benefit and reduced hospitalizations have also been shown for ARB therapy in patients intolerant to ACEI. The combination of ACEI and ARB may result in more reduction of LV size[99] and reduce the need for hospitalization more than either agent alone, although whether combination therapy further reduces mortality remains unclear.[99,100]

Diuretics are used for LV systolic dysfunction when there is evidence, or a prior history, of fluid retention.[97] The 2 major classes of diuretics differ in their pharmacologic actions. Loop diuretics are the preferred agents for patients with HF. Thiazide diuretics may be preferred in patients with hypertension, HF, and mild fluid retention, because of persistent antihypertensive effects. Low-dose spironolactone decreases morbidity and mortality in patients in NYHA class III or IV HF already taking ACEI.[97] Aldosterone antagonists should be initiated after titration of standard medical therapy. Because spironolactone and eplerenone can cause hyperkalemia, precautions should be taken to minimize the risk. In the Eplerenone Post-acute Myocardial Infarction Heart Failure Efficacy and Survival Study (EPHESUS) trial, the addition of eplerenone to standard care did not increase the risk of hyperkalemia when potassium was regularly monitored.[101] Digoxin can be used in patients who are symptomatic with atrial fibrillation and on maximal tolerated doses of the previously reported medications, because it can reduce symptoms, prevent hospitalizations, and increase exercise tolerance. However, the general use of digoxin in all patients with HF and low ejection fraction could be harmful.[102] In earlier studies comparing the combination of hydralazine and nitrates with placebo, the combination significantly reduced mortality in patients with HF who were not on ACEI or β-blockers.[103,104] These benefits were more pronounced in black patients with HF,[105] leading to a confirmatory large randomized trial in these patients.[106] Thus, the vasodilator combination is recommended for black patients who remain symptomatic despite optimal medical therapy.

Patients with HF and low ejection fraction who experience syncope of unclear origin have a high rate of subsequent sudden death and should also be considered for internal cardiac defibrillator placement.[107] Patients with low ejection fraction and no previous history of cardiac arrest or ventricular tachycardia also have a significant risk of sudden death. Therefore the current guidelines for internal cardiac defibrillator implantation recommend that all patients with cardiomyopathy (ischemic or nonischemic) and an LV ejection fraction of 35% or less despite optimal medical therapy should be considered for an internal cardiac defibrillator for primary prevention unless their prognosis is deemed to be end stage.[108–110] Approximately one-third of patients with low ejection fraction and class III to IV symptoms of HF manifest a QRS duration greater than 0.12 seconds, which represents abnormal cardiac conduction and has been associated with increased mortality in HF. This criterion has been used to identify patients with dyssynchronous ventricular contraction, which can require placement of biventricular pacemakers (cardiac resynchronization therapy [CRT]). When added to optimal medical therapy in patients who are persistently symptomatic, CRT has resulted in significant improvements in quality of life, functional class, exercise capacity, and ejection fraction in randomized trials.[111] In a meta-analysis of CRT trials, HF hospitalizations were reduced by 32% and all-cause mortality by 25%.[112]

Dietary instruction regarding sodium intake is recommended in all patients with HF. Dietary sodium restriction (2–3 g daily) is recommended for patients with HF.[113] Restriction of daily fluid intake to less than 2 L is recommended in patients with severe hyponatremia (serum sodium <130 mEq/L) and should be considered for all patients demonstrating fluid retention that is difficult to control despite diuretic use and sodium restriction.

Exercise training is known to reduce the debilitating symptoms of HF, such as breathlessness and fatigue.[114–116] A meta-analysis of exercise training trials has shown that exercise training is safe, improves survival, and extends hospitalization-free time.[117] A recent multicenter trial (Heart Failure: A Controlled Trial Investigating Outcomes of Exercise Training [HF-ACTION]) has shown nonsignificant reductions in all-cause mortality or hospitalization,[118] but significant improvements in self-reported health status compared with usual care without training.[119] Improvement occurred early and persisted over time.[119]

Atrial and ventricular arrhythmias

Atrial and ventricular arrhythmias, especially atrial fibrillation, are common in patients with HHD. Arrhythmias should be treated according to the guidelines published by the American College of Cardiology and the American Heart Association.[120,121]

Ischemic heart disease in the absence of significant epicardial CAD

Hypertension can cause ischemic heart disease in the absence of significant epicardial coronary stenosis. Common pathophysiologic mechanisms lead to changes of coronary vessels in HHD or in patients with established epicardial CAD; thus, prevention and reversal of these changes should be the goals of therapy for HHD. Recommendations for appropriate course of action are included in a statement of the American Heart Association.[122]

SUMMARY

HHD, a result of long-standing hypertension, is characterized by changes in the myocardial structure and function in the absence of other primary cardiovascular abnormalities. Although increased BP is the initiating stimulus, neurohormonal factors, particularly the renin-angiotensin system, play a key role in remodeling of cardiac chamber geometry and walls. Optimal antihypertensive therapy in the setting of therapeutic lifestyle changes is crucial in the prevention and control of HHD. Regression of LVH is achievable, and associated with improved prognosis. However, prevention of myocardial remodeling before LVH establishes would further increase the benefits to cardiac function and prognosis. Antihypertensive agents exhibit variable effectiveness in inducing LVH regression. Currently, renin-angiotensin system blocking agents seem to be the most effective approach for LVH regression and reverse remodeling in these patients.

REFERENCES

1. Kannel WB, Vasan RS, Levy D. Is the relation of systolic blood pressure to risk of cardiovascular disease continuous and graded, or are there critical values? Hypertension 2003;42(4):453–6.
2. Lewington S, Clarke R, Qizilbash N, et al. Age-specific relevance of usual blood pressure to vascular mortality: a meta-analysis of individual data for one million adults in 61 prospective studies. Lancet 2002;360(9349):1903–13.
3. World Health Organization. International statistical classification of diseases and related health problems 10th Revision. Diseases of the circulatory system. Chapter IX. Available at: http://apps.who.int/classifications/apps/icd/icd10online/. Accessed January 20, 2010.
4. Sugden PH. Mechanotransduction in cardiomyocyte hypertrophy. Circulation 2001;103(10):1375–7.
5. Baines CP, Molkentin JD. STRESS signaling pathways that modulate cardiac myocyte apoptosis. J Mol Cell Cardiol 2005;38(1):47–62.
6. Weber KT. Fibrosis and hypertensive heart disease. Curr Opin Cardiol 2000;15(4):264–72.
7. Berk BC, Fujiwara K, Lehoux S. ECM remodeling in hypertensive heart disease. J Clin Invest 2007;117(3):568–75.
8. Wolf-Maier K, Cooper RS, Banegas JR, et al. Hypertension prevalence and blood pressure levels in 6 European countries, Canada, and the United States. JAMA 2003;289(18):2363–9.
9. Levy D, Anderson KM, Savage DD, et al. Echocardiographically detected left ventricular hypertrophy: prevalence and risk factors. The Framingham Heart Study. Ann Intern Med 1988;108(1):7–13.
10. Kannel WB, Dannenberg AL, Abbott RD. Unrecognized myocardial infarction and hypertension: the Framingham Study. Am Heart J 1985;109(3 Pt 1):581–5.
11. Levy D, Larson MG, Vasan RS, et al. The progression from hypertension to congestive heart failure. JAMA 1996;275(20):1557–62.
12. Kalogeropoulos A, Georgiopoulou V, Kritchevsky SB, et al. Epidemiology of incident heart failure in a contemporary elderly cohort: the Health, Aging, And Body Composition study. Arch Intern Med 2009;169(7):708–15.
13. Butler J, Kalogeropoulos A, Georgiopoulou V, et al. Incident heart failure prediction in the elderly: the health ABC heart failure score. Circ Heart Fail 2008;1(2):125–33.
14. Lloyd-Jones D, Larson M, Leip E, et al. Lifetime risk for developing congestive heart failure: the Framingham Heart Study. Circulation 2002;106(24):3068–72.
15. World Health Report. Reducing risks, promoting healthy life. Geneva (Switzerland): World Health Organization; 2002. Available at: http://www.who.int/whr/2002/en/whr02_en.pdf. Accessed February 1, 2010.
16. Reichek N, Devereux RB. Left ventricular hypertrophy: relationship of anatomic, echocardiographic and electrocardiographic findings. Circulation 1981;63(6):1391–8.
17. Woythaler JN, Singer SL, Kwan OL, et al. Accuracy of echocardiography versus electrocardiography in detecting left ventricular hypertrophy: comparison with postmortem mass measurements. J Am Coll Cardiol 1983;2(2):305–11.
18. Okin PM, Wright JT, Nieminen MS, et al. Ethnic differences in electrocardiographic criteria for left ventricular hypertrophy: the LIFE study. Losartan Intervention for Endpoint. Am J Hypertens 2002;15(8):663–71.
19. Lee DK, Marantz PR, Devereux RB, et al. Left ventricular hypertrophy in black and white hypertensives. Standard electrocardiographic criteria overestimate racial differences in prevalence. JAMA 1992;267(24):3294–9.
20. Devereux RB, Reichek N. Echocardiographic determination of left ventricular mass in man. Anatomic validation of the method. Circulation 1977;55(4):613–8.
21. Devereux RB, Alonso DR, Lutas EM, et al. Echocardiographic assessment of left ventricular hypertrophy: comparison to necropsy findings. Am J Cardiol 1986;57(6):450–8.
22. Lang RM, Bierig M, Devereux RB, et al. Recommendations for chamber quantification: a report from the American Society of Echocardiography's Guidelines and Standards Committee and the Chamber Quantification Writing Group, developed in conjunction with the European Association of Echocardiography, a branch of the European Society of Cardiology. J Am Soc Echocardiogr 2005;18(12):1440–63.
23. Qin JX, Jones M, Travaglini A, et al. The accuracy of left ventricular mass determined by real-time three-dimensional echocardiography in chronic animal and clinical studies: a comparison with postmortem examination and magnetic resonance imaging. J Am Soc Echocardiogr 2005;18(10):1037–43.
24. Takeuchi M, Nishikage T, Mor-Avi V, et al. Measurement of left ventricular mass by real-time three-dimensional echocardiography: validation against magnetic resonance and comparison with two-dimensional and m-mode measurements. J Am Soc Echocardiogr 2008;21(9):1001–5.
25. Grothues F, Smith GC, Moon JC, et al. Comparison of interstudy reproducibility of cardiovascular magnetic resonance with two-dimensional

echocardiography in normal subjects and in patients with heart failure or left ventricular hypertrophy. Am J Cardiol 2002;90(1):29–34.
26. Edvardsen T, Rosen BD, Pan L, et al. Regional diastolic dysfunction in individuals with left ventricular hypertrophy measured by tagged magnetic resonance imaging–the Multi-Ethnic Study of Atherosclerosis (MESA). Am Heart J 2006;151(1): 109–14.
27. Raman SV, Shah M, McCarthy B, et al. Multidetector row cardiac computed tomography accurately quantifies right and left ventricular size and function compared with cardiac magnetic resonance. Am Heart J 2006;151(3):736–44.
28. Schlosser T, Mohrs OK, Magedanz A, et al. Assessment of left ventricular function and mass in patients undergoing computed tomography (CT) coronary angiography using 64-detector-row CT: comparison to magnetic resonance imaging. Acta Radiol 2007;48(1):30–5.
29. Schepis T, Gaemperli O, Koepfli P, et al. Comparison of 64-slice CT with gated SPECT for evaluation of left ventricular function. J Nucl Med 2006;47(8): 1288–94.
30. Flegal KM, Carroll MD, Ogden CL, et al. Prevalence and trends in obesity among US adults, 1999–2000. JAMA 2002;288(14):1723–7.
31. Sources of sodium among the US population, 2005–06. Available at: http://riskfactor.cancer.gov/diet/foodsources/sodium/#tables. Accessed February 10, 2010.
32. US Department of Health and Human Services, Centers for Disease Control and Prevention Atlanta (GA). Physical activity and health: a report of the surgeon general. Available at: http://www.cdc.gov/nccdphp/sgr/ataglan.htm. Accessed February 11, 2010.
33. Division of Adult and Community Health, National Center for Chronic Disease Prevention and Health Promotion, Centers for Disease Control and Prevention: National Fruit and Vegetable Program. Available at: http://apps.nccd.cdc.gov/5ADaySurveillance/. Accessed February 10, 2010.
34. Whelton PK, He J, Appel LJ, et al. Primary prevention of hypertension: clinical and public health advisory from The National High Blood Pressure Education Program. JAMA 2002;288(15):1882–8.
35. Collins R, Peto R, MacMahon S, et al. Blood pressure, stroke, and coronary heart disease. Part 2, Short-term reductions in blood pressure: overview of randomised drug trials in their epidemiological context. Lancet 1990;335(8693):827–38.
36. Kostis JB, Davis BR, Cutler J, et al. Prevention of heart failure by antihypertensive drug treatment in older persons with isolated systolic hypertension. SHEP Cooperative Research Group. JAMA 1997;278(3): 212–6.
37. Moser M, Hebert PR. Prevention of disease progression, left ventricular hypertrophy and congestive heart failure in hypertension treatment trials. J Am Coll Cardiol 1996;27(5):1214–8.
38. Jackson R, Lawes CM, Bennett DA, et al. Treatment with drugs to lower blood pressure and blood cholesterol based on an individual's absolute cardiovascular risk. Lancet 2005;365(9457): 434–41.
39. Ferrucci L, Furberg CD, Penninx BW, et al. Treatment of isolated systolic hypertension is most effective in older patients with high-risk profile. Circulation 2001;104(16):1923–6.
40. Expert Panel on Detection, Evaluation, and Treatment of High Blood Cholesterol in Adults. Executive Summary of The Third Report of The National Cholesterol Education Program (NCEP) Expert Panel on Detection, Evaluation, and Treatment of High Blood Cholesterol in Adults (Adult Treatment Panel III). JAMA 2001;285(19):2486–97.
41. Giles TD, Berk BC, Black HR, et al. Expanding the definition and classification of hypertension. J Clin Hypertens (Greenwich) 2005;7(9):505–12.
42. Mancia G, De Backer G, Dominiczak A, et al. 2007 guidelines for the management of arterial hypertension: the Task Force for the Management of Arterial Hypertension of the European Society of Hypertension (ESH) and of the European Society of Cardiology (ESC). J Hypertens 2007; 25(6):1105–87.
43. Wilson PW, D'Agostino RB, Levy D, et al. Prediction of coronary heart disease using risk factor categories. Circulation 1998;97(18):1837–47.
44. Falkner B, Gidding SS, Portman R, et al. Blood pressure variability and classification of prehypertension and hypertension in adolescence. Pediatrics 2008;122(2):238–42.
45. Geleijnse JM, Kok FJ, Grobbee DE. Impact of dietary and lifestyle factors on the prevalence of hypertension in Western populations. Eur J Public Health 2004;14(3):235–9.
46. Neter JE, Stam BE, Kok FJ, et al. Influence of weight reduction on blood pressure: a meta-analysis of randomized controlled trials. Hypertension 2003;42(5):878–84.
47. Stevens VJ, Obarzanek E, Cook NR, et al. Long-term weight loss and changes in blood pressure: results of the Trials of Hypertension Prevention, phase II. Ann Intern Med 2001;134(1):1–11.
48. Blair SN, Goodyear NN, Gibbons LW, et al. Physical fitness and incidence of hypertension in healthy normotensive men and women. JAMA 1984;252(4):487–90.
49. Appel LJ, Moore TJ, Obarzanek E, et al. A clinical trial of the effects of dietary patterns on blood pressure. DASH Collaborative Research Group. N Engl J Med 1997;336(16):1117–24.

50. Sacks FM, Svetkey LP, Vollmer WM, et al. Effects on blood pressure of reduced dietary sodium and the Dietary Approaches to Stop Hypertension (DASH) diet. DASH-Sodium Collaborative Research Group. N Engl J Med 2001;344(1):3–10.
51. Effects of weight loss and sodium reduction intervention on blood pressure and hypertension incidence in overweight people with high-normal blood pressure. The Trials of Hypertension Prevention, phase II. The Trials of Hypertension Prevention Collaborative Research Group. Arch Intern Med 1997;157(6):657–67.
52. Appel LJ, Espeland MA, Easter L, et al. Effects of reduced sodium intake on hypertension control in older individuals: results from the Trial of Nonpharmacologic Interventions in the Elderly (TONE). Arch Intern Med 2001;161(5):685–93.
53. Dietary guidelines for Americans. 6th edition. Washington, DC: US Department of Health and Human Services, US Department of Agriculture; 2005. Available at: http://www.health.gov/dietaryguidelines/dga2005/document/pdf/dga2005.pdf. Accessed February 11, 2010.
54. Centers for Disease Control and Prevention (CDC). Application of lower sodium intake recommendations to adults–United States, 1999–2006. MMWR Morb Mortal Wkly Rep 2009;58(11):281–3.
55. American Heart Association. IOM Committee on Strategies to Reduce Sodium Intake. March 30, 2009. Available at: http://americanheart.org/downloadable/heart/1240425252727AHA%20Statement%20to%20IOM%20on%20Strategies%20to%20Reduce%20Sodium%20Intake%20033009.pdf. Accessed February 10, 2010.
56. Frohlich ED, Chien Y, Sesoko S, et al. Relationship between dietary sodium intake, hemodynamics, and cardiac mass in SHR and WKY rats. Am J Physiol 1993;264(1 Pt 2):R30–4.
57. de Simone G, Devereux RB, Camargo MJ, et al. Influence of sodium intake on in vivo left ventricular anatomy in experimental renovascular hypertension. Am J Physiol 1993;264(6 Pt 2):H2103–10.
58. de Simone G, Devereux RB, Camargo MJ, et al. Reduction of development of left ventricular hypertrophy in salt-loaded Dahl salt-sensitive rats by angiotensin II receptor inhibition. Am J Hypertens 1996;9(3):216–22.
59. Chobanian AV, Bakris GL, Black HR, et al. Seventh report of the Joint National Committee on Prevention, Detection, Evaluation, and Treatment of High Blood Pressure. Hypertension 2003;42(6):1206–52.
60. Verdecchia P, Staessen JA, Angeli F, et al. Usual versus tight control of systolic blood pressure in non-diabetic patients with hypertension (Cardio-Sis): an open-label randomised trial. Lancet 2009;374(9689):525–33.
61. McNair A, Rasmussen S, Nielsen PE, et al. The antihypertensive effect of prazosin on mild to moderate hypertension, changes in plasma volume, extracellular volume and glomerular filtration rate. Acta Med Scand 1980;207(5):413–6.
62. Wilner KD, Ziegler MG. Effects of alpha 1 inhibition on renal blood flow and sympathetic nervous activity in systemic hypertension. Am J Cardiol 1987;59(14):82G–6G.
63. Matsui Y, Eguchi K, Shibasaki S, et al. Effect of doxazosin on the left ventricular structure and function in morning hypertensive patients: the Japan Morning Surge 1 study. J Hypertens 2008;26(7):1463–71.
64. Klingbeil AU, Schneider M, Martus P, et al. A meta-analysis of the effects of treatment on left ventricular mass in essential hypertension. Am J Med 2003;115(1):41–6.
65. Dahlof B, Devereux RB, Kjeldsen SE, et al. Cardiovascular morbidity and mortality in the Losartan Intervention For Endpoint reduction in hypertension study (LIFE): a randomised trial against atenolol. Lancet 2002;359(9311):995–1003.
66. Wachtell K, Lehto M, Gerdts E, et al. Angiotensin II receptor blockade reduces new-onset atrial fibrillation and subsequent stroke compared to atenolol: the Losartan Intervention For End Point Reduction in Hypertension (LIFE) study. J Am Coll Cardiol 2005;45(5):712–9.
67. Fogari R, Mugellini A, Destro M, et al. Losartan and prevention of atrial fibrillation recurrence in hypertensive patients. J Cardiovasc Pharmacol 2006;47(1):46–50.
68. Gonzalez A, Lopez B, Ravassa S, et al. Stimulation of cardiac apoptosis in essential hypertension: potential role of angiotensin II. Hypertension 2002;39(1):75–80.
69. ALLHAT Officers and Coordinators for the ALLHAT Collaborative Research Group, The Antihypertensive and Lipid-Lowering Treatment to Prevent Heart Attack Trial. Major outcomes in high-risk hypertensive patients randomized to angiotensin-converting enzyme inhibitor or calcium channel blocker vs diuretic: the Antihypertensive and Lipid-Lowering Treatment to Prevent Heart Attack Trial (ALLHAT). JAMA 2002;288(23):2981–97.
70. Wiysonge CS, Bradley H, Mayosi BM, et al. Beta-blockers for hypertension. Cochrane Database Syst Rev 2007;1:CD002003.
71. Bangalore S, Wild D, Parkar S, et al. Beta-blockers for primary prevention of heart failure in patients with hypertension insights from a meta-analysis. J Am Coll Cardiol 2008;52(13):1062–72.
72. Verdecchia P, Angeli F, Cavallini C, et al. Blood pressure reduction and renin-angiotensin system inhibition for prevention of congestive heart failure: a meta-analysis. Eur Heart J 2009;30(6):679–88.

73. Jamerson K, Weber MA, Bakris GL, et al. Benazepril plus amlodipine or hydrochlorothiazide for hypertension in high-risk patients. N Engl J Med 2008;359(23):2417–28.
74. Borzecki AM, Oliveria SA, Berlowitz DR. Barriers to hypertension control. Am Heart J 2005;149(5):785–94.
75. Osterberg L, Blaschke T. Adherence to medication. N Engl J Med 2005;353(5):487–97.
76. Mathew J, Sleight P, Lonn E, et al. Reduction of cardiovascular risk by regression of electrocardiographic markers of left ventricular hypertrophy by the angiotensin-converting enzyme inhibitor ramipril. Circulation 2001;104(14):1615–21.
77. Okin PM, Devereux RB, Harris KE, et al. Regression of electrocardiographic left ventricular hypertrophy is associated with less hospitalization for heart failure in hypertensive patients. Ann Intern Med 2007;147(5):311–9.
78. Okin PM, Devereux RB, Jern S, et al. Regression of electrocardiographic left ventricular hypertrophy during antihypertensive treatment and the prediction of major cardiovascular events. JAMA 2004; 292(19):2343–9.
79. Devereux RB, Dahlof B, Gerdts E, et al. Regression of hypertensive left ventricular hypertrophy by losartan compared with atenolol: the Losartan Intervention for Endpoint Reduction in Hypertension (LIFE) trial. Circulation 2004;110(11): 1456–62.
80. Okin PM, Hille DA, Kjeldsen SE, et al. Greater regression of electrocardiographic left ventricular hypertrophy during hydrochlorothiazide therapy in hypertensive patients. Am J Hypertens 2010;23 (7):786–93.
81. Agabiti-Rosei E, Trimarco B, Muiesan ML, et al. Cardiac structural and functional changes during long-term antihypertensive treatment with lacidipine and atenolol in the European Lacidipine Study on Atherosclerosis (ELSA). J Hypertens 2005;23(5):1091–8.
82. Bella JN, Palmieri V, Wachtell K, et al. Sex-related difference in regression of left ventricular hypertrophy with antihypertensive treatment: the LIFE study. J Hum Hypertens 2004;18(6):411–6.
83. Muller-Brunotte R, Edner M, Malmqvist K, et al. Irbesartan and atenolol improve diastolic function in patients with hypertensive left ventricular hypertrophy. J Hypertens 2005;23(3):633–40.
84. Terpstra WF, May JF, Smit AJ, et al. Long-term effects of amlodipine and lisinopril on left ventricular mass and diastolic function in elderly, previously untreated hypertensive patients: the ELVERA trial. J Hypertens 2001;19(2):303–9.
85. Brilla CG, Funck RC, Rupp H. Lisinopril-mediated regression of myocardial fibrosis in patients with hypertensive heart disease. Circulation 2000;102 (12):1388–93.
86. Diez J, Querejeta R, Lopez B, et al. Losartan-dependent regression of myocardial fibrosis is associated with reduction of left ventricular chamber stiffness in hypertensive patients. Circulation 2002;105(21):2512–7.
87. Ciulla MM, Paliotti R, Esposito A, et al. Different effects of antihypertensive therapies based on losartan or atenolol on ultrasound and biochemical markers of myocardial fibrosis: results of a randomized trial. Circulation 2004;110(5):552–7.
88. Warner JG Jr, Metzger DC, Kitzman DW, et al. Losartan improves exercise tolerance in patients with diastolic dysfunction and a hypertensive response to exercise. J Am Coll Cardiol 1999; 33(6):1567–72.
89. Setaro JF, Zaret BL, Schulman DS, et al. Usefulness of verapamil for congestive heart failure associated with abnormal left ventricular diastolic filling and normal left ventricular systolic performance. Am J Cardiol 1990;66(12):981–6.
90. Yusuf S, Pfeffer MA, Swedberg K, et al. Effects of candesartan in patients with chronic heart failure and preserved left-ventricular ejection fraction: the CHARM-Preserved Trial. Lancet 2003;362 (9386):777–81.
91. Ahmed A, Rich MW, Fleg JL, et al. Effects of digoxin on morbidity and mortality in diastolic heart failure: the ancillary digitalis investigation group trial. Circulation 2006;114(5):397–403.
92. Cleland JG, Tendera M, Adamus J, et al. The Perindopril in Elderly People with Chronic Heart Failure (PEP-CHF) study. Eur Heart J 2006;27(19): 2338–45.
93. Massie BM, Carson PE, McMurray JJ, et al. Irbesartan in patients with heart failure and preserved ejection fraction. N Engl J Med 2008;359(23): 2456–67.
94. Aldosterone Antagonist Therapy for Adults With Heart Failure and Preserved Systolic Function (TOPCAT). Available at: http://clinicaltrials.gov/ct2/show/NCT00094302. Accessed June 29, 2010.
95. Paulus WJ, Tschope C, Sanderson JE, et al. How to diagnose diastolic heart failure: a consensus statement on the diagnosis of heart failure with normal left ventricular ejection fraction by the Heart Failure and Echocardiography Associations of the European Society of Cardiology. Eur Heart J 2007;28(20):2539–50.
96. Shah SJ, Gheorghiade M. Heart failure with preserved ejection fraction: treat now by treating comorbidities. JAMA 2008;300(4):431–3.
97. Jessup M, Abraham WT, Casey DE, et al. 2009 focused update: ACCF/AHA Guidelines for the Diagnosis and Management of Heart Failure in Adults: a report of the American College of Cardiology Foundation/American Heart Association Task Force on Practice Guidelines: developed in

collaboration with the International Society for Heart and Lung Transplantation. Circulation 2009; 119(14):1977–2016.

98. McAlister FA, Wiebe N, Ezekowitz JA, et al. Meta-analysis: beta-blocker dose, heart rate reduction, and death in patients with heart failure. Ann Intern Med 2009;150(11):784–94.

99. Wong M, Staszewsky L, Latini R, et al. Severity of left ventricular remodeling defines outcomes and response to therapy in heart failure: Valsartan heart failure trial (Val-HeFT) echocardiographic data. J Am Coll Cardiol 2004;43(11):2022–7.

100. McMurray JJ, Ostergren J, Swedberg K, et al. Effects of candesartan in patients with chronic heart failure and reduced left-ventricular systolic function taking angiotensin-converting-enzyme inhibitors: the CHARM-Added trial. Lancet 2003; 362(9386):767–71.

101. Pitt B, Bakris G, Ruilope LM, et al. Serum potassium and clinical outcomes in the Eplerenone Post-Acute Myocardial Infarction Heart Failure Efficacy and Survival Study (EPHESUS). Circulation 2008;118(16):1643–50.

102. Georgiopoulou VV, Kalogeropoulos AP, Giamouzis G, et al. Digoxin therapy does not improve outcomes in patients with advanced heart failure on contemporary medical therapy. Circ Heart Fail 2009;2(2): 90–7.

103. Cohn JN, Archibald DG, Ziesche S, et al. Effect of vasodilator therapy on mortality in chronic congestive heart failure. Results of a Veterans Administration Cooperative Study. N Engl J Med 1986;314(24):1547–52.

104. Cohn JN, Johnson G, Ziesche S, et al. A comparison of enalapril with hydralazine-isosorbide dinitrate in the treatment of chronic congestive heart failure. N Engl J Med 1991;325(5):303–10.

105. Carson P, Ziesche S, Johnson G, et al. Racial differences in response to therapy for heart failure: analysis of the vasodilator-heart failure trials. Vasodilator-Heart Failure Trial Study Group. J Card Fail 1999;5 (3):178–87.

106. Taylor AL, Ziesche S, Yancy C, et al. Combination of isosorbide dinitrate and hydralazine in blacks with heart failure. N Engl J Med 2004;351(20):2049–57.

107. Knight BP, Goyal R, Pelosi F, et al. Outcome of patients with nonischemic dilated cardiomyopathy and unexplained syncope treated with an implantable defibrillator. J Am Coll Cardiol 1999;33(7): 1964–70.

108. Bardy GH, Lee KL, Mark DB, et al. Amiodarone or an implantable cardioverter-defibrillator for congestive heart failure. N Engl J Med 2005;352(3):225–37.

109. Moss AJ, Zareba W, Hall WJ, et al. Prophylactic implantation of a defibrillator in patients with myocardial infarction and reduced ejection fraction. N Engl J Med 2002;346(12):877–83.

110. Kadish A, Dyer A, Daubert JP, et al. Prophylactic defibrillator implantation in patients with nonischemic dilated cardiomyopathy. N Engl J Med 2004; 350(21):2151–8.

111. Abraham WT, Fisher WG, Smith AL, et al. Cardiac resynchronization in chronic heart failure. N Engl J Med 2002;346(24):1845–53.

112. McAlister FA, Stewart S, Ferrua S, et al. Multidisciplinary strategies for the management of heart failure patients at high risk for admission: a systematic review of randomized trials. J Am Coll Cardiol 2004;44(4):810–9.

113. Paterna S, Gaspare P, Fasullo S, et al. Normal-sodium diet compared with low-sodium diet in compensated congestive heart failure: is sodium an old enemy or a new friend? Clin Sci (Lond) 2008;114(3):221–30.

114. Experience from controlled trials of physical training in chronic heart failure. Protocol and patient factors in effectiveness in the improvement in exercise tolerance. European Heart Failure Training Group. Eur Heart J 1998;19(3):466–75.

115. McKelvie RS, Teo KK, Roberts R, et al. Effects of exercise training in patients with heart failure: the Exercise Rehabilitation Trial (EXERT). Am Heart J 2002;144(1):23–30.

116. Hambrecht R, Niebauer J, Fiehn E, et al. Physical training in patients with stable chronic heart failure: effects on cardiorespiratory fitness and ultrastructural abnormalities of leg muscles. J Am Coll Cardiol 1995;25(6):1239–49.

117. Piepoli MF, Davos C, Francis DP, et al. Exercise training meta-analysis of trials in patients with chronic heart failure (ExTraMATCH). BMJ 2004; 328(7433):189.

118. O'Connor CM, Whellan DJ, Lee KL, et al. Efficacy and safety of exercise training in patients with chronic heart failure: HF-ACTION randomized controlled trial. JAMA 2009;301(14):1439–50.

119. Flynn KE, Pina IL, Whellan DJ, et al. Effects of exercise training on health status in patients with chronic heart failure: HF-ACTION randomized controlled trial. JAMA 2009;301(14):1451–9.

120. Fuster V, Ryden LE, Cannom DS, et al. ACC/AHA/ESC 2006 guidelines for the management of patients with atrial fibrillation—executive summary: a report of the American College of Cardiology/American Heart Association Task Force on Practice Guidelines and the European Society of Cardiology Committee for Practice Guidelines (Writing Committee to Revise the 2001 Guidelines for the Management of Patients With Atrial Fibrillation). J Am Coll Cardiol 2006;48(4):854–906.

121. Zipes DP, Camm AJ, Borggrefe M, et al. ACC/AHA/ESC 2006 guidelines for management of patients with ventricular arrhythmias and the prevention of sudden cardiac death: a report of the American

College of Cardiology/American Heart Association Task Force and the European Society of Cardiology Committee for Practice Guidelines (Writing Committee to Develop Guidelines for Management of Patients With Ventricular Arrhythmias and the Prevention of Sudden Cardiac Death). J Am Coll Cardiol 2006;48 (5):e247–346.

122. Rosendorff C, Black HR, Cannon CP, et al. Treatment of hypertension in the prevention and management of ischemic heart disease: a scientific statement from the American Heart Association Council for High Blood Pressure Research and the Councils on Clinical Cardiology and Epidemiology and Prevention. Circulation 2007;115(21):2761–88.

Index

Note: Page numbers of article titles are in **boldface** type.

Cardiol Clin 28 (2010) 693–697
doi:10.1016/S0733-8651(10)00100-1
0733-8651/10/$ – see front matter

United States
Postal Service

Statement of Ownership, Management, and Circulation
(All Periodicals Publications Except Requestor Publications)

1. Publication Title Cardiology Clinics	2. Publication Number 0 0 0 - 7 0 1	3. Filing Date 9/15/10
4. Issue Frequency Feb, May, Aug, Nov	5. Number of Issues Published Annually 4	6. Annual Subscription Price $264.00
7. Complete Mailing Address of Known Office of Publication (*Not printer*) (*Street, city, county, state, and ZIP+4®*) Elsevier Inc. 360 Park Avenue South New York, NY 10010-1710		Contact Person Stephen Bushing Telephone (Include area code) 215-239-3688

8. Complete Mailing Address of Headquarters or General Business Office of Publisher (*Not printer*)

Elsevier Inc., 360 Park Avenue South, New York, NY 10010-1710

9. Full Names and Complete Mailing Addresses of Publisher, Editor, and Managing Editor (*Do not leave blank*)

Publisher (*Name and complete mailing address*)

Kim Murphy, Elsevier, Inc., 1600 John F. Kennedy Blvd. Suite 1800, Philadelphia, PA 19103-2899

Editor (*Name and complete mailing address*)

Barbara Cohen-Kligerman, Elsevier, Inc., 1600 John F. Kennedy Blvd. Suite 1800, Philadelphia, PA 19103-2899

Managing Editor (*Name and complete mailing address*)

Catherine Bewick, Elsevier, Inc., 1600 John F. Kennedy Blvd. Suite 1800, Philadelphia, PA 19103-2899

10. Owner (*Do not leave blank. If the publication is owned by a corporation, give the name and address of the corporation immediately followed by the names and addresses of all stockholders owning or holding 1 percent or more of the total amount of stock. If not owned by a corporation, give the names and addresses of the individual owners. If owned by a partnership or other unincorporated firm, give its name and address as well as those of each individual owner. If the publication is published by a nonprofit organization, give its name and address.*)

Full Name	Complete Mailing Address
Wholly owned subsidiary of	4520 East-West Highway
Reed/Elsevier, US holdings	Bethesda, MD 20814

11. Known Bondholders, Mortgagees, and Other Security Holders Owning or Holding 1 Percent or More of Total Amount of Bonds, Mortgages, or Other Securities. If none, check box ☐ None

Full Name	Complete Mailing Address
N/A	

12. Tax Status (*For completion by nonprofit organizations authorized to mail at nonprofit rates*) (*Check one*)
The purpose, function, and nonprofit status of this organization and the exempt status for federal income tax purposes:
☐ Has Not Changed During Preceding 12 Months
☐ Has Changed During Preceding 12 Months (*Publisher must submit explanation of change with this statement*)

13. Publication Title: Cardiology Clinics

14. Issue Date for Circulation Data Below: May 2010

15. Extent and Nature of Circulation		Average No. Copies Each Issue During Preceding 12 Months	No. Copies of Single Issue Published Nearest to Filing Date
a. Total Number of Copies (*Net press run*)		1767	1543
b. Paid Circulation (By Mail and Outside the Mail)	(1) Mailed Outside-County Paid Subscriptions Stated on PS Form 3541. (*Include paid distribution above nominal rate, advertiser's proof copies, and exchange copies*)	673	582
	(2) Mailed In-County Paid Subscriptions Stated on PS Form 3541 (*Include paid distribution above nominal rate, advertiser's proof copies, and exchange copies*)		
	(3) Paid Distribution Outside the Mails Including Sales Through Dealers and Carriers, Street Vendors, Counter Sales, and Other Paid Distribution Outside USPS®	322	302
	(4) Paid Distribution by Other Classes Mailed Through the USPS (e.g. First-Class Mail®)		
c. Total Paid Distribution (*Sum of 15b (1), (2), (3), and (4)*)		995	884
d. Free or Nominal Rate Distribution (By Mail and Outside the Mail)	(1) Free or Nominal Rate Outside-County Copies Included on PS Form 3541	100	71
	(2) Free or Nominal Rate In-County Copies Included on PS Form 3541		
	(3) Free or Nominal Rate Copies Mailed at Other Classes Through the USPS (e.g. First-Class Mail)		
	(4) Free or Nominal Rate Distribution Outside the Mail (Carriers or other means)		
e. Total Free or Nominal Rate Distribution (Sum of 15d (1), (2), (3) and (4)		100	71
f. Total Distribution (Sum of 15c and 15e)		1095	955
g. Copies not Distributed (See instructions to publishers #4 (page #3))		672	588
h. Total (Sum of 15f and g)		1767	1543
i. Percent Paid (15c divided by 15f times 100)		90.87%	92.57%

16. Publication of Statement of Ownership

If the publication is a general publication, publication of this statement is required. Will be printed in the **November 2010** issue of this publication. — Publication not required

17. Signature and Title of Editor, Publisher, Business Manager, or Owner

Stephen R. Bushing – Fulfillment/Inventory Specialist — Date: September 15, 2010

I certify that all information furnished on this form is true and complete. I understand that anyone who furnishes false or misleading information on this form or who omits material or information requested on the form may be subject to criminal sanctions (including fines and imprisonment) and/or civil sanctions (including civil penalties).

FPO

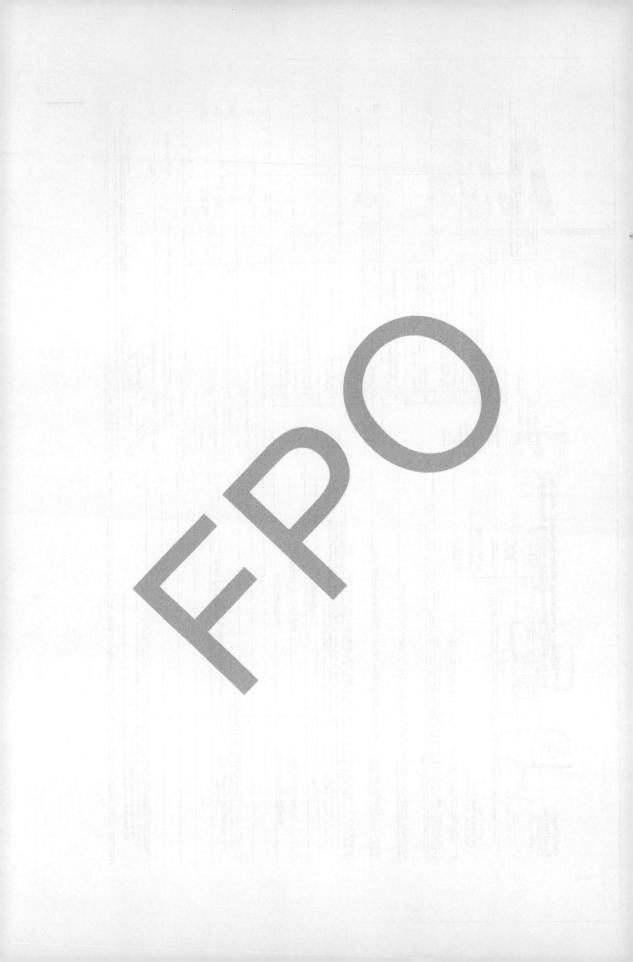

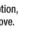

Printed and bound by CPI Group (UK) Ltd, Croydon, CR0 4YY
03/10/2024
01040359-0015